Palgrave Texts in Counsellinç

Series Editors
Arlene Vetere
Family Therapy and Systemic Practice
VID Specialized University
Oslo, Norway

Rudi Dallos
Clinical Psychology
Plymouth University
Plymouth, UK

This series introduces readers to the theory and practice of counselling and psychotherapy across a wide range of topical issues. Ideal for both trainees and practitioners, the books will appeal to anyone wishing to use counselling and psychotherapeutic skills and will be particularly relevant to workers in health, education, social work and related settings. The books in this series emphasise an integrative orientation weaving together a variety of models including, psychodynamic, attachment, trauma, narrative and systemic ideas. The books are written in an accessible and readable style with a focus on practice. Each text offers theoretical background and guidance for practice, with creative use of clinical examples.

Arlene Vetere, Professor of Family Therapy and Systemic Practice at VID Specialized University, Oslo, Norway.

Rudi Dallos, Emeritus Professor, Department of Clinical Psychology, University of Plymouth, UK.

More information about this series at
http://www.palgrave.com/gp/series/16540

Kasia Kozlowska · Stephen Scher ·
Helene Helgeland

Functional Somatic Symptoms in Children and Adolescents

A Stress-System Approach to Assessment and Treatment

Foreword by George P. Chrousos

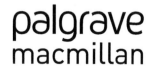

Kasia Kozlowska
The Children's Hospital at Westmead
Disciplines of Child & Adolescent Health,
and of Psychiatry
University of Sydney Medical School
Sydney, NSW, Australia

Stephen Scher
McLean Hospital
Department of Psychiatry
Harvard Medical School
Belmont, MA, USA

Helene Helgeland
Department of Child and Adolescent
Mental Health in Hospitals
Oslo University Hospital
Oslo, Norway

ISSN 2662-9127 ISSN 2662-9135 (electronic)
Palgrave Texts in Counselling and Psychotherapy
ISBN 978-3-030-46183-6 ISBN 978-3-030-46184-3 (eBook)
https://doi.org/10.1007/978-3-030-46184-3

Cover illustration: Alfio Scisetti/Alamy Stock Photo

This Palgrave Macmillan imprint is published by the registered company Springer Nature Switzerland AG
The registered company address is: Gewerbestrasse 11, 6330 Cham, Switzerland

Endorsements

'*Functional Somatic Symptoms in Children and Adolescents*, at the intersection of mind-body medicine, is a must-read for clinicians across pediatrics, psychiatry, neurology, psychology, social work, and allied rehabilitation disciplines involved in diagnosing and treating children and adolescents with functional symptoms. The authors have done a masterful job of linking together emerging cutting-edge biology with case-based discussions and practical treatment suggestions to aid the development of a mind-body program. Functional disorders are common in pediatrics, and this book is a major advance in bringing this set of conditions out of the shadows and into mainstream educational and clinical initiatives.'
    —David L. Perez, MD, MMSc, *Massachusetts General Hospital,*
Harvard Medical School

'A uniquely creative, well-informed, and authoritative account that uses the latest scientific and clinical research to inform clinical assessment and treatment of functional symptoms and syndromes in children and young people. The authors' stress-system model for understanding these experiences is complemented by the extensive use of clinical vignettes that are integrated into an overarching clinical framework that will prove useful for trainees and the broad range of clinicians addressing these problems in their own practices.'

—Elena Garralda, MD, MPhil, FRCPsych, FRCPCH, *Emeritus Professor of Child and Adolescent Psychiatry, Imperial College London*

'This is the book that clinicians, researchers and educators concerned with children and adolescents with functional somatic symptoms have been waiting for. For clinicians treating these children—both paediatricians and mental health professionals—this is a "must-have" book. Until very recently, research in this field has been sparse, and in the absence of a clear understanding of these symptoms, it has been difficult for clinicians to provide good, persuasive explanations to children and their distressed parents. The frequent result has been extensive medical assessments, trips to doctor after doctor, and an increasing likelihood that the symptoms would become chronic. Advances in research methodologies now set a neuroscience basis for functional somatic symptoms as reflecting disturbances of neurophysiological regulation. In this context, the book sets forth the important and clinically useful stress-system model for functional somatic symptoms. It also provides the knowledge and skills for clinicians to understand both the complexities in the neurophysiological dysregulation and how to communicate this understanding to patients and families. *Functional Somatic Symptoms* is an impressive and important book that should become a basic work of reference for multidisciplinary health professionals concerned with the role of disturbances of neurophysiological regulation in children and adolescents with functional somatic symptoms.'

—Trond H. Diseth, MD, *Professor of Child and Adolescent Psychiatry, University of Oslo, Norway*

'In this superb book Kozlowska and colleagues have provided a much-needed roadmap for accelerating our understanding of functional somatic symptoms. It describes important scientific developments while also maintaining a strong clinical focus relevant to medicine, nursing, social work, psychology, psychiatry, and other fields of health care.'

—Leanne Williams, PhD, *Professor of Psychiatry and Behavioral Sciences, Director of Center for Precision Mental Health and Wellness, Stanford University*

'Help is on the way for stressed and traumatized children (and their families) suffering from functional somatic symptoms, thanks to this great book for pediatricians, medical specialists, and mental health providers still confused by those children's "medically unexplained" symptoms and unable to help them heal. In this brilliant, compassionate, and eminently practical resource, Kozlowska and her colleagues have distilled decades of clinical experience and integrated many areas of research—from attachment relationships and adverse childhood experiences to the neurobiology of the stress-system encompassing the circadian clock, autonomic nervous system, inflammatory/immune system, and hypothalamic-pituitary-adrenal axis. They explain the "unexplained" and provide the map and toolbox for professionals to effectively apply their stress-system approach as individuals and teams. Everyone who works with children presenting with functional somatic symptoms, from pain and fatigue to non-epileptic seizures, will greatly benefit from reading this landmark book and putting its wisdom and practices into action.'

—James W. Hopper, PhD, *Independent Consultant & Cambridge Health Alliance, Harvard Medical School*

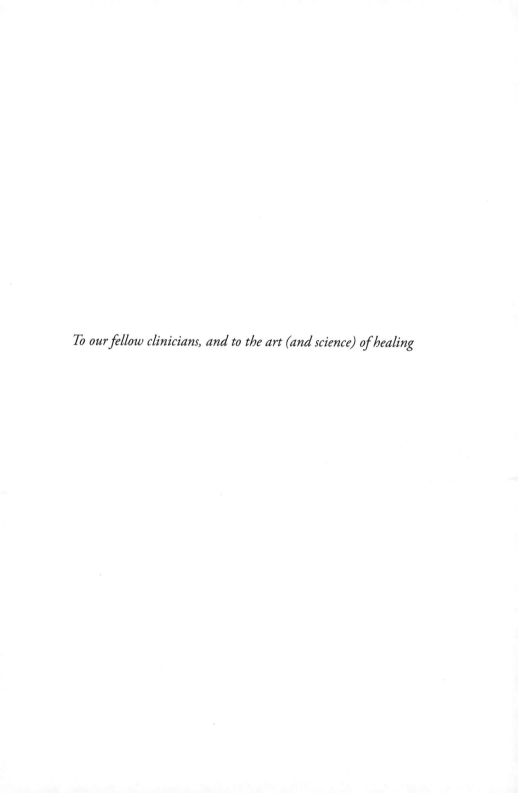

To our fellow clinicians, and to the art (and science) of healing

Foreword

I am delighted to write the foreword to this brilliant book, *Functional Somatic Symptoms in Children and Adolescents: A Stress-System Approach to Assessment and Treatment*, by Kasia Kozlowska, Stephen Scher, and Helene Helgeland. The book has three major sections: the clinical encounter; the stress system and the generation of functional somatic symptoms; and the treatment of these symptoms.

We humans and our societies are the most complex systems we know of in our surrounding universe, and a book such as this one provides a precious distillation of what is important in helping us understand how we feel, how our feelings are generated, and how we could influence them to palliate our suffering. Like all other complex systems, we exist in a dynamic equilibrium that requires energy to be sustained. This is what Walter Cannon called *homeostasis*, an equilibrium that is constantly disturbed by *stressors* and corrected by *adaptive responses*. Homeostasis has lower and upper limits; within the range of these limits, stressors are benign and the system 'us' remains in a state of harmless harmony. Stressors that push this homeostatic range on either side of its limits are not benign, and the system 'us' is *in stress*.

Aristotle spoke first of the unity of mind and body, while Epicurus later described *eustatheia* or *eustasis* as the mind and body's harmonious balance. This was over two thousand years before the Cartesian fallacy of a separate mind and body. Nowadays, it has become emphatically clear that our entire organism is an 'extended brain'. The complex system 'us' has its own complex subsystems that are activated when our homeostasis is threatened. These are the highly intertwined stress and immune/inflammatory systems. The former sounds the general alarm leading to the classic 'fight', 'flight', and 'freezing' responses, while the latter is activated when potentially injurious substances threaten the organism. The stress system thus generates the *stress syndrome*, while the immune/inflammatory system generates the *sickness syndrome*. The so-called 'functional symptoms' are primarily manifestations of the classic stress and sickness syndromes; these manifestations occur in children and adolescents, as well as in adults, in whom they have been called 'medically unexplained/unexplainable symptoms' (MUS); these are, in fact, quite explainable, as amply described in this book.

The book focuses on the functional symptoms of children and adolescents, which include not only those described as adult MUS but also other functional symptoms that pertain to all ages. These refer to stress-induced changes that influence both the interoception and exteroception functions of the brain, and include gastrointestinal, neurological, neuromuscular, perceptional, and other symptoms—all manifestations associated with suffering. Naturally, the pain and fatigue systems of the brain, as well as the reward system, are major players in the generation of suffering and functional symptoms of children, adolescents, and adults. Similarly, the biological circadian clock is involved—explaining the frequent association of these symptoms with the time of the day and night. These concepts are all well integrated in the book and help with the understanding of the pathophysiology of functional symptoms and the rationale for their treatment. The secret is obviously the management of stress and, through it, the alleviation of psychic and bodily pain.

I believe this erudite but also clearly and cogently written book will be of major service to children and adolescents and to the alleviation of overall human suffering. I congratulate the authors for a job greatly done.

George P. Chrousos, MD, MACP, MACE, FRCP
Professor of Pediatrics and Endocrinology, Emeritus
Holder, UNESCO Chair on Adolescent Health Care
Director, University Research Institute of Maternal and Child
Health and Precision Medicine
National and Kapodistrian University of Athens, Medical School
Aghia Sophia Children's Hospital
Athens, Greece

Acknowledgments

With three separate authors and three separate paths to the writing of this book, we beg the reader's indulgence in opening these acknowledgments with our three separate stories.

Kasia Kozlowska. The beginnings of this book are connected, in two ways, with The Royal Alexandra Children's Hospital—now renamed The Children's Hospital at Westmead—and the lives and work of various talented clinicians who worked there. Initially, in the 1960s, Dr. J. Denby Bowdler, a paediatric radiologist at the hospital, invited my father—also a paediatic radiologist—to leave Poland, a country that lay behind the Iron Curtain, to emigrate to Australia and join the hospital's medical staff. Dr. Bowlder died in 1976, when I was still a child; these acknowledgments provide an opportunity to recognize his role in profoundly changing the lives of me and my family. The Royal Alexandra Children's Hospital came back into the story in 1994, when I was introduced to the problem of functional somatic symptoms during my placement as child psychiatry fellow for Dr. Kenneth Nunn, then head of the hospital's Department of Psychiatry. In response to his experiences with a series of patients with debilitating functional somatic symptoms, Dr. Nunn had the foresight to develop an inpatient rehabilitation program—now known as the Mind-Body Program—for children with functional somatic symptoms.

When I started working with Dr. Nunn, I had no inkling that, a decade later, I would pick up the baton from him and continue the process of running and developing the program, which was facilitated by the progressive emergence of scientific literature pertaining to functional somatic symptoms. I am also indebted to Dr. Nunn for his support in my early efforts in academic writing, for his decision to create space in the department calendar for academic research, and for his encouragement to undertake an epidemiology study (published in 2007) regarding functional neurological symptoms, and to Dr. Katrina Williams and Donna Rose for their advice to fold my ongoing research into a PhD program at the University of Sydney Medical School (with Lea Williams, Kerri Brown, Loy McLean, and Angie Claussen as supervisors).

Another key figure who supported the Mind-Body Program and my work in it was Sister Margaret English. Before joining the Department of Psychological Medicine of The Royal Alexandra Children's Hospital as a clinical nurse consultant, Margaret had been the charge sister of the hospital's Hall Ward, a general paediatric ward, for many years; in addition to running the ward with supreme competence, she was as astute in observing and managing the hospital system as she was about children and their families. Margaret supported the Mind-Body Program from its inception until her retirement in 2013.

Also deserving of recognition are the dedicated clinicians who have been working at my side on the mind-body team: Catherine Chudleigh, Catherine Cruz, Grace Garber, Nicola Gray, Amanda Jenkins, Melissa Lim, Georgia McClure, Judy Longworth, and Blanche Savage. And because of the particular character of the *mind-body* problems that we addressed, the team regularly relied on the expertise, generously provided of the hospital's medical, nursing, and allied health staff and the staff in the hospital school: Gretel Butler, Dawn Carnevale, John Collins, Russell Dale, Victor Fung, Paul Gibbons, Deepak Gill, Wendy Griffiths, Clare Harb, Natasha Haynes, Amy Hickey, Sean Hogan, Michelle Lorentzos, Samantha Mihailovich, Fiona Nelson, Robert Ouvrier,

Simon Paget, Marilyn Paull, Peter Procopis, Anthony Pullen, Reena Rampersad, Bindu Sankaran, Samantha Soe, Elizabeth Sweeney, Sue Towns, Fiona Wade, Richard Webster, and Mercedes Wilkinson.

Finally, I thank Ali Asadi-Pooya, Selma Aybek, Alan Carson, Katherine Gill, Katrin LaFaver, W. Curt LaFrance, Timothy Nicholson, David Perez, Susannah Pick, Jon Stone, and Valerie Voon for involving me in various collaborative projects aimed at increasing our knowledge of functional neurological disorder.

Stephen Scher. I feel privileged to have had an ongoing, though ad hoc, role in the Mind-Body Program's efforts to frame and disseminate their research on functional somatic symptoms. In this context, I was fortunate to have had the opportunity to work on two major academic journals, the *American Journal of International Law* and *Harvard Review of Psychiatry* (with the latter continuing to this day), in the capacity of Senior Editor. In that role, and for nearly two (overlapping) decades at each journal, I was able to work with leading scholars, from all over the world, to articulate the results of their research simply, directly, and transparently. These skills are ones that find expression, too, in the present book.

Helene Helgeland. It has been my good fortune to have encountered inspiring mentors and teachers whose competence and wisdom were crucially important in shaping me as a person and enabling me to find my professional path. Included in this context are Bjørg Antonsen at Innlandet Hospital Trust, for helping to guide my development into a child and adolescent psychiatrist and clinician, Hanne Kristensen at the Regional Centre for Child and Adolescent Mental Health, Eastern and Southern Norway, for her skillful supervision of my research on children with functional abdominal pain, Trond H. Diseth and Helene Gjone at Oslo University Hospital, for teaching me the importance of a holistic biopsychosocial understanding of the individual child and for taking me in as a colleague, and Inger Helene Vandvik, a retired professor of child and adolescent psychiatry at Oslo University Hospital (and also my mother-in-law) for generously sharing her expertise and wisdom, and for reminding me of the importance of a clinical perspective. Finally, I would like to express my gratitude to the first and second authors, who generously and unreservedly have included me on their journey with this book. Their goodwill, friendliness, and hospitality have helped me to prosper and develop both personally and professionally.

* * *

Clinical teaching and more formal professional presentations have enabled the first author to learn, by trial and error, how best to present complex materials to interested and highly motivated, but not therefore expert, audiences. In addition to many presentations in and around her home state of New South Wales, venues have included the following: Lady Cilento Children's Hospital in Brisbane (via Susan Wilson), Women's and Children's Hospital in Adelaide (via Mark Pertini), Alfred Hospital in Melbourne (via Jack Kirszenblat), Australian Association of Family Therapy and Williams Road Family Therapy Centre in Melbourne (via Sophie Holmes), and Faculty of Child and Adolescent Psychiatry of the Royal Australian and New Zealand College of Psychiatrists (Julian Katz Oration; via Fiona Wagg). Venues in Norway have included, through the support of Trond H. Diseth, Finn Berset, and Hans-Petter Fundingsrud, the University of Oslo, the Cato Centre, and Tromsø University Hospital. In Portugal, arrangements and support for teaching were provided by Teresa Goldschmidt, Inês Pinto, and Simon Wilkinson, along with Carla Maia. All these teaching efforts have deepened the material and extended our capacity to present it (we hope) both simply and clearly.

In preparing this book, we have profited clinically, and most directly, from our opportunities to treat hundreds of patients with functional somatic symptoms. We also thank the children and families who have given us consent to use their stories (in deidentified form) in teaching and also in this book. The clinicians in our teams, as well as Janet Baker and Katherine Knight, have been most generous in helping us present various amalgam vignettes. Michelle Corke and Rasha Howari, currently Fellows in Psychiatry, provided probing feedback regarding the use of the stress-system model in clinical practice.

The relentless enthusiasm, encouragement, and goodwill of our readers of draft chapters kept this book moving along and maintained our spirits as we addressed their concerns and worked to achieve the proper focus and balance for clinicians. Odd Fyhn and Ingvild Damskog read every chapter, and Pascale Carrive, Bronwen Elliott, Aaron Fobia, and David Lamberth all provided feedback on numerous chapters. We also thank Maryllor (Lor) De, Rebecca Low, and Sister Veronica Chandler for their help with the illustrations; Danae Laskowski for allowing us to use and build on her version of the traffic light system safety plan; Patrician Crittenden for allowing us to use a visual representation of the Dynamic-Maturational Model of attachment and adaptation; and Alicja Kozlowska for her help in preparing the final manuscript. Finally, we thank Bhupinder Thind for her support in locating materials, some quite obscure, from libraries all over New South Wales.

We are indebted to the many friends and colleagues who have discussed these issues with us in conferences, over coffee or dinner, in the hallway, or by email or telephone, sometimes in response to drafts or articles of various sorts that we have sent to them. In this context Michael Bowden, Kevin Bragg, Hege Bruun-Hanssen, Max Cornwell, Megan Chambers, Douglas Drossman, Sue Foley, Lesley Hanney, Karen Hazell Raine, Philip Hazell, Marek Jantos, Sloane Madden, Hugh and Maxine Martin, John Morris, Carolyn Quadrio, Jean Starling, Beverly Turner, the late Danielle Vandenberg, Joanna Walton, and Andrea Worth deserve special thanks. Finally, Rudi Dallos and Arlene Vetere—the editors of the Palgrave Texts in Counselling and Psychotherapy series—have been remarkably supportive and generous in reviewing drafts and passing on their various criticisms, insights, and concerns.

Finally, we have been lucky to have been guided through the publication process itself by such talented editors at Macmillan and Palgrave. Early on, Peter Hooper moved the process forward with his clear focus on bringing a potentially longer book within the framework of the Counselling and Psychotherapy series. Later on, Beth Farrow and Joanna O'Neill provided ongoing advice and support as we prepared our final text. Their efforts have made the book both stronger and more accessible to clinicians.

Contents

List of Online Supplements

List of Figures

List of Tables and Text Boxes

1

A Brief Introduction

Abstract This chapter sets the scene for the rest of the book. Across time and across cultures, functional somatic symptoms have presented under many different guises, been given many different names, and been conceptualized in many different ways. Theories and speculation have therefore abounded, but without any firm scientific foundation. It is only very recently that scientists have come to learn enough about the body—and about the stress system, in particular—that a scientifically grounded understanding of functional somatic symptoms and their treatment is beginning to take shape. After a few brief paragraphs about such background matters, this chapter turns to the three authors themselves and how each of them came to be involved in the issues addressed in this book. The hope is that readers will see parts of themselves in these stories and also, in the process, come to consider how they each came to be involved in this intriguing and challenging field.

Electronic supplementary material The online version of this chapter (https://doi.org/10.1007/978-3-030-46184-3_1) contains supplementary material, which is available to authorized users.

Every day in hospitals, doctors' surgeries, and school sick bays around the world, children (including adolescents) present with what have come to be known as *functional somatic symptoms*. These symptoms are ones that cannot be explained by an identifiable disease process—even after an extensive medical assessment has been done. They reflect, instead, disturbances of neurophysiological regulation that cause the child to suffer physical discomfort (e.g., pain, dizziness, or nausea) or disruptions of various kinds (e.g., irregular bowel or bladder function), to experience disturbances of motor or sensory processes or capacities (e.g., paralysis, loss of vision, or seizure events), or to lose the sense of health and well-being (e.g., exhaustion, general malaise, or fatigue).

In contemporary medicine, doctors use the term *functional* to distinguish such disorders or symptoms from those that are caused by an objectively identifiable disease process (Roenneberg et al. 2019). In hospital corridors one might therefore hear doctors saying that the neurological symptoms or abdominal pain or hearing loss is functional rather than organic. What they're communicating is that standard medicines will not work; some other approach is required. The term *functional somatic symptoms* thus parallels how *functional* is used in medical contexts: to borrow from Mayou and Farmer (2002, p. 265), it assumes 'only a disturbance in bodily functioning', with no further implication regarding causation. It is important to note, too, that the word *functional* as used in this book has *no connection* to how the word is used within the fields of clinical psychology or family therapy, where the clinician may, for example, conceptualize a symptom or dynamic as having a function for the child within the family system.

In this book our use of the term *functional* moves beyond the functional/organic distinction to take into account recent advances in neuroscience. As the reader will see in the following chapters, the 'disturbance[s] in bodily function' underlying functional somatic symptoms involve disturbances in neurophysiological regulation. These disturbances (resulting in too much activation, too little activation, or aberrant patterns of activation) are the result of cumulative or, in some cases, acute stress, either physical or psychological. And these changes in neurophysiological regulation are themselves often accompanied by discernible changes in structure on a cellular or tissue level (not just function; see Chapters 4 and 8, and Online Supplements 4.2, 4.3, and 8.2).

Throughout history—and in today's contemporary medicine—functional somatic symptoms have been given many different names and been classified, by different medical specialties, in many different ways (for more about terminology, see Online Supplement 1.1). Throughout this book we use the term *functional somatic symptoms* as an umbrella term that includes all the different types of functional symptoms that occur across all body systems and that present to doctors who work across the full range of medical specialties.

Because functional somatic symptoms occur more frequently in girls than in boys, we generally use the pronoun *she* to reflect this clinical reality.

The Goal of This Book

The goal of this book is to communicate our current understanding of functional somatic symptoms and how best to treat them. The audience includes any clinician—whether in medicine, nursing, social work, psychology, psychiatry, or other fields of health care—who works with children experiencing functional somatic symptoms. These clinicians know that until very recently, research on functional symptoms has been sparse and that the knowledge base about functional illnesses has lagged behind developments seen in the rest of medicine. These clinicians have also experienced the challenges of trying to explain functional symptoms to children and their distressed families. They have witnessed the efforts of parents struggling to understand why their previously well child has become so sick. They have seen families who have gone from doctor to doctor, in search of help and an explanation that makes sense to them—just to be told that there is nothing wrong and that the physical exam and test results are normal. In an effort to explain what's wrong, these clinicians have found themselves with little choice but to use language derived from models of dissociation and conversion (from more than a century ago) or somatization and psychogenesis (from the early 1990s). But when patients and their families ask what these words mean, and what exactly the underlying mechanisms are, clinicians have typically been at a loss.

The good news is that advances in research methodologies have emboldened researchers to become interested in functional somatic symptoms yet again; the neuroscience of functional somatic symptoms is beginning to take shape. In this context, the present book sets forth the *stress-system model for functional somatic symptoms*. This model has been developed over the past decade through the research and clinical experience of the first author (KK). Building upon her own work and the work of other neuroscientists, the model brings together what is known about such symptoms and defines an approach to understanding and treating them in children and adolescents.

About the Authors

In this section (in the voice of the first author), we discuss how each of us came to be engaged in the problems addressed in this book. What has been apparent to all three of us is that the paths of engagement with functional somatic symptoms, like the symptoms themselves, are diverse and idiosyncratic. The many different dimensions of the problems engage clinicians in different ways. Our hope is that, in the descriptions of our three stories, readers will find that their own paths of engagement mirror and, in various ways, interweave with ours.

For interested readers, Online Supplement 1.3 contains a reference list for the work of individuals who are mentioned in this chapter.

The First Author: Kasia Kozlowska

The three co-authors of this book each came to this field through different routes. Speaking for myself as first author and as a child and adolescent psychiatrist, I had my initial encounters just over 25 years ago with patients experiencing functional somatic symptoms. It was during a six-month placement as a child psychiatry fellow at The Royal Alexandra Hospital for Children in Sydney, Australia. In 1994, Dr. Kenneth Nunn (my then supervisor) had established an inpatient treatment program for children with functional symptoms—now known as the Mind-Body

Program—in response to the presentation of children with functional paralysis of the legs. As a member of a multidisciplinary team that treated these patients—and in the role of the children's individual therapist—I was in much the same position as health professionals are even now. How should one conceptualize such problems, which occupy what seems to be a middle ground between the mind (as in psychiatry/psychology) and the body of standard, biological medicine? And how does one treat such problems effectively? These questions demanded answers, but what they tended to generate were more and more puzzles.

During the two-year training period to become a child and adolescent psychiatrist, I also became acquainted with different psychological theories, including the work of psychoanalysts Sigmund Freud and Melanie Klein, both of whom put particular emphasis on the role that infantile fantasies—generated from unconscious internal conflicts—played in child development and the emergence of psychopathology. I saw these theories as no better than weakly founded speculation. My aversion was particularly strong regarding Freud's construction of sexual abuse as an internal psychic conflict (rather than as involving real events in the lives of children and young women) and Klein's emphasis on the central role of parental figures in children's fantasy lives (rather than parents' actual impact on their real lives). From my contact with Dr. Carolyn Quadrio—a child and adolescent psychiatrist and my supervisor in family therapy—I was well aware that sexual abuse and ongoing family conflict were not only common but could seriously compromise children's health and well-being.

Disillusioned by psychoanalytic models, I also questioned Freud's theory of conversion—namely, that unacceptable mental contents (usually unconscious sexual conflicts) were transformed, or converted, into somatic symptoms. This conception of functional somatic symptoms, which influenced the third and fourth editions of the US-based *Diagnostic and Statistical Manual of Mental Disorders* (DSM-III and -IV), was the one that I was obliged to learn and to use for documenting diagnoses. But if the conversion hypothesis was correct, then what were the biological mechanisms by which it happened? The psychoanalytic models couldn't even hint at an answer. And why focus exclusively on imagined events or internally created conflicts as generating

conversion symptoms? Real-life, external events can generate psychological responses that are just as strong as, or even stronger than, internally
generated events or conflicts. If internally generated phenomena are
enough to trigger conversion symptoms, why couldn't mental phenomena tied in with external events do the same?

My child psychiatry training—unlike that of the third author (HH;
see below)—had an Anglo-American bias. I have no memory of having
been taught anything about Pierre Janet's dissociation model, developed
in France in the late nineteenth and early twentieth centuries, which
better acknowledged that functional somatic symptoms and dissociative
symptoms arose when patients had experienced terror or severe stress,
illness, or fatigue.

My deep reservations about models of thinking that were available
in the early 1990s continued during my first job as a child psychiatrist,
working as team leader of the preschool program at a child psychiatry unit
(Arndell Children's Unit, Royal North Shore Hospital). A key strength of
the unit was its family orientation and its family admissions program; a
multidisciplinary team worked with the family to help the parents manage their own emotional states, thereby enabling the family to help the
distressed child to regulate more effectively. When this family-based intervention was successful, the child's behavioural, emotional, or somatic
symptoms would actually just melt away. What was also evident was that
most of the children referred to the program had developed emotional,
behavioural, or functional somatic symptoms in the context of family
conflict, loss events, mental illness in the family, or maltreatment. Many
were quite distressed—even traumatized—by these experiences, and in the
supportive environment that we provided in the unit, the children were
able to communicate their experiences both verbally and in imaged form
(Kozlowska and Hanney 2001; Hanney and Kozlowska 2002). After a
thorough family assessment, it was usually clear to the treatment team that
the children's experiences were real and tangible, and that their symptoms
needed to be understood and treated against that background.

In this context, it was not surprising that I was drawn to the work
of John Bowlby, who believed that psychoanalysis needed to open itself
to scientific debate and inquiry and who contended that psychoanalysis
neglected the role of loss and trauma events. Bowlby's scientific enquiry

took the form of empirical observation of what happened to young children when they were separated from their mothers and put in the care of strangers. The research findings and the ideas emanating from these findings were articulated in *Attachment and Loss*, whose three volumes were published from 1969 to 1980. In Bowlby's view, children's development and their emotional, behavioural, and somatic problems are shaped by the quality of their emotional bonds with attachment figures and by adverse life events such as separation, loss, trauma, and maltreatment.

Bowlby's work, along with that of Mary Ainsworth (who had worked in Bowlby's research unit at the Tavistock Clinic in the early 1950s and later collaborated with him as an equal colleague), set the stage for a further development of attachment theory, the Dynamic-Maturational Model of attachment and adaptation (DMM). This model was being elaborated in the 1990s and 2000s by Patricia (Pat) McKinsey Crittenden, a developmental psychologist and attachment researcher who was herself a student of Ainsworth's. In 1996, soon after finishing my child psychiatry training, I had the good fortune to attend a daylong lecture by Pat. From that time and continuing through 2015, I worked together with a wonderful group of clinicians from around the world, helping Pat to gather the clinical materials that enabled her to fill in the model's details (Crittenden 2006). Pat's 1999 monograph, *Danger and Development: The Organization of Self-Protective Strategies*, influenced me profoundly. Against this background—which included many hours spent under Pat's astute clinical eye watching children interact with attachment figures—I came to realize that the child's close relationships shape biological regulation processes (Francis and Meaney 1999) and that the chronic disruption of what are normally comfortable and nurturing attachments could disrupt those processes. Most importantly for the purposes of this book, I also came to realize that chronic or severe stress, including but not limited the stress and danger associated with disrupted attachment relationships, contributes to the emergence of functional somatic symptoms.

Also in the mid-1990s, when I was still a young child/adolescent psychiatrist, I came across the work of Bruce Perry and Frank Putnam, two American child psychiatrists who were engaged both in clinical work with traumatized children and in neuroscience research. Their published works engraved in my mind the idea that developmental experiences—including those with attachment figures—help shape the organization and function of the developing body and brain.

And in 1998, when I started working at The Children's Hospital at Westmead, I read *The Web of Life: A New Synthesis of Mind and Matter*, by Fritjof Capra, a physicist and a systems theorist. In contrast to family therapists, who applied systems thinking to relationships and to the family, Capra applied it to all living systems—beginning with the level of the cell. This extended way of applying systems thinking enabled me to conceptualize the problems of my patients as involving different system levels—governed by different laws and representing different levels of complexity—while being at the same time interrelated and interdependent. By using systems thinking I was able to shift my attention back and forth between system levels to identify and address different issues: the brain and body, the mind, the child's attachment relationships, the family, and the school. What this meant in practice was that I could apply all the skills that I had learnt in my training—my skills as a doctor, as a psychiatrist, as an attachment clinician, and as a psychotherapist and family therapist—without prioritizing one system level as being more important than another.

From my family therapy training I had retained an interest in the work of Milton Erickson, an American psychiatrist who specialized in medical hypnosis and family therapy. In my mind I held an image of Erickson sitting in front of a crackling fire talking with patients and bringing about positive change in their lives by his use of metaphor and suggestion (see also Chapter 15). In 2002, I enrolled in a two-year course in clinical hypnosis so that I could use hypnosis in my own work and also better understand the writings of Janet and other clinicians who had used hypnosis with patients with functional somatic symptoms.

Around that same time, I also became acquainted with the work of Antonio Damasio, a neurologist and neuroscientist whose clinical work led him to be interested in the neurobiology of consciousness, emotions, and feelings. Damasio wrote, 'Emotions play out in the theater of the body. Feelings play out in the theater of the mind. As we shall see, emotions and the host of related reactions that underlie them are part of the basic mechanisms of life regulation; feelings also contribute to life regulation, but at a higher level' (Damasio 2003, p. 28). For me, Damasio's work solidified the idea that psychological, emotional, and behavioural phenomena were all embedded in a biological substrate. So, when I began to see a lot of children with functional somatic symptoms—referred by paediatricians describing the problems as *psychogenic*—my basic assumption was that the functional symptoms were embedded in a biological substrate, a substrate that we did not, as yet, understand (Kozlowska 2005).

It was from this neuroscience perspective that, in 2006, I began my PhD on functional neurological disorder (FND), with the neuroscientist Dr. Leanne Williams as my primary supervisor. The PhD research program was a series of studies that looked at various biological markers in children and adolescents presenting with FND.

As I was working on the PhD, I came across the work of Hans Selye (1907–1982), an endocrinologist who introduced the idea of the *stress response* and, with it, the word *stress*—including *le stress, der stress, lo stress, el stress,* and *o stress*—into our vocabulary across cultures and languages (Selye 1956). According to Selye's broad definition, stress (or a stressor) is any event, whether physical, chemical, or psychological, that causes the body to activate an adaptive (or in some cases, maladaptive) response. The stress response includes the many different ways in which the body responds or adapts to the myriad challenges, ranging from the negligible to the catastrophic, that we encounter as part of our daily lives—what Selye called *the stress of life.* Selye highlighted that mild, brief, and controllable states of stress could be perceived as pleasant or exciting, and could function in a positive way to facilitate the individual's emotional, physical, or cognitive health and subjective well-being. By contrast, more severe, protracted, or uncontrollable stress—exceeding a tolerable threshold and associated with distress rather than pleasure, excitement, or goal-associated determination—could have a different outcome. In particular, it could lead to a stress response that had a negative effect on the individual's well-being and that, over time, could result in what Selye called *diseases of adaptation.* For a fuller account of Selye's work and that of other scientists who laid the foundations for the stress-system model presented in this book, see Online Supplement 1.2.

During this same period of working on my PhD, I also came across the work of George Chrousos, an endocrinologist and neuroscientist. Together with colleagues, Chrousos had introduced the idea of the *stress system* as a systemic framework for looking at the diverse, interrelated biological systems that underpin stress-related illnesses (Chrousos et al. 1988). According to Chrousos, the stress system comprises a set of overlapping and interrelated hormonal, neural (autonomic nervous system), immune-inflammatory, and brain systems involved in mediating the brain-body stress response and underpinning the body's ability to regulate itself in response to the stress of life. Chrousos defined stress as 'a state of disharmony, or threatened homeostasis' and introduced the term *stress-system disorders* (for Selye's *diseases of adaptation*), which he conceptualized as arising from hyper- or hypo-activation of the stress system (Chrousos and Gold 1992, p. 1245).

I realized that Chrousos's overarching stress-system framework provided a systemic way of thinking about a broad range of functional somatic symptoms. This realization was confirmed by the data that emerged from the studies that made up my PhD: the children with FND showed activation of all components of their stress systems. My clinical team and I incorporated this way of thinking into our daily clinical practice; some examples of our clinical work were published in the *Harvard Review of Psychiatry* as 'Stress, Distress, and Bodytalk: Co-constructing Formulations with Patients Who Present with Somatic Symptoms' (Kozlowska 2013). Building upon my PhD research, these clinical results, and the work of other neuroscientists, I presented a more fully elaborated *stress-symptom model for functional neurological symptoms* in a 2017 contribution to the *Journal of the Neurological Sciences* (Kozlowska 2017).

Since that time, other prominent clinicians and scientists have influenced my work and thinking. Of special note on the clinical side are Peter Levine, Kathy Kain, Pat Ogden, and Richard Gevirtz, who have developed bottom-up interventions for working with patients in psychotherapy. In this context, and in order to hone my own clinical skills in bottom-up somatic interventions, I completed Levine's three-year Somatic Experiencing psychotherapy training and Kain's 16-day Touch Skills for Therapists course (training in somatic awareness and tactile skills for trauma resolution). Of special note on the research side are Bruce

McEwen, who looked at the biological cost, over time, of an overactivated stress system, and Michael Meaney, whose research established the foundation for understanding how a child's early-life experiences become biologically embedded in the brain and body. For interested readers, Online Supplement 1.2 summarizes, within a historical framework, key aspects of their work and that of other scientists whose work has contributed to my understanding of the stress system.

The Second Author: Stephen Scher

The second author, Stephen Scher, joined this journey just over a decade ago, when my article 'Healing the Disembodied Mind: Models of Conversion Disorder' was being finalized for publication in the *Harvard Review of Psychiatry*. His close, acute attention to the article (as Senior Editor) helped me to sort out various conceptual and linguistic problems, and it also began an ongoing conversation about mind and body. But his own interest in these problems far antedates our work together on that article. Beginning with his undergraduate work in philosophy and continuing through his PhD work in the same field, one of his primary interests was philosophy of mind, at the centre of which—going back to the seventeenth-century writings of Descartes—was the mind-body problem. His PhD dissertation, 'Freedom and Determinism in Kant's *Critique of Practical Reason*' (Scher 1977), was itself a historical study of this problem, and his clinical work on medical ethics in hospitals affiliated with Harvard Medical School was a response to what he perceived as an all-too-narrow focus on the intellect in trying to understand how health professionals learnt to think and act ethically. That line of thinking, years later, ultimately led to the publication—with me as co-author—of *Rethinking Health Care Ethics*, our Open Access book in which we follow the logic of his initial insights to develop an approach in which clinical ethics is literally embodied in each clinician's own history and his or her own thoughts, emotions, and actions (Scher and Kozlowska 2018). In a wonderful way, that book might be understood as coming full circle to our original encounter—that is, to an embodied mind, as it were, that enables clinicians to better understand and advance their own ethical thinking, feeling, and acting.

The Third Author: Helene Helgeland

The story of Helene Helgeland's involvement in this book is more complex. My initial contact with Helene, a child/adolescent psychiatrist in Norway, dates from 2015, when she invited me, via email, to give a series of talks at Oslo University Hospital in 2017. Those led to additional series of talks in 2018 and 2019—at the Cato Center in Son, at Tromsø University Hospital in Tromsø, and again in Oslo—and also to some further collaboration, including this book. Her own interest in the problems addressed in this book dates from around 2000, when she was working as a psychiatrist in a child and adolescent outpatient clinic.

Early on, it was Helene's impression that patients with functional somatic symptoms were almost absent from the clinic's patient population and also that very few were referred to their clinic because of such problems. But then—inspired by her husband, Per Olav Vandvik, a physician who was conducting research on functional abdominal pain in adults—she started asking her patients about the presence of abdominal pain. To her surprise, she discovered that not only abdominal pain but also other nonspecific somatic symptoms such as headache, nausea, and musculoskeletal pain were common among her young patients. In some, the symptoms had a huge impact on their daily functioning.

Helene soon realized—no doubt, like many readers of this book—how very little she knew about functional somatic symptoms and how very little she had learnt about this patient group as a medical student. She also realized that the majority of her colleagues both in general and mental health care had little knowledge—and often little interest—in these patients. Once a disease process was excluded, many paediatricians felt that they had finished up with such patients and felt no further responsibility for treatment. And many mental health clinicians, in turn, dismissed these patients because they did not show any obvious psychological symptoms such as anxiety and depression. Even when clinicians moved past these threshold obstacles, the baseline problem was still the same: what is happening to these patients? The clinicians themselves typically felt helpless, and their relations with patients and families often deteriorated, triggering anxiety, worries, anger, and misunderstandings.

Helene then embarked on the path that ultimately led to our acquaintance and to her work as a co-author. The first step was the research on her

PhD—on functional abdominal pain in children. In reading the international research literature she became increasingly interested in clinical hypnosis as an effective treatment for children with functional abdominal pain. Another source of inspiration at that time was her mother-in-law—Dr. Inger Helene Vandvik—a child and adolescent psychiatrist who has been one of the pioneers promoting the implementation of clinical hypnosis in paediatric patients in Norway (Helgeland 2018); in 2008, Dr. Vandvik established a one-year professional education program for using hypnosis clinically with children and adolescents. The program continues today under the leadership of Helene and her colleague Maren Lindheim (Lindheim and Helgeland 2017).

Although Helene's own knowledge and clinical experience continued to grow, she remained acutely aware that few health professionals had the understanding and capacity to help patients with functional somatic symptoms. To change the situation, it was necessary, she realized, to disseminate knowledge not only to health professionals but also to health authorities, decision makers, and the general population. In 2014, when Norway established its National Advisory Unit on Psychosomatic Disorders in Children and Adolescents, Helene joined the effort and recognized it as her opportunity to make a difference. Her searches of the literature led her to me. What was especially valuable for her (and other professionals in Norway) was that my articles presented both a well-developed clinical approach to treating functional somatic symptoms and a comprehensive model that integrated emerging research evidence on the underlying neurophysiological mechanisms.

What Connects Us Together as Authors

Finally, what also ties the three authors together is our interest in the well-being of the person as a whole, whether this be the well-being of our patients and their families, our teams, or our students. We try to support, and to promote the growth of, the whole person in our practice of medicine as a healing art (Cassell 2013), in working collaboratively with colleagues and respecting their moral voices (Scher and Kozlowska 2018), and in our mentoring of students and trainees when they spend time in our programs.

What the three of us hope is that, with our different but overlapping perspectives, knowledge, and skill sets, we have been able to put together a book that communicates what we know in a way that makes it accessible and usable by health professionals. With good luck, the presentation will engage the reader, and the trip through the pages will be both rewarding and a source of pleasure. We hope that after reading this book, all clinicians will hold in mind the many ways that physical and psychological stress can affect the child's body and compromise her health and well-being.

In an effort to make this material on functional somatic symptoms most accessible to the reader, we have divided the book into three parts representing the three overarching intellectual and clinical challenges that the clinician needs to address: (Part I) Children with Functional Somatic Symptoms: The Clinical Encounter; (Part II) Mind, Body, and the Science of Functional Somatic Symptoms; and (Part III) The Treatment of Functional Somatic Symptoms. For interested readers we also provide additional references—and references to basic science articles—in Online Supplement 1.3 for each of the chapters of the book.

* * *

In this closing paragraph we would like to address the limitations of the book. First, because the book's primary audience is mental health clinicians—and because we often try to articulate ideas in a way that can also be used to talk to children and families—we have tried to simplify the neurobiology as much as possible. But in simplifying the neurobiology we lose some of the detail and some of the complexity, and our neuroscientist colleagues may find the simplification a bit frustrating. Second, we have had to put a boundary around what we cover and what we do not cover in this book. The child's pattern of presentation may involve other comorbid, stress-related disorders such as anxiety, depression, and post-traumatic symptoms. Early-childhood stress also increases the risk for medical disorders such as diabetes, cardiovascular disease, inflammatory diseases, and obesity. Limitations on length do not allow us to discuss the interplay of functional somatic symptoms with these comorbidities. Third, knowledge about functional somatic symptoms and the processes underlying them is rapidly evolving. Much is becoming known and much is unknown. In this context, this book should be understood as just one step in the larger story.

References

Capra, F. (1997). *The Web of Life: A New Synthesis of Mind and Matter.* London: Flamingo.

Cassell, E. J. (2013). *The Nature of Healing: The Modern Practice of Medicine.* Oxford: Oxford University Press.

Chrousos, G. P., & Gold, P. W. (1992). The Concepts of Stress and Stress System Disorders: Overview of Physical and Behavioral Homeostasis. *JAMA, 267,* 1244–1252.

Chrousos, G. P., Loriaux, D. L., & Gold, P. W. (1988). Preface. In G. P. Chrousos, D. L. Loriaux, & P. W. Gold (Eds.), *Mechanisms of Physical and Emotional Stress.* New York: Plenum Press (Advances in Experimental Medicine and Biology, Vol. 245).

Crittenden, P. M. (1999). Danger and Development: The Organization of Self-Protective Strategies. *Monographs for the Society for Research on Child Development, 64,* 145–171.

Crittenden, P. M. (2006). The Dynamic-Maturational Model of Attachment. *Australian and New Zealand Journal of Family Therapy, 27,* 106–115.

Damasio, A. R. (2003). *Looking for Spinoza: Joy, Sorrow, and the Feeling Brain.* Orlando, FL: Harcourt.

Francis, D. D., & Meaney, M. J. (1999). Maternal Care and the Development of Stress Responses. *Current Opinion in Neurobiology, 9,* 128–134.

Hanney, L., & Kozlowska, K. (2002). Healing Traumatized Children: Creating Illustrated Storybooks in Family Therapy. *Family Process, 41,* 37–65.

Helgeland, H. (2018). Meeting Our Mentors: Dr. Inger Helene Vandvik. *International Society of Hypnosis Newsletter, 43,* 17–19. https://www.ishhypnosis.org/wp-content/uploads/2018/07/ISH_201806.pdf.

Kozlowska, K. (2005). Healing the Disembodied Mind: Contemporary Models of Conversion Disorder. *Harvard Review of Psychiatry, 13,* 1–13.

Kozlowska, K. (2013). Stress, Distress, and Bodytalk: Co-constructing Formulations with Patients Who Present with Somatic Symptoms. *Harvard Review of Psychiatry, 21,* 314–333.

Kozlowska, K. (2017). A Stress-System Model for Functional Neurological Symptoms. *Journal of the Neurological Sciences, 383,* 151–152.

Kozlowska, K., & Hanney, L. (2001). An Art Therapy Group for Children Traumatised by Parental Violence and Separation. *Clinical Child Psychology and Psychiatry, 6,* 49–78.

Lindheim, M. O., & Helgeland, H. (2017). Hypnosis Training and Education: Experiences with a Norwegian One-Year Education Course in Clinical Hypnosis for Children and Adolescents. *American Journal of Clinical Hypnosis, 59,* 282–291.

Mayou, R., & Farmer, A. (2002). ABC of Psychological Medicine: Functional Somatic Symptoms and Syndromes. *BMJ, 325,* 265–268.

Roenneberg, C., Sattel, H., Schaefert, R., Henningsen, P., & Hausteiner-Wiehle, C. (2019). Functional Somatic Symptom. *Deutsches Ärzteblatt International, 116,* 553–560.

Scher, S. (1977). Freedom and Determinism in Kant's *Critique of Practical Reason.* PhD dissertation, Brown University.

Scher, S., & Kozlowska, K. (2018). *Rethinking Health Care Ethics.* Singapore: Palgrave Macmillan. https://www.palgrave.com/us/book/9789811308291.

Selye, H. (1956). *The Stress of Life.* New York: McGraw-Hill.

Part I

Children with Functional Somatic Symptoms: The Clinical Encounter

Part I—Chapters 2 and 3—describes the child and family's experience in the health care system, including the clinical encounters between the family and the paediatrician, and between the family and the mental health clinician. By immersing the reader in the diverse dimensions of the clinical encounter, these chapters aim to help the reader to appreciate and understand the encounter from the full range of relevant perspectives: the child, family, paediatrician, and mental health clinician.

Chapter 2 highlights the important role of the paediatrician in the process of establishing a therapeutic relationship and creating a secure base for the child and family and for their later encounter and dealings with the mental health clinician. The chapter underscores the importance of including functional somatic symptoms in paediatric teaching curricula to ensure that the next generation of paediatricians has the necessary skills to assess functional somatic symptoms, to discuss and explain the symptoms and their clinical findings in a clear and respectful way, to provide a positive diagnosis, and to support the child and family to find a way through the health care system. Chapter 2 will also help the mental health clinician to understand the difficulties that the child and family may encounter in their path through the health care system and what experiences—good or bad—may be brought to the assessment interview in the mental health setting.

Chapter 3 is about the assessment process with the mental health clinician or multidisciplinary team. It describes the assessment interview, the co-construction of a formulation, and the process of negotiating an agreement about the treatment process. This chapter aims to help mental health clinicians to connect with the problem of functional somatic symptoms and to recognize their own patients in the vignettes describing the clinical encounter. The authors hope that these preliminary clinical chapters will help mental health clinicians recognize that their training has actually given them the requisite clinical skill set for working with children with functional somatic symptoms. What is also needed, however, is a broadening of perspective. Brain, body, and mind need to be understood as deeply integrated, with stress—whether physical or psychological—having systemic effects on all of them.

Taken together, these two chapters set the stage for Part II on the science of functional somatic symptoms and Part III on the treatment of such symptoms. What we hope is that the clinician will come to realize that by using systems (biopsychosocial) thinking—the bread and butter of working with children and families—to both conceptualize and treat functional somatic symptoms, those symptoms will, in effect, fade away. That is, as the dysregulated physiological state associated with severe stress dissipates, so will the symptoms. The authors also hope that these introductory clinical chapters communicate that working with children with functional somatic symptoms is rich and rewarding: good work can change people's lives.

2

Going to See the Paediatrician

Abstract The paediatrician has a central role as a gatekeeper both in diagnosing functional somatic symptoms and in directing the child and family onto a path toward health and well-being. In addition to determining that the child's symptoms are not caused by a disease process, the paediatrician provides the child and family with a positive diagnosis that sits under the umbrella of functional somatic symptoms. In so doing, the paediatrician validates the child's symptoms; the family feel relieved and validated; and the child and family are ready to accept referral to a mental health clinician—or to a multidisciplinary team that treats functional somatic symptoms. In this way, the paediatrician contributes to the creation of a *secure base* from which the child, family, and mental health clinician can feel safe enough to explore the various factors that contributed to the child's presentation. By contrast, when the clinical encounter with the paediatrician does not go well, the distressed family may end up consulting doctor after doctor, health professional

---

Electronic supplementary material The online version of this chapter
(https://doi.org/10.1007/978-3-030-46184-3_2) contains supplementary material,
which is available to authorized users.

after health professional. As time passes, new symptoms arise; the child's presentation gathers layer upon layer of complexity; and the child's symptoms may become chronic and more difficult to treat.

The Visit to the Doctor

When a child (including an adolescent) with functional somatic symptoms sees the doctor—the family doctor, paediatrician, or paediatric specialist in neurology, cardiology, rheumatology, or gastroenterology—she and her family are commonly told that all the tests are normal and that the physical and neurological examinations are also normal. But the paediatrician also needs to validate the child's symptoms (by giving a positive diagnosis), to explain that the symptoms are related to a temporary disturbance in body function (rather than to some serious disease), and to link up the family with appropriate help. When that all happens, the child and family are already moving along the path of recovery; early diagnosis and treatment are associated with good health outcomes (see following vignette of Amalia and summary of outcome data in Online Supplement 2.1).

Amalia was a 12-year-old girl who was training to be a gymnast. Eight months earlier Amalia had landed badly in a fall. Because of ongoing pain in her neck and some twitching in the muscles of her right hand, she had to wear a neck collar prescribed by her orthopaedist. After three months her symptoms had fully resolved, and she slowly returned to her gymnastics training. More recently, Amalia again twisted her neck in a fall. Although repeated medical examinations were unable to find any medical problem, Amalia continued to experience headache and fatigue. Two weeks later she presented to the emergency department with leg weakness and an unsteady gait. Reassessment by the orthopaedic team—which included a blood screen, X-rays, and a head scan—led to a referral to the neurology team. The paediatric neurologist did a careful neurological examination, explained that Amalia's tests were all clear, and that the neurological examination indicated a functional neurological disorder (FND). She explained that in FND the structure of the muscles, nerves, and bones was *all good* but that the function had been disrupted. She also explained that FND was commonly triggered by physical or emotional stress—in Amalia's case, her fall and twisting injury—and that two-thirds of children with FND also suffered from comorbid pain. She described to Amalia and her family the neurological tests that she had done and how they enabled her to assess whether Amalia's nervous system was intact. She told Amalia and the family that FND needed treatment and that, with treatment, most children recovered. She told Amalia and the family about the hospital's Mind-Body Program for treating FND, run by Psychological Medicine. Amalia and her family connected with the mind-body team, and Amalia successfully completed the standard, two-week admission to the Mind-Body Program (daily physiotherapy, psychotherapy, hospital school, and weekly family sessions). During the admission her walking difficulties resolved; she started on some melatonin to help manage her disturbed sleep; and she learnt and began to implement specific strategies to manage her pain. Amalia then returned to school and continued working with a psychologist to improve and maintain her mind-body regulation strategies (see Chapters 14 and 15). No other contributing factors were identified in Amalia's history.

The Paediatrician as Gatekeeper

The Need for a Clear Diagnosis: Establishing a Secure Base

The paediatrician acts as gatekeeper. As such, the paediatrician needs to take a thorough clinical history and to conduct a good physical examination; to undertake any tests that are necessary to exclude other medical conditions; and to identify any concomitant medical factors that are part of the child's presentation. And in the following conversation with the child and family, the paediatrician needs to explain that the child's pattern of symptoms and signs has a name (a positive diagnosis)—for example, functional abdominal pain or functional neurological disorder—and that specific treatment is generally required, potentially including referral to a clinician or team that treats functional disorders. Online Supplement 2.1 provides the reader with more information about the positive diagnosis.

As gatekeeper, the paediatrician establishes *safety* for both the family and the mental health clinician. The paediatrician confirms that the child is medically safe—that the child does not have an organic condition that needs to be treated using contemporary medical or surgical interventions—and that it is safe and appropriate for the mental health clinician to proceed with a treatment intervention. In this way, the paediatrician contributes to the creation of a *secure base* from which the child, family, and mental health clinician can feel safe enough to explore the various factors that contributed to the child's presentation (see Chapter 3). We borrow this idea from Mary Ainsworth, who noted how the mother can serve as a safe base, or relationship, from which the child can 'explore the world … under circumstances in which danger is absent' (Ainsworth 1967, p. 346), and from John Byng-Hall, who used the idea of safe base in working with families (Byng-Hall 1995).

The Sequelae of Diagnostic Uncertainty

If the paediatrician has not established this safe, secure base for the family, the child and family are unable to let go of the nagging fear that some organic disease process may have been missed. Assailed by this nagging fear, the child and family will struggle to accept a referral to a clinician/team who treat functional symptoms within a psychological setting, and will find it difficult to accept a formulation and treatment plan pertaining to a functional rather than organic illness.

Likewise, if the mental health clinician senses the absence of an adequate medical assessment or if the clinician has not been provided with a clear functional diagnosis, the clinician will also feel unsafe or, at the very least, lacking a proper mandate for proceeding with treatment. Concern that the child has not been adequately assessed medically—and that an organic condition may have been missed—may lead the clinician herself to encourage the family to obtain a new, comprehensive assessment, along with whatever tests and investigations are required. As we will see below, such additional referrals can contribute to a never-ending process of doctor visits.

Addressing Diagnostic Uncertainty Head-On

Unfortunately, there are times when the gatekeeping encounter with the paediatrician does not go well, as we see in the following four vignettes. The first vignette of Lola demonstrates that providing a positive diagnosis is very different from telling the child and family what the symptoms *are not*. Stating that all the tests are normal, that the symptoms are non-organic, that the pain is not from the heart, or that the problem is not asthma or not epilepsy conveys no information about what the problem *is*, and fails to recognize the child's symptoms as real. It also leaves the family in a state of confusion, anxiety, and not-knowing. The vignette of Lola highlights that the mental health clinician may need to liaise with the paediatrician to ensure that this final step of the medical assessment process is completed.

> Lola was a 13-year-old girl who presented to hospital with intermittent shaking in her right arm that sometimes progressed to a non-epileptic seizure (more generalized shaking; NES). Lola was investigated by the neurology team. At the family assessment interview with the mind-body team, Lola's family reported that the doctor from the referring neurology team had told them that the symptoms were *not organic, not caused by epilepsy*, and *not harmful*. When the first author (KK) asked the family if Lola had been given a diagnosis, the family looked confused and replied that no diagnosis had been given. A phone call to the neurology doctor, with the family present in the room, confirmed a diagnosis of functional neurological disorder, or FND—of which NES is a subset. Once the diagnosis was confirmed and then communicated to the family, the mind-body team could explain the implications of the diagnosis and elaborate the treatment that needed to be implemented. In a subsequent conversation, the doctor who had seen the child and family—who was training to be a neurologist—admitted that she had struggled to provide a positive diagnosis of FND because doing so made her anxious. The first author suggested that shadowing another neurologist—one who had mastered this task—might help the training neurologist overcome her anxiety and become proficient in this clinical skill.

In the following vignette of Evie, we see how a positive diagnosis allowed Evie to let go of the nagging thought that an organic disease process has been missed by all the doctors who had assessed her pain. Evie suffered from with intermittent pain in her chest—called *precordial catch syndrome*—which subjectively felt like a bursting bubble (Gumbiner 2003; University of Wisconsin–Stevens Point Health Service 2005). Precordial catch pain is a functional somatic symptom thought to be caused by tension patterns in muscle and fascia tissues that sit within the chest cavity. Until the positive diagnosis was given, Evie did not feel safe—a secure base had not been achieved—and she was unable to accept the referral to, or to engage with, the mind-body team.

> Evie was a 15-year-old girl who presented with intermittent pain in her chest—called *precordial catch syndrome*. Sometimes the pain became unbearable and would trigger a non-epileptic seizure, or NES. Evie had had a difficult time in the health care system. In the previous hospital, where she had been fully and extensively investigated by multiple specialists, the doctors had diagnosed NES. They also gave Evie the distinct impression, however, that her symptoms of pain and the NES were all in her head. On her subsequent presentation to our hospital (and the mind-body team), Evie remained preoccupied with her recurring chest pains and was plagued by thoughts that the paediatrician's medical assessment may have missed a disease process. For example, Evie spoke about her previous cardiology consult with sarcasm: 'She [the cardiology fellow] did not know. She said that she thinks it is not the heart. So, what if the doctors don't know? What if they have gotten it wrong?' But, after a senior paediatrician at our hospital provided the diagnosis of precordial catch syndrome, and after Evie had read the fact sheet about that syndrome, she accepted both the diagnosis and the unwelcome reality that she would need to learn to manage the pain. With the safe base thus created for Evie and her family, Evie began to engage effectively with the mind-body team. She collaborated in the history-taking process and in co-constructing a formulation (see Chapter 3), and she then got on with the task of implementing mind-body strategies that enabled her both to manage the precordial catch pain and to avert her NES. Evie and her parents also implemented family interventions that enabled them to resolve tensions in their relationships. A clear, positive diagnosis of both precordial catch syndrome and NES had enabled Evie both to accept the symptoms and to engage in the therapeutic intervention that helped her return to health and well-being.

Premature Referrals

The third and fourth vignettes demonstrate that, when the paediatrician as gatekeeper refers the child too early—prior to the completion of a comprehensive medical assessment—and therefore fails to create a safe, secure base for the child, family, and mental health clinician, serious organic conditions can be missed, potentially leading to serious harm.

When the first author was a junior consultant—and had not yet leant to stand her ground when determining whether referrals had been properly worked up medically—she was pressured by the referring neurologist to fit in a family assessment for Martha, a 13-year-old adolescent. Martha was presenting with an unusual array of neurological symptoms, which the neurologist assumed to be functional. The mind-body team's family assessment did not yield any particular story or pattern, even after much gentle, but lengthy, probing. Two days later a head scan, ordered prior to the referral but conducted after the family interview, revealed that Martha's symptoms were caused by a brain tumour.

Ian was a 15-year-old boy referred by a general paediatrician for the treatment of NES. On screening the referral, the mind-body team noticed that the medical workup was incomplete; the paediatrician had not done an electroencephalograph (EEG), the gold-standard test for distinguishing epileptic from non-epileptic seizures. Despite our request for an EEG, the paediatrician refused because she had seen the seizures events and was sure of her diagnosis of NES. During the family assessment interview with Ian and his family, the first author noted the stereotypic nature of the events over a period of ten years—a characteristic of epileptic seizures. After completing the interview she referred Ian for an EEG herself and briefed the neurology team that her provisional diagnosis was that of epileptic seizures. An EEG confirmed epilepsy, and an MRI showed a seizure focus—a scar in the brain. After surgical removal of the scar, the seizures ceased.

The Loss of Trust and the Spiral into Chronicity

As we have already seen, when the clinical encounter with the paediatrician goes well, it is the first, forward-looking step toward a favourable outcome. The child and family are able to take the fork in the road that leads to health and well-being. We also need to track what happens, however, when the encounter does not go well and the child and family take the fork in the road that spirals into chronicity.

If the paediatrician provides no positive diagnosis and, with no adequate explanation, refers the child and family to a mental health clinician, the family may leave the doctor's office baffled and distressed or even angry. Their eyes tell them that their child's *body* is ill: the child is shaking, or having seizures, or struggling to walk, or experiencing disabling pain, or too exhausted to do anything. It is difficult for them to believe that the findings of the medical examination are normal, that nothing is wrong. If the paediatrician has suggested that the symptoms may be caused by emotional or psychological distress, or that an emotional trauma may have caused the debilitating symptoms, the family may emphasize that the child has grown up in a loving home and that emotional trauma is not part of the family story. In other cases, the family may note that their child's somatic symptoms started after a common infection or illness, or after a physical injury, sprain, fall, or bump on the head, and that no psychological stress has occurred (see, for example, the vignette of Amalia, above). In any event, whereas most families see the logic of bringing in a physiotherapist, the suggested need to bring in a mental health clinician might be experienced as a rejection and taken as proof that the doctor thinks the symptoms are not real. The child—and her parents—may feel that the doctor does not understand. They are likely to feel hopeless, angry, and dismissed (see following vignette of Samantha).

> Samantha, a 10-year-old girl, lived with her father, paternal grandparents, and one younger sibling. As a child she had been exposed to domestic violence between her parents and to considerable family upheaval. At school, Samantha was an engaged, compliant student who had good relationships with her teachers and peers. At the beginning of year 5 in school, following a nasty viral infection, Samantha developed recurring headaches that slowly became chronic, with the consequence that the pain in her head was constant. Two months later, Samantha began to experience dizziness, shaking, and jerking. Over a six-month period, Samantha had frequent presentations to her local doctor and her local emergency department. She was repeatedly examined, including via an EEG (to exclude epilepsy) and a head scan. She and the family were

repeatedly told that everything was normal, that the doctors could find nothing wrong. Because the problem was conceptualized as *psychological*, Samantha was referred to the community mental health team for treatment. Since the mental health team believed that functional neurological symptoms pointed to a history of sexual abuse, they kept asking Samantha and her family questions whose aim was to uncover sexual abuse. This naturally upset Samantha and her family, who discontinued their contact with the mental health team after a few sessions.

Six months later the shaking and jerking culminated in non-epileptic seizures, or NES. A diagnosis of *pseudoseizures* (an old term for NES) was given. Samantha interpreted the diagnosis to mean that she was *making the seizures up*. On another occasion, the diagnosis of *psychogenic NES* was given. This time Samantha interpreted the diagnosis to mean that she was *psycho* (i.e., crazy). Because the seizure events were occurring many times a day, Samantha became wheelchair-bound. Her family insisted that she use the wheelchair to keep from falling and hitting her head. After one frightening seizure—in the ninth month of her illness—Samantha was taken by ambulance to the local hospital for treatment. Because the family refused to take Samantha home, insisting that something had to be done, the hospital transferred Samantha to the first author's tertiary care hospital for 24-hour EEG monitoring. At the hospital Samantha was assessed by the neurology team—who gave Samantha and the family a clear diagnosis of NES and chronic complex pain. The neurology team also told the family that these illnesses were common and that the mind-body team in Psychological Medicine ran a specialized program for NES. With reluctance, the family agreed to meet the mind-body team because they were now desperate for Samantha to receive treatment (see Chapter 3 for this family's clinical encounter with the mind-body team).

When the family is unable to understand or accept the diagnosis provided by the paediatrician, the child and family may simply move on to another doctor. And each new doctor, not knowing what else to do, orders the same (or even further) tests—which simply fuels the family's anxiety and serves to perpetuate the child's symptoms.

This process of never-ending doctor visits—fuelled by inadequate clinical encounters—has unfortunate consequences. The anxiety experienced by both the family and child is likely to increase. Anxiety in parents may also lead to catastrophizing about the child's symptoms and increased vigilance; they begin to *look out* for the symptoms, to pay the symptoms more and more attention, and to respond to the symptoms with caregiving behaviours. This constellation of parental behaviours has the effect of increasing symptom intensity and frequency. Moreover, as the child's parents become more anxious, so does the child. In the absence of a clear diagnosis, some children may worry that they never will recover or that they have a life-threatening illness. Anxiety is a powerful top-down activator of the stress system—further amplifying symptom intensity, increasing symptom frequency, and often contributing to the generation of new, additional functional somatic symptoms. The children's book *Malte and Malte's Stomach* has beautiful illustrations about the child and family's journey through the medical system (Toscano 2016).

As time goes on, the somatic symptoms will begin to impair the child's functioning. The child will miss school and stop exercising. Connections with friends, as well as all the benefits that these relationships provide, will deteriorate. With social isolation and a progressively sedentary lifestyle that leads to deconditioning, a range of body systems will become more dysregulated and shift even further toward a non-healthy brain-body state. With each shift, the child will become sicker and sicker, and may develop new symptoms—a vicious cycle of ever-progressing illness. At this point, much will need to be done to help the child regain her physical well-being and conditioning. Eventually, even if emotional symptoms had not been part of the child's original presentation, the child may become very distressed, and her mood may be affected. In addition, her sleep may now be disturbed, with the consequence that she experiences no relief from the symptoms day or night.

Family interactions will also have changed. The child is now disconnected from her life outside the family and overly connected—in a way that is not appropriate to developmental stage—with one or both parents and with any siblings in the family who have adopted a caregiving role. The situation pushes the child into a sick role and also changes the parents' behavioural expectations for their child. These patterns of relating together, where the child signals her symptoms and distress, and the parents respond to the signalling, will have stabilized into a pattern that is difficult to break and that creates a barrier to getting well. Additional work will be needed to help the family change their patterns of relating, and to adopt ones that promote the recovery process.

Working in a children's hospital, we have seen many children and families who have walked this complicated pathway, the spiral to chronicity, because they were unable to find (or in some cases, accept) help within the existing medical system.

Going from Doctor to Doctor: How a Child Can Collect Multiple Diagnoses

If the child's functional somatic symptoms disrupt function in multiple body systems and if the child and family end up seeing a number of doctors—each with a specialty oriented toward a particular body system—the child may accumulate many specialty-specific *positive* functional diagnoses from different specialists, which can seriously confuse the family (see vignette of Paula, below). If the doctor is unable to explain that these diagnoses are interrelated and that they all sit under the umbrella of functional somatic symptoms, then the family will remain confused.

Eleven-year-old Paula, in year 5 at school, fell while playing soccer and was diagnosed with a hairline fracture in the lateral epicondyle of the right femur that caused severe pain in the knee. The fracture healed, though Paula continued to experience intermittent pain. She found it difficult to sleep, and as time went on, even a bump to the leg near the knee would cause pain that lingered for weeks, often requiring the use of crutches. That same year, Paula's maternal grandfather—with whom she was very close—was diagnosed with cancer; his visible physical decline was an ongoing stress.

Two years later, an orthopaedic surgeon diagnosed Paula's problem as chronic regional pain syndrome (CRPS Type 1). On an outpatient assessment, our hospital's Pain Team rejected the diagnosis of CRPS and used the terms *chronic pain* or *complex pain* to describe the problem. With weekly physiotherapy and hydrotherapy, both the pain and Paula's walking got better. During that year, however, Paula's *paternal* grandfather—whom Paula did not know well—died from cancer. And, given that her *maternal* grandfather's health continued to deteriorate, the death was a distressing reminder that he was dying, too.

A year later (year 8), Paula was bullied at school. Again, her sleep became disturbed. And after one particular instance of bullying—being pushed while trying to close a door—she developed left arm weakness and pain. Later that same year, over a period of months, Paula developed bilateral weakness in the legs, a persistent headache, and musculoskeletal pain that migrated all over her body; the pattern of pain kept changing over time. As Paula became less and less mobile, and spent more time in her bed, she developed symptoms of dizziness—especially on standing up from bed—and fatigue, as well as intermittent nausea, abdominal pain, and loss of regular bowel motions. Sometimes her body lost control: her heart thumped, she sweated, and she felt breathless and faint. The symptoms were worse when the stress at school was worse, and they remitted when the stress eased. During this time, Paula's parents took her to see many different specialists for her various symptoms. In the respective specialist reports, the neurologist presented a diagnosis of FND; the psychiatrist, conversion disorder and generalized anxiety disorder; the gastroenterologist, functional gut disorder; and the rheumatologist, amplified musculoskeletal pain syndrome (Sherry 2000) and probable postural orthostatic tachycardia syndrome (POTS) secondary to physical deconditioning (Wells et al. 2018).

At the first author's hospital, the Pain Team continued to see the problem (as per its initial assessment) as chronic or complex pain accompanied by intermittent functional neurological symptoms, but the Pain Team also recognized that Paula was becoming progressively more debilitated; effectively bed-bound, she was unable to mobilize around the house for more than five minutes at a time. The family, now very worried about Paula's fatigue, had begun to wonder if Paula might also be suffering from chronic fatigue syndrome.

Because of Paula's progressive debilitation, the Pain Team referred her for admission to the hospital's Mind-Body Program. In the weeks prior to initial assessment by the mind-body team, Paula developed another new symptom—intermittent loss of vision in the left eye—and an ophthalmologist told the family that the problem was non-organic. During the assessment itself, it became apparent that the profusion of diagnoses made the family confused and gave them the impression that Paula—now 15 years of age and in year 9—was suffering from a combination of disorders from which recovery was unlikely.

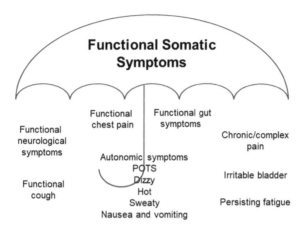

Fig. 2.1 The wide-ranging functional diagnoses that fall under the umbrella term *functional somatic symptoms* (© Kasia Kozlowska 2019)

To overcome the confusion that multiple medical diagnoses can create, some researchers and clinicians have suggested the use of a unifying diagnosis, such as *bodily distress syndrome* (or *disorder*) (for references see Online Supplement 1.1). The key problem is that this unifying terminology is not currently integrated across the two key diagnostic systems, the *International Classification of Diseases* and *Diagnostic and Statistical Manual of Mental Disorders* (for more detail about terminology, see Online Supplement 1.1). In this book we have chosen the term *functional somatic symptoms* as the unifying term for the broad range of functional somatic symptoms that we see in our child and adolescent patients (see Fig. 2.1). For a description of our use of the term, see Chapter 1.

The Problem That Multiple Specialty-Specific Diagnoses Pose for Professionals

Specialty-specific diagnoses also pose problems for professionals, potentially compromising their ability to communicate with each other and to provide mutually complementary care. Specialists from one specialty (e.g., neurology) may not be up to date with the specialty-specific diagnoses used by their colleagues from other fields (e.g., gastroenterology). Specialist also tend to work in a blinkered sort of way—addressing problems pertaining, for example, only to the gut, nervous system, heart, or ear, nose, and throat. Consequently, when a specialist makes a functional diagnosis related to his or her particular medical specialty, the specialist may not even recognize the diagnosis as being functional, may fail to make links to, or even inquire about, potential symptoms in other organ systems, or may fail to communicate the interrelated nature of all functional diagnoses to the child and the family.

The vignette of Louisa (below) demonstrates how the phenomenon of specialization within modern medicine—and the loss of holistic care—can also create confusion between specialists, and how difficult it can be, even for teams who work in the field of functional somatic symptoms, to reach conceptual clarity. The vignette is also a good example of a system intervention that takes place within the health care system—to build a common way of thinking about the child's problems between all the professionals involved in a child's care.

When referred to our Mind-Body Program, Louisa, an 11-year-old girl in year 6 at school, was experiencing symptoms of anxiety, depression, fatigue, disturbed sleep, and buzzing in the left ear that was described in the referral letter as tonic tensor tympani syndrome. Louisa had a long history of separation anxiety and intermittent functional abdominal pain, which had been worse when Louisa was bullied in year 4. When Louisa's first ear, nose, and throat specialist and his team were unable to treat her ear problem effectively using various recommended therapies for tinnitus (for references see Online Supplement 1.3), she proceeded to be seen by a long series of other ear, nose, and throat specialists and pain specialists, each of whom had issued a specialty-specific diagnosis. A second ear specialist had diagnosed tinnitus, another hyperacusis, and a pain specialist had used the diagnosis of chronic ear pain. Nevertheless, despite the long list of medical consultations, Louisa's health and function had not improved.

Our review of Louisa's medical history suggested that her sensitivity to sound and her pain in the ear were consistent with a functional disorder. In this context, we read the neuroscience literature about tinnitus and discovered that in cases where tinnitus—which is uncommonly reported by children presenting to our program—is *not* associated with any damage in the auditory apparatus, it *is* associated with increased activity in the brain stress systems (see Chapter 11), a finding that parallels those in other functional disorders (see Chapter 11).

With this information in hand, and through a series of telephone calls over a two-week period to each of the health professionals previously involved in Louisa's care, we all came to the same conclusion (though only after considerable probing by the mind-body team): despite the different terminology and what appeared to be ongoing disagreements about what exactly was happening to Louisa, all the specialists agreed that Louisa's various symptoms and difficulties were best conceptualized under the umbrella of functional somatic symptoms with comorbid anxiety.

In the above vignettes of Paula and Louisa, we see that the medical professionals had focused narrowly on what they saw as specialists, and that all had generated specialty-specific diagnoses and treatment recommendations. What they had all failed to recognize was that the symptoms that they were focusing on were interconnected not only with other functional somatic symptoms but with other stress-related disorders, such as anxiety, depression, and post-traumatic stress disorder.

Putting It All Together

One way of understanding the myriad terms that doctors have used to talk about functional somatic symptoms—both now and in previous eras (for a terminological history reaching back to Ancient Greece, see Online Supplement 1.1)—is through the parable of the blind men who tried, each through a single touch, to determine the true nature of an elephant. Depending upon the specific part that each had access to, the elephant was considered to resemble, for example, a snake (trunk) or fan (ear) or rope (tail) or wall (body) or tree (leg). In much the same way, each set of terms that has been used, over time, to refer to functional somatic symptoms reflects some portion of the truth (Fig. 2.2).

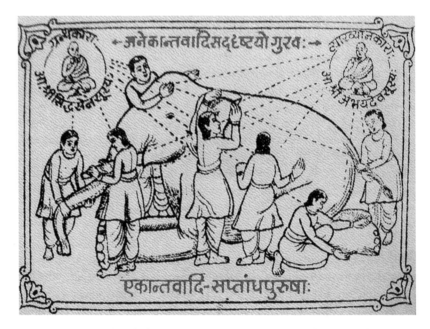

Fig. 2.2 The parable of the seven blind men and the elephant. This parable comes from the Indian tradition, where it was used to highlight the multi-sided, multifaceted nature of truth. This particular image is taken from Siddhasena's *Sanmatitarkaprakaraṇa* (1986), an Indian text from the fifth century. [Siddhasena Divākara, Jayasundaravijaya, and Abhayadeva. (1986). *Sanmatitarkaprakaraṇa* (Prathamāvṛtti ed.). Dholakā, Gujarāta: Divyadarśana Ṭrasṭa.] (*Source* Romana Klee via Wikimedia Commons CC-BY-SA)

The Role of the Support Group

The use of speciality-specific diagnoses has led to the growth of support groups for specialty-specific conditions. Some of the children and families who present for assessment and treatment of functional somatic symptoms will have searched the internet for information and will have accessed support from such groups. Our clinical experience is that some support groups are primarily health focused and serve to support the child and family with the process of getting well. Other support groups are symptom focused, however, and by focusing on symptoms—rather than the process of getting well—these groups may lead the child and family further down the spiral into chronic illness.

An additional problem is that many support groups are made up predominantly of patients whose symptoms have become chronic and who have, in effect, had to adjust to and accept the experience of being chronically unwell. Those who have gotten well have returned to their ordinary lives and have no need of ongoing support. Consequently, if a child and family make contact with such a support group when the child first presents, the child will get the erroneous message that the condition is always chronic. This erroneous message, in and of itself, will affect the child and family's expectations, and will make it less likely that the child will return to health and well-being (see Chapter 12 for a discussion of expectations).

In sum, families face ongoing challenges in managing and assessing the information that they and their child might obtain via the internet or via support groups. Just how they address these challenges will continue to affect the child and family's willingness and capacity to engage effectively with mental health professionals.

* * *

In this chapter we have discussed the important role of the paediatrician (or other doctor)—as gatekeeper—in both diagnosing functional somatic symptoms (a positive diagnosis) and in referring the child and family for appropriate treatment. As gatekeeper, the paediatrician establishes *safety* for both the family and the mental health clinician. The paediatrician confirms that the child is medically safe and that it is safe and appropriate for the mental health clinician to proceed with a treatment intervention. In this way, the paediatrician contributes to the creation of a *secure base* from which the child, family, and mental health clinician can explore the various factors that contributed to the child's presentation (see Chapter 3).

References

Ainsworth, M. D. S. (1967). *Infancy in Uganda: Infant Care and the Growth of Love*. Baltimore, MD: Johns Hopkins Press.

Byng-Hall, J. (1995). *Rewriting Family Scripts*. London: Guilford Press.

Gumbiner, C. H. (2003). Precordial Catch Syndrome. *Southern Medical Journal, 96*, 38–41.

Sherry, D. D. (2000). An Overview of Amplified Musculoskeletal Pain Syndromes. *Journal of Rheumatology. Supplement, 58,* 44–48.

Toscano, L. (2016). *Malte Og Maltes Mave* [Malte and Malte's Stomach]. Copenhagen, Denmark: Komiteen for Sundhedsoplysning [Committee for Health Education].

University of Wisconsin–Stevens Point Health Service. (2005). *Precordial Catch Syndrome.* https://www.uwsp.edu/Stuhealth/Documents/Other/Precordial%20catch.Pdf.

Wells, R., Spurrier, A. J., Linz, D., Gallagher, C., Mahajan, R., Sanders, P., et al. (2018). Postural Tachycardia Syndrome: Current Perspectives. *Vascular Health and Risk Management, 14,* 1–11.

3

The Family Assessment Interview: The Narrative, Formulation, and Discussion of Treatment Options

Abstract The clinical encounter with the mental health clinician—or multidisciplinary team—typically begins in the family assessment interview, where engagement and rapport building between the clinician and the family take place through a series of therapeutic processes. First comes the process of generating a narrative. The child or adolescent and family present, roughly chronologically, the family genogram (which gives a bird's-eye view of the family story across three generations), the child's developmental history, and the story of the child's symptoms. This process provides the clinician with key information: the story of the family's adverse experiences and those of the child (ACEs); how the family and child managed such experiences; and a working understanding of the factors that have shaped the child's stress system. This therapeutic conversation also provides the child and family with the experience of being listened to and heard. Second comes the process of co-constructing a formulation: the narrative told by the child and family is framed through the lens of the stress-system model. Thus

Electronic supplementary material The online version of this chapter (https://doi.org/10.1007/978-3-030-46184-3_3) contains supplementary material, which is available to authorized users.

© The Author(s) 2020   **37**
K. Kozlowska et al., *Functional Somatic Symptoms in Children and Adolescents*, Palgrave Texts in Counselling and Psychotherapy,
https://doi.org/10.1007/978-3-030-46184-3_3

interpreted within the neurobiology of brain, body, and mind, the child's symptoms take on new meaning. They come to be understood by the child and family as reflecting activation or dysregulation of the stress system in response to physical and psychological stress. Third come the discussion and rationale regarding the mind-body interventions that are needed to target the identified areas of dysfunction. Fourth comes the therapeutic contract. Once the family interview has been completed—and rapport and a shared understanding of the problem have been established—the clinician and family are in a good position to work together as a team to enable the child to get back on the road to health.

The Family Assessment Interview

For the mental health clinician, the family assessment interview is usually the first encounter with the child (including the adolescent) presenting with functional somatic symptoms and with her family (Kozlowska et al. 2013). Some children and families will come to the assessment in the wake of a positive experience within the health care system. They will have seen a doctor or paediatrician who completed the medical assessment with skill and empathy, and who, in a timely manner, provided the child and family with a clear diagnosis and explanation. In this scenario, the paediatrician has already created a *secure base* from which the child, family, and mental health clinician can feel safe enough to explore the various factors that contributed to the child's presentation (see Chapter 2). These families will come to the family interview with an open stance keen to do whatever is necessary to help the child get better.

Other children and families will come to the assessment in the wake of a negative experience within the health care system (see the vignette of Samantha in Chapter 2). They will have seen a doctor or paediatrician who did not understand functional somatic symptoms, who was irritated by them, or who felt too anxious to give a positive diagnosis and talked only about the diagnoses that the child did not have (diagnoses of exclusion). Alternatively, the child and family may have experienced throwaway remarks made by an ambulance driver, nurse, or accident and emergency doctor who perceived the symptoms as not being part of 'real medicine' (see the vignette of Samantha in Chapter 2). In this scenario, the child and family may have been knocked about in the medical system and may bring with them memories of negative interactions with health care providers, as well as experiences of feeling unheard, dismissed, or even derogated (see Text Box 3.1). They will come to the family interview with a defensive stance, ready to defend the child or themselves from further put-downs. The *secure base* from which the child, family, and mental health clinician can feel safe enough to explore the various factors that contributed to the child's presentation has yet to be established.

Text Box 3.1. Examples of derogatory comments made by health care workers—Reported by families to the first and third authors' clinical teams, or reported in the literature

'They are false seizures'
'She's faking it'
'Stop looking for attention'
'She is just making it up for attention'
'Attention seeker'
'Drama queen'
'Putting on episodes'
'Hypochondriac'
'Leave her at home on the bed and let her have it [the episode]'
'The problem is supratentorial'
'It's all in the head'
'He's doing his dying-swan act again'
'I know you're are faking it; snap out of It'
'Life is a bucket of shit; put a lid on it'
'Wanting attention from mummy and daddy'
'Waste of government time and funding'
'I am grabbing my coworker and walking out'
'To save her [the patient] the embarrassment, I will take her [in the ambulance]'
'Time wasters' (Worsely et al. 2011)
'Fakers' (Worsely et al. 2011)
'Should be shot' (Worsely et al. 2011)

To make things more complicated, the family may find the family assessment interview challenging for other reasons. The interviewer may touch upon events that the family would prefer to leave in the past. The interviewer may see temporal connections between events in the family story and patterns of response in the child's body—phenomena that may have, to date, been uncoupled and that, in some cases, the family would prefer to remain that way. Connecting the story of the child's body to the story of the challenges and adversities in her life can be difficult and emotionally painful. Because families differ in their inherent capacities and preparedness to manage the interview process and to make connections between the family story and the story of the child's body, the process of generating a narrative—and engaging with the family— may be straightforward, fraught with difficulty, or anywhere in between.

In this context, establishing rapport—the therapeutic relationship— and a secure base with the child and family should be considered the primary goals of the family assessment interview. The clinician (or in some settings, the multidisciplinary team) needs to engage the child and family, and to connect with them in a constructive way that looks to the future. While the first interview with the child and family can be set up and run in many different ways—the way we run the interview being just one possible way (Kozlowska et al. 2013)—the sections below highlight some key elements. The overarching goal is to increase the probability that the assessment process will set the stage for the child, family, and clinician to work together with 'mutual confidence, respect and acceptance' (Sattler 1992, p. 404). For a discussion of different assessment formats, see Online Supplement 3.1.

When Repair Is Needed

When the family steps into the clinic room, the clinician can make no assumptions about the family's experience through the health care system. To highlight just how difficult the situation might be, we pick up the story of Samantha (see Chapter 2). In the normal course of events, any repair pertaining to adverse experiences in the health care system takes place as part of the normal assessment process (see following sections). Samantha's story highlights how the repair process may need to take priority and may need to be dealt with upfront.

Samantha entered the clinic room with her father, younger brother, and paternal grandparents (who lived with the family). They were glaring at the clinician—and other members of the multidisciplinary team—with hostility, and Samantha's father stated outright, 'There is nothing wrong with our family, and we won't be answering any of your stupid questions.' It was clear from the outset that the family were hurt and angry, and that the assessment interview could not proceed in the usual manner. In this context, the clinician made a statement acknowledging that many families whose child was seeking treatment for non-epileptic seizures (NES) had reported *horrendous* experiences in the medical system. She invited Samantha and her family to tell her what had happened to them.

Samantha wept with anger as she recounted how different professionals had treated her. The ambulance officer had sternly told her, 'Stop it! I know you're putting it on.' The emergency department doctor had taken her father aside and told him that 'Samantha is faking it.' A nurse had told Samantha that life was a 'bucket of shit' and that she should 'put a lid on it'. The paediatrician who examined her concluded that the seizures—he called them *pseudoseizures* and said they were *psychogenic*—functioned as a means of avoiding school. Samantha's impression was that the paediatrician thought *she was not quite right in the head*. When the family was subsequently interviewed by the local mental health service, they were grilled in an effort to elicit a history of *sexual abuse*.

The clinician (and team) listened to the above story—calmly, patiently, and with no effort to hurry it or avoid the unpleasant details. Gravely, and with sadness, the clinician told the family that most medical and paramedical staff knew little or nothing about NES because this area of medicine had been largely neglected. The clinician then explained that the word *pseudoseizure* referred to the fact that NES could look just epileptic seizures but that on the electroencephalogram (EEG) they did not have the signature spike pattern of epilepsy. So, the word *pseudo* did not mean *fake*. It just meant *not epileptic*. The clinician also explained that the word *psychogenic* was still used by some neurologists and others because—in the past—it had been thought that NES were psychological in origin. But now we know better. NES are caused by stress on the body and brain. The stress could be physical (e.g., an illness or pain) or psychological (e.g., bullying at school, stress in relationships, or painful or stressful memories about past events). For this reason NES have also been referred to as *stress seizures*. They were very common, and the team saw a new patient with NES every one or two weeks.

Now, Samantha and her family were listening.

The clinician also told Samantha that the words *malingering* and *factitious*, referred to people who were putting it on. But neither of these words applied to Samantha. Her diagnosis was NES and chronic/complex pain.

At this point in the interview, an hour had passed, and the clinician decided to offer the family a *formulation* based on the information that the family had offered on their own, without being directly asked. The clinician began the formulation from the most biological factor that she could identify since the family had expressively communicated that they found discussion of family issues difficult. The clinician said that from what the family had told her, it seemed that several biological factors were contributing to Samantha's NES. First, Samantha had reached puberty, and it was well known that female sex hormones increased risk for NES. In all available studies, females have been more prone than males to develop NES. The reason is that female stress hormones up-regulate the stress system, which is made up of the various brain-body systems that activate in response to stress.

Second, the clinician had noticed that Samantha had been breathing very fast during the assessment, at 28 breaths or more per minute. The clinician said that some kids hyperventilated when their stress systems were switched on. She explained that in a study that the team had completed, 50 percent of the children with NES triggered their symptoms with hyperventilation. The family told the clinician that they had also noticed that Samantha hyperventilated. The grandfather said that he was always telling her to calm herself down.

Third, the clinician—a doctor—asked Samantha if it was OK if she felt her neck and back for any tension patterns. This examination elicited significant discomfort and identification of trigger points in the muscles of the neck and shoulder region (for references see Online Supplement 1.3). Everyone could see Samantha's response to the palpation of her tense muscles. The clinician told Samantha and the family that chronic tension in the muscles of the head and neck contributed to chronic headache and needed to be addressed if Samantha's headache was to get better.

Fourth, Samantha had been suffering from chronic pain. The clinician noted that pain can also up-regulate the brain-body stress systems and contribute to NES. The family nodded and said that Samantha had been in a lot of pain and that they had noticed that the pain made her distressed.

At this point in the interview the family volunteered yet another stress. They said that the Samantha had been very traumatized by her mother's violent outbursts and that memories of that trauma continued to play on her mind. When these memories were triggered, Samantha was unable to sleep, and the family thought that this lack of sleep could also be contributing to her NES.

The clinician confirmed that both the trauma-related memories and the lack of sleep functioned to up-regulate the brain-body stress systems, making Samantha even more prone to NES.

The team then offered the family either a place in the inpatient Mind-Body Program or, if they preferred, outpatient therapy in their local community (in which case the Mind-Body Program could serve as a backup). Samantha was relieved that the NES could be treated. The family chose the outpatient option. The team did a careful handover of the case, and Samantha—after some hard work with her psychologist—returned to health and well-being.

The Narrative: Building a Therapeutic Relationship via the Storytelling Process

In the normal course of events—when the usual interview structure can be used—the therapeutic relationship can be built via the storytelling process. For the first author (KK) and her team, the storytelling process begins with the construction of the family genogram. The genogram gives a bird's-eye view of the family story across three generations. It identifies the family medical history, mental health history, and key family events, including births, deaths, separations, feuds, illnesses, and hospitalizations, along with their impact on the child. As the interview progresses, it is the clinician's job to make sure that key family events that were identified in the genogram are woven into the fabric of the narrative. The genogram brings into focus—through visual representation—key points in the family story that may need to be further discussed (McGoldrick et al. 2008). For example, if the genogram shows that the child's parents separated when the child was five, then—when the story reaches age five, and if the family fails to mention the separation—the interviewer needs to ask a question about the separation and its impact on the child and family.

Once the genogram is complete, the clinician conducting the interview asks the family to tell the story of the child's development and her symptoms. The clinician tracks the child's story in temporal order, starting with a brief account—usually from the child's mother—of the child's early developmental history, starting from conception. Was the child a planned child? How was the pregnancy? Was the family generally doing well, or was it, for example, conflicted, disrupted, or unsettled, during the pregnancy? Did the delivery go well? Did self-regulation milestones—feeding, sleeping, settling, connecting with others—go well in the first year of life? Were other milestones normal? Was the family doing well also? Did the child have any separation anxiety as a preschooler? What was she like in the preschool years? Did she make friends? Were there any family events or health issues? And so on, and so on. In the normal course of events, the family will take over the telling of the story, with the interviewer asking the odd question, to help the family think about the manner in which the child and her body responded to family events.

As the story moves into the school years, the clinician involves the child—and siblings—in the storytelling process more and more. From the time that the child attended preschool or kindergarten, the clinician tracks the story by school years to scaffold the child's memory and to anchor life events in the context of school years marked by specific teachers, classes, or classroom friends. At some point, the story merges into the story of the child's functional somatic symptoms. Throughout the storytelling process, the clinician maintains the story's temporal order—'put that on hold, we haven't gotten to year 5 yet'—and encourages the child to tell as much of the story as possible. Along the way, the clinician obtains additional details about the symptoms and asks questions that connect the symptoms to the context in which they occurred—to the year at school, to any important events at school, at home, or in the broader family or social context, and to the family's experience with the medical system. The questions help the family— while they are telling their story—to make connections between the child's symptoms and context.

The storytelling process has a number of important functions. First, the family need to know that their concerns have been heard and that the clinician fully appreciates the child's clinical presentation and the worries about the child's health. Being heard and being understood are particularly important for families who have been dismissed by the health care system. It is common for these families to have experienced distress in their efforts to obtain health care, and these adverse experiences need to be heard and acknowledged, enabling the events to be put into the past so that healing can take place.

Second, the story needs to include sufficient details about possible adverse childhood experiences (ACEs) that took place before the child's symptoms began to appear. This information is essential if the interviewer is to put together a picture—from the perspective of the child's body—of the factors that have shaped the child's stress system over time.

Third, the story needs to include sufficient details about the child's symptoms and the associated medical investigations. Only against that background can the interviewer be confident that the requisite medical assessment is complete and be in a position to think about the symptoms from a neurobiology perspective (see Chapters 4–12). In a multidisciplinary team, the clinician with a medical background is likely to be best suited to pursue this aspect of the assessment.

Fourth, using the child's body as the beacon, the interviewer needs to ask questions about the symptoms that help build a context around the symptoms: what was happening in the child's life when the symptoms arose? The process of context building is facilitated if the clinician has helped the family tell the story in temporal order, enabling the symptoms to be ordered along a time line that also marks other events in the child's and family's lives. In this context, the clinician needs to keep control of the temporal order of the interview, asking family members to put information on hold, until the correct time frame is reached in the storytelling process. Maintaining the time line is crucial in helping the family make connections—in making meaning—between events in the child's life and the child's symptoms. Most families compartmentalize and medicalize the symptoms, and fail to connect them with the distress associated with adverse life events. Through this process the story often shifts from a story of the symptoms to a story of how the child's body responded—via the symptoms—to various events in the child's and family's life stories.

Fifth, if the child's symptoms are longer-standing rather than acute, the interviewer needs to determine how the child and family have been managing or adapting to the illness, including such matters as the attention given to the symptoms and the impact of the illness on school attendance, physical activity, and engagement with peers.

We see all of these factors at work in the following case study of Paula, the 15-year-old bed-bound girl with a four-year history of functional somatic symptoms whom we first met in Chapter 2.

Case Study: Paula

Establishing a Therapeutic Relationship

The hospital's Pain Team referred Paula to Psychological Medicine, to be assessed for admission into the Mind-Body Program run by the first author.

Paula came to the family assessment interview with her older brother and her parents. The interview took two hours and involved construction of a family genogram (including medical history across three generations), the family telling the story of Paula's development and Paula's symptoms, the formulation, and a conversation about a treatment contract for the mind-body admission.

The genogram signalled that the family constellation was uncomplicated, that there was a history of terminal cancer on both sides of the family, and that Paula and her brother were very close to the maternal grandfather, who was dying. There was also a mental health history on the mother's side of the family (see Fig. 3.1), signalling a potential risk for Paula. The interviewer noted that the illnesses of both grandfathers in a time frame that intersected with Paula's own illness would need to be woven into the family story, as would the impact of those illnesses not only on Paula but on the family. The interviewer also noted that the miscarriage that had occurred before Paula had been conceived, coupled with Paula's need to be admitted to the neonatal intensive care unit (NICU) after she was born—may have set up a dynamic in which Paula's mother was acutely sensitive about health issues that came up with Paula.

The storytelling processing itself, as briefly summarized above, began with a question about Paula's conception. Everyone laughed and said that Paula was a very wanted baby. Paula's mother was asked briefly about the pregnancy and delivery. Paula had been a premature baby (30 weeks gestational age) and had spent one week in the NICU. On discharge from the NICU and in the first year of life, Paula had been able to regulate in terms of sleeping, feeding, and eating (breastfed for two years). She had demonstrated short-lived separation anxiety on going to preschool at three years of age.

The family gave the story clearly, and they conveyed the sense that everything had been tracking well right into primary school. As school came into focus, the interviewer suggested that Paula should now be able to access memories; progressively, and assisted when necessary by her parents and brother, Paula became the main storyteller. Paula related that she had been a physically active school-age child who enjoyed the outdoors. Although she always had some difficulties with making friends, she managed to maintain a friendship group who, like her, were interested in reading and in writing scripts for movies and plays. The interviewer then tracked Paula's health concerns by using her body as a beacon. In addition to asking detailed questions about Paula's symptoms, the interviewer made sure that the family saw how the symptoms were related to the context in which they had occurred (e.g., physical injury, illness concerns regarding the two grandfathers, and bullying).

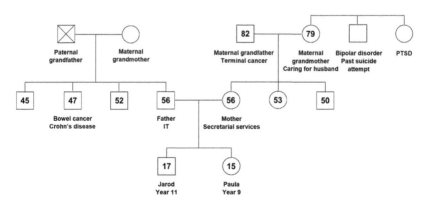

Fig. 3.1 Paula's genogram (© Kasia Kozlowska 2019)

When Paula told about the fracture in the lateral epicondyle of her right femur—at 11 years of age (year 5 in school)—the interviewer commented, 'Physical injuries are a stress for the body, so the fracture was the first major stress that your body had to deal with.' When Paula teared up when her maternal grandfather's illness was mentioned, the interviewer took time to explore the impact of the illness on all members of the family. When Paula teared up again when alluding to the bullying at school, the interviewer asked her to describe the bullying in detail to make sure that everyone in the family was aware of the extent of her distress. The interviewer also asked for details about how Paula's body had responded to the bullying. At the appropriate moments in the story, the interviewer interwove questions about the death of the paternal grandfather, the deteriorating health of the maternal grandfather, and the emotional responses of the family. The emergence of multiple symptoms—limb weakness, persistent headache, intermittent abdominal pain, and musculoskeletal pain that migrated all over her body—suggested that Paula's body had not been coping with the cumulative stress. Then the interviewer tracked the family's interactions with the medical system, their increasing anxiety and confusion pertaining to the many different diagnoses given by different medical specialists (see Chapter 2), the efforts by Paula and the family to manage her symptoms, Paula's being bullied at school, and her increasing functional impairment. Finally, taking into account Paula's decreased exercise and her withdrawal to her bed, the interviewer tracked symptoms of autonomic dysregulation and fatigue, as well as the emergence of panic attacks.

Co-constructing a Formulation

During the assessment process the ongoing effort to consolidate the therapeutic relationship continues via the process of co-constructing the formulation. In this context, the narrative told by the child and family is framed through the lens of the stress-system model (see Chapters 4–12). What happens, in effect, is that the story told by the family (i.e., what the child and the family know) is melded together with the meaning of that story from the perspective of the body (i.e., what the clinician knows). The two narratives, brought together, merge into a new, shared formulation. In the case of Paula and her family, the formulation was both articulated verbally and shown visually using visual metaphors. This example shows how the clinician (KK) went about the process of weaving the family story into a formulation picking up on the issues that she (the clinician) had marked as being relevant (and that, along with many other issues, will be discussed in much more detail in Part II on the neurobiology of functional somatic symptoms).

The formulation, which incorporates material that the reader will encounter in Part II, went as follows:

Thank you all for telling us the story of the symptoms so clearly. So now let me share with you my understanding of Paula's symptoms. Even though Paula's presentation is very complex, all of Paula's symptoms reflect activation and dysregulation of the brain-body stress systems. The stress system includes all the systems in the brain and body that activate when the body senses threat and danger. The body does not distinguish between stress that is physical (like Paula's epicondyle fracture and the physical bullying that Paula experienced) and emotional stress (like the verbal bullying that Paula experienced and her distress about her maternal grandfather's illness and physical deterioration). The body responds to all types of stress with activation of the stress system. So, I am going to draw the stress system for you (circles metaphor of the stress system; see Fig. 3.2).

First, the bottom circle represents the hypothalamic-pituitary-adrenal (HPA) axis. The HPA axis activates with stress. It uses signal molecules—hormones—to communicate. The final product of activating the HPA axis is the release a stress hormone called cortisol. Cortisol is involved in energy regulation and adaptation to stress. It ensures that the body system has sufficient energy resources to deal with the stress. We know that Paula's HPA axis got switched on because activation of the HPA axis disturbs sleep. And Paula described really clearly how her sleep was disturbed both after the fracture and at the time of the bullying. Cortisol also facilitates stress responses in the brain, which we shall talk about in a bit.

The coloured circles on the left represent the autonomic nervous system—another component of the stress system (circles metaphor of the stress system; see Fig. 3.2). The autonomic system regulates body arousal on a second-by-second basis. It regulates all the organs inside the body,

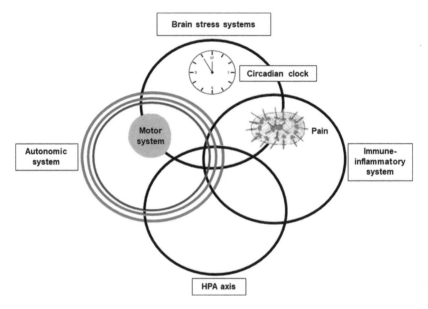

Fig. 3.2 Circles metaphor of the stress-system model for functional somatic symptoms. Online Supplement 4.4 depicts a version of the circles metaphor that can be printed out (© Kasia Kozlowska 2013)

including the heart. Let me show you [the interviewer draws and explains the functional diagram of the autonomic system and the symptoms associated with its activation; see Fig. 6.1]. We know that Paula's autonomic system is activated and dysregulated because the diagnosis of postural orthostatic tachycardia syndrome (POTS) (see Chapter 6) involves too little blue/restorative-parasympathetic activity (allowing heart rate to increase) and too much red/sympathetic activity (through which heart rate increases even more on standing). This is why Paula feels dizzy when standing up. And Paula's symptoms of nausea are activated by the purple/defensive parasympathetic, which switches on the gut's defensive programs, including the nausea program. The loss of regular bowel function also shows that the blue/restorative parasympathetic is not working well and that the red/sympathetic is switched on too high: the red/sympathetic switches off the gut and can cause constipation.

Now here things get even more complicated. The red/sympathetic system works hand in hand with the motor respiratory system (part of the motor system, the pink ball in the circles metaphor of the stress system;

see Fig. 3.2). During the interview—when Paula got teary—I counted her respiratory rate. It was 35 breaths per minute. This means that when Paula's body gets aroused—when the sympathetic system gets switched on—she also switches on the respiratory muscles, and she hyperventilates (as confirmed later on a hyperventilation challenge; see Fig. 3.3). Activation of the sympathetic system (which causes the heart to thump and the sweatiness that Paula experiences), as well as hyperventilation (which contributes to Paula's dizziness), also occurs during Paula's panic attacks. Hyperventilation contributes to dizziness because when people hyperventilate, they blow off too much carbon dioxide and lower the carbon dioxide concentration in the blood. The brain hates this. Low carbon dioxide makes the brain arteries constrict. This decreases blood flow and causes dizziness. Some people will even faint from hyperventilation.

Now we still need to talk about Paula's other symptoms: weakness in the limbs; intermittent loss of vision; chronic migrating pain; and pervasive sense of fatigue. In our diagram of the stress system, these symptoms involve the brain stress systems, which are represented by the top circle (circles metaphor of the stress system; see Fig. 3.2). Within the brain a number of regions activate in response to stress, threat, and danger—whether the threat is physical or emotional (see Chapter 11). The stress systems in the brain also activate in response to the negative emotions such as those that emerged, for example, when Paula was being bullied or when she was thinking about her grandfather who is dying (see Chapter 12). Then we also have the brain regions that process other experiences:

- *Pain maps* process pain.
- *Motor-processing regions* process motor function.
- *Sensory-processing regions* process sensory function.
- *Energy- and fatigue-processing regions*, also known as the *fatigue alarm system* or *fatigue alarm* (and still not well defined), regulate the use of energy (including feelings that represent fatigue).

Now, the brain stress systems are supposed to *switch on* when the danger occurs and then to *switch off* once the danger has passed. However, we know from imaging studies of patients with chronic pain, functional neurological symptoms, or other functional somatic symptoms that the brain stress systems *fail to switch off*. What happens, instead, is that these regions become overactive and over-dominant [the interviewer draws a large red ball]. In this state, the brain stress systems can disrupt motor-processing regions and cause motor symptoms—like the weakness

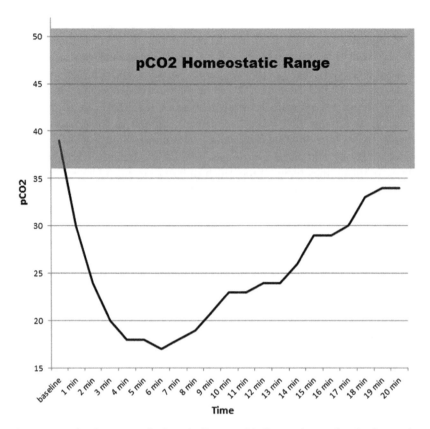

Fig. 3.3 Paula's hyperventilation challenge. This figure shows that in the resting state she was breathing at a healthy respiratory rate that kept her arterial CO_2, or pCO_2, within the homeostatic range. When Paula was asked to hyperventilate voluntarily, her pCO_2 dropped, as it should. However, when Paula was asked to stop hyperventilating, she was unable to do so. She continued to hyperventilate, and her pCO_2 did not return to baseline (the homeostatic range). The hyperventilation challenge was consistent with clinical observations that Paula hyperventilated when thinking about distressing life events, that she had trouble regulating her breathing when her system was activated as part of a panic attack, and that the poorly regulated breathing contributed to her symptoms of dizziness and fatigue (© Kasia Kozlowska 2019)

in the legs that Paula has experienced (see Fig. 11.2). The brain stress systems can also disrupt sensory-processing regions and cause sensory symptoms—like the visual loss that Paula has experienced (see Fig. 11.3).

And they can amplify pain by keeping the pain map switched on (see Fig. 11.5). In this way, the pain becomes chronic and can be triggered by a minor physical or emotional stress, and the pain can do odd things like migrate all over the body. That's something you all already know because you have observed the pain migrating around Paula's body. In addition, activation of the brain stress systems involves an increased use of energy, and many patients experience increased feelings of fatigue.

We are almost done. But I have forgotten to tell you about three things. This clock image represents the circadian clock (see Fig. 3.2). The circadian clock regulates the sleep cycle. When the circadian clock is dysregulated—as it is in Paula's case—it means that the brain misses out on all the restorative processes that are supposed to take place at night. Disturbed sleep also contributes to activation of the stress system—nothing is ever allowed to switch off—plus disturbed sleep increases pain. So, sorting out sleep is going to be very important.

And then, we have the immune-inflammatory system—the last component of the stress system (see Fig. 3.2). This system is very important because it contributes to chronic pain. In chronic pain this system is switched on, and immune-inflammatory cells in the body secrete pro-inflammatory substances that keep pain nerves activated, thereby signalling pain. One such cell type is the *macrophage* (see Fig. 9.1). Macrophages normally go around the body cleaning up debris and secreting anti-inflammatory molecules. But when they are switched into defensive mode—as happens in chronic pain—they secrete pro-inflammatory molecules that maintain pain. Exercise helps macrophages to switch into healthy restorative mode, in which they secrete anti-inflammatory molecules that decrease pain. But *lack* of exercise causes macrophages to switch into *defensive* mode. So, the fact that Paula is so deconditioned and that she is not doing any exercise is contributing to activation of the immune-inflammatory system—cells like the macrophage—and is keeping the pain maps activated. Reintroducing exercise is therefore going to be very important, too.

Finally, we come to the role of the mind. The way we use our minds can either switch on the stress system or help it settle (see Chapter 12). Paula told me that she worries about the symptoms. Sometimes she even worries that she will be sick forever. She can even visualize herself as an invalid in a wheelchair when she grows up. Every time she worries or brings up that image, she uses her mind to switch on the stress system top-down. This top-down activation of the stress system just makes things worse. Another factor that makes symptoms worse is attention. Every time Paula pays attention to the pain, it will intensify. Every time mum asks about the pain, watches out for it, or is experienced by Paula as worrying about it, the pain will also intensify. So, changing how we all focus our attention will be another important part of the intervention.

Now that we have finished our explanation of the stress system and its interactions with other brain regions, you can see that, although the different specialists have used different names for different symptoms, all the symptoms arise from an interrelated process: the activation and dysregulation of the stress system. [At this point the interviewer may write down the different words different specialists use and include some other words that the family is likely to run across.] Next, we are going to talk about treatment options. But before we go on, do you have any other questions?

Depicting the Treatment Process via Visual Metaphor

If the child and family accept the formulation—the story of their child's illness through the lens of the stress-system model—then the conversation moves onto treatment. The family's acceptance (or lack thereof) is usually communicated quite clearly. The tension in the room suddenly disappears. A parent may let out a sigh of relief. Faces brighten. Often someone in the family articulates their felt sense of relief: the relief that comes with understanding what is happening for the child and her body. Sometimes, if someone in the family had an *aha! moment*, they will share this new understanding. Sometimes the family will acknowledge that the neurobiology is very complex and thank the clinician for taking the time to explain it to them.

For some families it can be helpful to depict the process of treatment via a visual metaphor. In Figs. 3.4 and 3.5, the treatment process is represented visually using the circles metaphor and the castle-fortress metaphor, respectively. The figures depict that the clinician—and child and family—will be working together to choose interventions that will shift the child's stress system from an activated, dysregulated, incoherent state (a stress system in defensive mode) back to a more regulated, more coherent state, and to a more healthy way of functioning (a stress

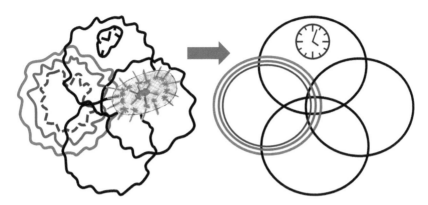

Fig. 3.4 Treatment depicted using the circles metaphor of the stress-system model for functional somatic symptoms. Using the circles metaphor, the treatment process can be conceptualized as involving a shift from a dysregulated state—with stress-system components being overactivated, underactivated, out of harmony with other components, or out of synchrony with the circadian rhythm—to a regulated state that supports health and well-being (© Kasia Kozlowska 2017)

Castle in defensive mode   **Castle in restorative mode**

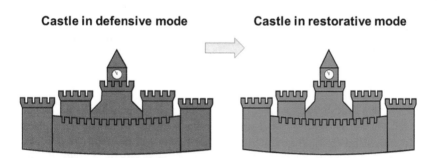

Fig. 3.5 Treatment depicted using the castle-fortress metaphor of the stress system model for functional somatic symptoms. Using the castle-fortress metaphor, the treatment process can be conceptualized as involving a shift from a castle-fortress in defensive mode (denoted by the colour red)—where battle towers are manned to protect the castle-fortress from attack—to a castle-fortress in peace time (denoted by the colour blue) (© Kasia Kozlowska 2017)

system in restorative mode). The stress system in defensive mode supports the generation of functional somatic symptoms, whereas a stress system in restorative mode supports health and well-being and is not compatible with the generation of functional somatic symptoms.

If specific factors have been identified as contributing to stress-system activation, these can be written in above the visual representation, with large arrows that depict their role in activating the stress system. For example, in Paula's case, bullying at school, worry about the deterioration of her maternal grandfather, ruminating and catastrophizing about school, and parental attention to the symptoms would all be written into the visual representation, highlighting the role of these factors in activating Paula's stress system.

Rationale for the Interventions That Make Up Treatment

The conversation then moves onto the rationale for using certain interventions in the treatment program. The treatment rationale builds directly on the neurobiology of the stress system, as previously discussed with the family. Sometimes, the rationale for certain interventions has already been addressed during the formulation itself, as when we discussed with Paula the need for her to start mobilizing again. In offering Paula an admission into our inpatient program, we also explained the various other interventions that would be implemented as part of the program. The conversation went as follows:

> Now let's talk about treatment—what needs to happen for Paula to get well. As you know, the Pain Team are really keen that Paula is given a place in our Mind-Body Program. And we are happy to offer Paula two weeks in the program. But let us tell you about the program so that Paula can decide if it is something she wants to do. [The program is described in detail by a member of the team.] Paula will come into the adolescent medicine ward for two weeks to learn the program. After completing those two weeks, she will then need to take the program home and continue it, with the support of the family, for the next 12 months, or even longer. She will need to build some components of the program—for example, the regulation strategies and the regular exercise—into her life for the long term.

Earlier, when we discussed the neurobiology of Paula's symptoms, we saw that they all involve the activation and dysregulation of the stress system. Treatment of functional somatic symptoms—using body-mind interventions—aims to help Paula switch off the stress system and to regulate the stress system better. Because Paula has been sick such a long time, we shall use every intervention and strategy we know—at the same time—to help her stress system regulate better. Here is the plan that I have in my mind:

- Right after admission, we shall do a blood test to check Paula's iron level, vitamin B12, vitamin D, and a few other things that weren't checked before. We shall also perform a hyperventilation challenge to see how significant Paula's hyperventilation is and how well she is able regulate her breathing. Paula will also do a standing test for the POTS, so we can see how her body regulates heart rate and blood pressure when she stands up from a lying-down position on waking up in the morning. We always make sure that the medical assessment is complete and that all the boxes are ticked. [This final set of tests found that Paula was iron deficient—ferritin level 4 μg/L (reference range 10–150 μg/L). This iron deficiency contributed to her fatigue. The hyperventilation challenge confirmed Paula's hyperventilation (see Fig. 3.3). The standing test for POTS revealed that the autonomic dysregulation was severe and needed active treatment to stabilize (see Table 3.1). Paula's standing test showed (1) a minimum heart rate increase of 38 beats per minute, and a maximum increase of 64 beats per minute, on standing, and (2) no substantial change in blood pressure within ten minutes. In children, an increase in heart rate of >40 beats per minute is consistent with orthostatic intolerance.]
- Our first immediate intervention will be to stabilize Paula's sleep—the circadian clock—to harness all the restorative processes that take place at night. Good sleep will help Paula's body regulate. No one can regulate without good sleep. Paula can start the sleep intervention at home while she is waiting for a bed in the Mind-Body Program. You need to put together a timetable that marks bedtime and getting up time. Paula will need to go to bed at the same time every day and also get up at the same time. She will need to sit in the sun in the morning—on waking up—for about an hour. We shall also use melatonin—the natural substance that the brain secretes—to help regulate her sleep. If these measures are not sufficient, there are other things we can do (see Chapter 5). [In the end, Paula's sleep was regulated with 9 mg melatonin and 25 mg quetiapine.]

Table 3.1   Paula's heart rate and blood pressure values on the Standing Orthostatic
Tolerance Test (© Kasia Kozlowska 2019)

Time period	Blood pressure	Heart rate
Baseline (lying down)	117/68	84
1 minute (standing)	124/80	135
2 minutes (standing)	132/85	128
3 minutes (standing)	132/86	128
4 minutes (standing)	127/82	132
5 minutes (standing)	112/79	122
6 minutes (standing)	111/87	146
7 minutes (standing)	124/85	128
8 minutes (standing)	93/66	126
9 minutes (standing)	115/90	126
10 minutes (standing)	121/88	126

- Our second intervention during the admission will be to treat the
  POTS (the dysregulation of the autonomic system) with body strategies: increasing fluid intake, taking salt tablets, using stockings, and
  implementing slow-breathing strategies that help increase blue/par-
  asympathetic function and decrease red/sympathetic function [point
  out the relevant nerves on Fig. 6.1]. If these strategies are not enough,
  there are other things we can do (e.g., treatment with propranolol)
  (van der Zalm et al. 2019). The treatment should help Paula's symptoms of dizziness on standing and, over time, her energy levels. [In
  the end, treatment for POTS included salt tablets, increased water
  intake, and pressure stockings; the slow-breathing strategies were
  incorporated into the broader strategy for improving Paula's capacity
  for self-regulation (see next item).]
- Paula will work with [name of psychologist] to work out what
  mind-body strategies she is able to use to help regulate her body and
  her stress system. [In the end, Paula's key bottom-up strategies were
  slow breathing, muscle relaxation, and shifting attention away from
  pain to sensations that were pleasant.]
- Paula will also need to work with [name of psychologist] to determine
  how she contributes to the symptoms with her mind, as by worrying,
  ruminating, catastrophizing, and so on. [Basic cognitive-behavioural
  interventions were used to address these issues and, in combination
  with mindfulness interventions, were continued with a psychologist
  after discharge.]

– During the first week of the admission—as we get to know Paula better—we shall also decide if Paula will need medication (a selective serotonin reuptake inhibitor [SSRI]) to treat her severe anxiety, or whether mind-body strategies will be sufficient. We are raising the potential need for medication now because Paula is very ill and because we know—from the information about Paula's panic attacks—that her anxiety is quite severe. You also need to know that anti-anxiety medication can be helpful in treating POTS (Rowe 2014). [We found that Paula's anxiety was overwhelming and completely incapacitating. Alongside mind-body strategies, she was treated with fluoxetine 20 mg (increased slowly from 2.5 mg in the morning, in 2.5 mg increments) and quetiapine 6.25 mg in the morning, which helped take the edge of her anxiety and helped her get to the hospital school.]

– Paula will work with the physiotherapist on a daily basis to set up an exercise program that she can take home. The exercise will help the POTS, anxiety, and deconditioning, and it will help shift Paula's macrophages into restorative mode—which, in the long term, will help decrease Paula's pain. [Paula continued an exercise program that was monitored by an external physiotherapist and that her parents also continued to oversee.]

– Paula will go to the hospital school every morning. During the afternoon, she can either attend school or the adolescent group—whichever she prefers. She can use the school to practice her strategies for the pain and fatigue, and to build up her energy levels, enabling her to resume attending her own local school. [Paula returned to her own school, full time, on discharge.]

– There is no visiting during the day, when Paula is busy with the program. Visiting hours are limited to the hours after she has completed that day's program. There is no program on the weekend; Paula will have a gate pass from hospital to go home for Saturday night. Because attention to symptoms makes the symptoms worse, we ask the family, when together with Paula, to practice not asking about symptoms but to ask about what Paula did that day (if in the hospital) or to engage in some other activities. Paula is also to practice not talking about the symptoms. She can, however, boast to everyone about what she is doing to manage the symptoms.

– We will have a weekly family meeting to track how Paula is doing and to begin the process of helping everyone in the family make the necessary changes that will support Paula's health and well-being in the long term.

- We expect that at some point during the admission, Paula might have some difficult days—might feel exhausted and unable to go on. If that happens, we shall use it as opportunity for the family to see how Paula (and they) will manage days that are difficult and that feel like a setback. [Paula's temporary setback came after she jarred her arm while travelling on a bus with her father while returning home from a Saturday night concert. The bus had stopped suddenly, activating high-intensity back pain and panic attacks, and Paula wanted to retreat to bed. While recovering from this setback, Paula was encouraged to use her various strategies (as described above) with increased frequency, and she attended the hospital school in a wheelchair, soon graduating to pushing it herself. Within a few days, she returned to the point of progress where she had been a few days earlier. The episode also functioned as a trial run for Paula's mother—a coaching exercise—as to what she needed to do when Paula had a setback at home.]
- Finally, Paula's present diet is low in fruit, vegetables, yogurt, and meat. So, Paula needs to start improving her diet while she is waiting for the hospital admission. A healthy diet has to be part of any program for getting well. [The family also opted to incorporate probiotics into Paula's daily intake.]

Therapeutic Contract

After the treatment has been discussed, a therapeutic contract needs to be agreed, including the following: confirmation that the child wants to come into the Mind-Body Program and that the parents consent to all components of the program; the goals that the child has to meet before the admission itself; the time frame of the admission; the program structure; and discussion and negotiation of any potentially 'sticky' points. The contract also involves discussion as to what will happen with outpatient treatment afterward—for example, with referral or handover back to local services. At this time of negotiating a therapeutic contract, the family has the option of deciding whether they want to take up the offer of inpatient treatment or, instead, whether they would like the team to help them set up a program with resources from their local community. The team also has the option of withdrawing the offer of an inpatient admission if the family do not agree to core components of the treatment program or if the child or family are not sufficiently motivated. In the latter situation, the offer of the program—with its specific, defined conditions—remains open to the child and family in the future.

Occasionally, we admit a child into our Mind-Body Program with only the parents' consent (and contract)—even if the child does not want to come into the program. This is sometimes necessary because the child, due to severe anxiety, will not cooperate with any aspect of treatment or because the lack of cooperation is part of the presenting picture. In this scenario the intervention begins by establishing a therapeutic environment in which the child is given multiple opportunities to engage with different therapists within the program—the nursing staff, psychotherapist, physiotherapist, and school staff—on a daily basis. In these scenarios, the child is, if necessary, taken to the school classroom on her bed.

The Outcome of the Mind-Body Admission for Paula

The overall treatment program involved both a preadmission intervention—Paula had to reach some goals before admission into the hospital program—and a two-week admission to the Mind-Body Program itself, which was extended to three weeks because of Paula's significant level of deconditioning (since she had been sick for so long). The interventions implemented prior to admission included the following: re-establishing a normal sleep-wake cycle, along with an hour of sun exposure immediately after arising; establishing a healthy diet, with regular meals; and establishing an exercise routine as part of the process of gradual reconditioning (initially, for example, by implementing short walks outside the house to the front gate of the garden). The interventions implemented during her program are those that were discussed with the family above. After completion of the hospital program, Paula took the program home with her and continued to implement it with the help of her parents, a psychologist, a local physiotherapist, and her general practitioner. Her pain and fatigue resolved to a large extent; her anxiety continued to be challenging to manage; and she had a number of time-limited relapses of functional neurological symptoms (leg weakness and vision loss). But she continued to persevere with the program and to attend school—and stay connected to her friendship group—just as she had done in the hospital setting.

* * *

In this chapter we have examined how multidisciplinary teams engage with children with functional somatic symptoms and their parents through the therapeutic process of a family assessment interview. As we have seen through our discussion of Paula, the assessment interview serves multiple purposes. Among other things, it assists the family in telling the story of the symptoms in relation to the broader story of the events and challenges that occurred in the life of the child and family; it facilitates a shared understanding of those events and challenges; it enables the co-construction of a formulation by looking at the information provided by the family through the lens of the stress-system model; it provides a rationale for treatment; and it facilitates the articulation of a therapeutic contract through which everyone agrees to work together before, during, and after the period of the mind-body intervention. We hope that clinicians working in a broad range of clinical settings will be able to adapt some of the ideas presented in this chapter to their own way of working and to the needs of their own clinical contexts and practice

References

Kozlowska, K., English, M., & Savage, B. (2013). Connecting Body and Mind: The First Interview with Somatizing Patients and Their Families. *Clinical Child Psychology and Psychiatry, 18,* 223–245.

McGoldrick, M., Gerson, R., & Petry, S. (2008). *Genograms: Assessment and Intervention.* New York: Norton.

Rowe, P. C. (2014). *General Information Brochure on Orthostatic Intolerance and Its Treatment.* Baltimore, MD: Chronic Fatigue Clinic, Johns Hopkins Children's Center. http://www.dysautonomiainternational.org/pdf/RoweOIsummary.pdf.

Sattler, J. M. (1992). *Assessment of Children*. San Diego, CA: Jerome M Sattler, Publisher.

Van Der Zalm, T., Alsma, J., Van De Poll, S. W. E., Wessels, M. W., Riksen, N. P., & Versmissen, J. (2019). Postural Orthostatic Tachycardia Syndrome (POTS): A Common but Unfamiliar Syndrome. *Netherlands Journal of Medicine, 77,* 3–9.

Worsely, C., Whitehead, K., Kandler, R., & Reuber, M. (2011). Illness Perceptions of Health Care Workers in Relation to Epileptic and Psychogenic Nonepileptic Seizures. *Epilepsy & Behavior, 20,* 668–673.

Part II

Mind, Body, and the Science of Functional Somatic Symptoms

Part II—Chapters 4–12—is about the neurobiology of functional somatic symptoms. Chapter 4 introduces the reader to the stress system and the stress-system model for functional somatic symptoms. The remaining chapters in Part II discuss the various interacting components of the stress system, along with some other factors that, though not specifically elements of the stress system, have a substantial impact on the stress system and on functional somatic symptoms themselves.

Although the idea of the stress system now seems a familiar one, it is only recently that stress has been conceptualized in terms of a neurobiological system: in 1986, a group of scientists—the child endocrinologist George Chrousos and his colleagues—formulated the notion of the stress system as a framework for analysing the neurobiological mechanisms involved in the body's response to physical and emotional stress (Chrousos et al. 1988). In this book the stress system serves as a framework for thinking about functional somatic symptoms and the many different factors that affect the body, brain, and mind—the system levels that contribute to the generation of functional somatic symptoms in children and adolescents.

Our clinical experience is that children and families find the stress-system model useful because it provides a concrete and straight-forward way—accompanied by visual representations—of talking about what is happening to the child in her body, brain, and mind. When the model is used in daily clinical work, families often experience an aha! moment when they begin to understand the different factors that interact on the body, brain, and mind system levels to generate functional somatic symptoms. Sometimes the explanation provided to the child and family draws on medical knowledge that is well established. Other times the conversations rely on current developments or upon current hypotheses that reflect the thinking of leaders in the field. Either way, children and families are relieved to know that functional somatic symptoms are the focus of current research, and they like to hear—in simple terms—where the field is up to. All of a sudden, symptoms that appeared mysterious, that could not be explained, or that were explained as being psychosomatic have clear and more straightforward explanations—sometimes hypothetical—as to underlying mechanisms involving body, brain, and mind.

In contrast to the commonly held belief that children with functional somatic symptoms and their families are difficult to engage, we have found that the children and families who come seeking treatment at our respective services become very involved in the process of sharing the story of the somatic symptoms and in co-constructing a formulation. Families are, indeed, typically eager to engage in the treatment process so that their child can get well. Likewise, clinicians who have come to training sessions about the stress-system model of functional somatic symptoms—or who have come to learn the model during a clinical placement—have found this way of working with patients and families to be both helpful and empowering. As one such trainee noted:

> I am pleased to say that using the stress-system explanation for non-epileptic seizures and chronic pain syndrome has made a drastic difference in how my patients and their families understand and engage in treatment. It's almost transformative in the sense that families feel

their child is finally being taken seriously and their symptomatology has a very real and robust pathophysiological basis. To them it's the difference between being blamed for 'a symptom in their head' versus having their very distressing symptoms being validated and treated.

Another trainee observed:

As the child and family gain an understanding of the stress-system model during formulation, they will volunteer new information—stressors and symptoms—that fit into their growing understanding of their own experience of this process.

In this context, the chapters in Part II will give the reader a good basic grounding in the neurobiology of the stress system and functional somatic symptoms, along with an introduction to the research literature, with additional references available in Online Supplement 1.3. The chapters also provide the reader with some visual resources that can be used to communicate, in a very simple way, the complex biological processes involved in the body's response to stress. The hope and expectation is that familiarity with this scientific material will provide the foundation for readers to use the stress-system model in their clinical work with children and their families—as further elaborated in Part III, on treatment.

Reference

Chrousos, G. P., Loriaux, D. L., & Gold, P. W. (1988). Preface. In G. P. Chrousos, D. L. Loriaux, & P. W. Gold (Eds.), *Mechanisms of Physical and Emotional Stress*. New York: Plenum Press (Advances in Experimental Medicine and Biology, Vol. 245).

4

The Stress-System Model for Functional Somatic Symptoms

Abstract This chapter introduces the reader to the stress-system model for functional somatic symptoms through the personal journey of the first author. The stress-system model provides clinicians with a framework for thinking about the neurobiology of functional somatic symptoms and for explaining them to children and their families. The components of the brain-body stress system—the neurobiological systems that regulate body state—include the circadian clock, hypothalamic-pituitary-adrenal axis, autonomic nervous system, immune-inflammatory system, and brain stress systems that underpin salience detection, arousal, pain, and emotional states. All components of the stress system are interconnected and form part of a larger, integrated system that ensures effective energy regulation, promotes health and survival, and protects the individual from a broad range of threats. When the stress system—or one or more components of the stress system—is activated too much, too little, too long,

Electronic supplementary material The online version of this chapter (https://doi.org/10.1007/978-3-030-46184-3_4) contains supplementary material, which is available to authorized users.

or in aberrant ways, or when it fails to return to baseline function, then functional somatic symptoms may arise.

As every mental health clinician knows, a good clinical assessment requires one to listen carefully to the child (including the adolescent) and family, and to piece together the story behind the clinical presentation. After listening to patients' stories for some years, I (the first author, KK) realized that my own observations of children with functional somatic symptoms ran contrary to the assumptions and myths that shaped clinical thinking and practice in the late 1990s, which is when I began my clinical practice as a child psychiatrist. I also realized that my observations of the child and her functioning in the family rarely matched those of the family. Over the years, as I puzzled about these recurring discrepancies, conducted my own research, and read countless research and clinical articles about patients with functional somatic symptoms, I came to recognize the central importance of *stress*. All of this clinical work and research comes together in the stress-system model for functional somatic symptoms, the focus of this book.

The easiest way to understand this model is to retrace my path and to review the discrepancies, puzzles, and clinical phenomena that led me both to recognize the centrality of stress and to use it as a foundation for understanding functional somatic symptoms. This retracing takes us through the first half of the chapter; the shared work of the three authors (KK, SS, HH) begins again with the section 'Embodied Family History'. Additional references for this chapter are available in Online Supplement 1.3.

Clinical Observations About the Role of Stress

The Consistent Presence of Stress in the Family Story

When I first learnt about functional somatic symptoms, they were seen as a reflection of stress and distress (Taylor 1986; Maisami and Freeman 1987), which is actually how I see them now. But importantly, there was also a lingering belief, dating to the work of Sigmund Freud, that unusually adverse life events—such as abuse, maltreatment, or incidents involving serious trauma—were the main factors contributing to and triggering the symptoms (see Online Supplement 1.3). A product of this belief was that clinicians spent a lot of time probing for, and asking about, the existence of such events. As might be expected, this process often made the family uncomfortable—and also reluctant to engage in treatment. For example, in the story of Samantha in Chapter 2, engagement with the mental health team and Samantha failed because the team was intent on looking for a history of sexual abuse—and they kept asking questions about potential sexual abuse—when sexual abuse was not, in fact, part of Samantha's story.

Recent research has presented a more complicated picture of how functional somatic symptoms emerge. As originally thought, there *is* an association between functional somatic symptoms and maltreatment early in life or exposure to serious trauma (Afari et al. 2014). Children who have been sexually abused have a higher lifetime prevalence of somatic symptoms or syndromes (see studies listed in Online Supplement 1.3). Likewise, individuals traumatized by war have higher rates of functional somatic symptoms. For example, Holocaust survivors from World War II—who suffered from a combination of intense stress, severe physical deprivation, and loss of loved ones when they were children or young adults—have a higher prevalence of functional gastrointestinal symptoms, fibromyalgia, chronic/complex pain, and other nonspecific somatic symptoms (dizziness, exhaustion, and weakness), often comorbid with depression and post-traumatic stress disorder (see studies listed in Online Supplement 1.3). Finally, adolescent Cambodian refugees—fleeing from the more than two decades of ongoing strife in that country—also experienced high rates of somatic symptoms, with headache and dizziness being the most common (Mollica et al. 1997). Interestingly, orthostatic symptoms, including dizziness, were some of the most common functional somatic symptoms experienced by soldiers from the American Civil War (1861–1864) (see Online Supplement 1.1).

Nevertheless, my clinical experience with children presenting with functional somatic symptoms, as well as my own research and that of others over the past 20 years, indicated that exposure to extreme stress was not actually necessary—or even common. Most of the children and families that I saw had stories that were full of relatively common, but also surely adverse, life events—such as physical illness, death of a grandparent, especially intense athletic training, or conflict in the family or at school (including bullying)—that had occurred in relatively close proximity to one another and that seemed to have had a cumulative effect on the child over time. Very often a minor physical event—viral illness, minor fall or twisting injury, knock on the head by a ball, or medical intervention or illness—or a relatively minor psychological event had precipitated the functional presentation. A small handful of children and families *did* report maltreatment (physical or sexual abuse, or serious neglect), family conflict that had gotten out of control (domestic violence), or some other especially traumatic event, but these circumstances were uncommon. The typical pattern that came up time and again was that of cumulative, normative stress events. The family and child reported that the child had coped with event 1, had coped with event 2, had coped with event 3, but had then, following event 4, suddenly developed debilitating functional somatic symptoms that had had precipitated the presentation to hospital.

After hearing many, many stories, it became clear to me that the origin of the functional somatic symptoms was associated with the overall burden of *chronic* or *repeated* stress—whether physical or emotional. It also seemed that the brain did not adhere to mind-body dualism and that physical stress events could trigger the illness just as easily as emotional events. As we got better at documenting trigger events in our studies, we found that about half our patients presented with physical triggers and half with emotional triggers, usually in the context of chronic or repeated stress (Kozlowska et al. 2011).

Research over the last 20 years has highlighted the important role of commonplace adverse life events. In particular, results from the Adverse Childhood Experiences Study (ACE Study) (Redding 2003; Felitti et al. 1998) showed that *household dysfunction*—situations such as the child's mother being treated violently, mental illness of a family member, substance abuse, parental separation or divorce, and imprisonment of a household member—played a central role in health and disease. Early research using this broader framework focused on the association between adverse childhood experiences and common physical health (ischaemic heart disease, cancer, chronic lung disease, skeletal fractures, and liver disease) and mental health (alcoholism, drug abuse, depression, and suicide attempts) conditions (see studies listed in Online Supplement 1.3). More recent studies have confirmed the long-observed association between adverse childhood experiences and functional somatic symptoms and syndromes (see studies listed in Online Supplement 1.3). In our own studies of children with functional neurological disorder (FND) and chronic/complex pain, antecedent illness or injury, family conflict, and bullying in the school and peer contexts have also consistently emerged as additional important antecedents (Kozlowska et al. 2011; McInnis et al. 2020).

The Parents Said 'Our Child Is Fine', but the Child's Body Did Not Agree

When telling their story, the parents and the child reported that, even though the child had experienced one difficulty after another, the child had coped and seemed to be *fine*. I found, however, that when the child's story was tracked via the child's body—the response of the body being used as the beacon by which the child's wellness was gauged—a different picture emerged (Kozlowska et al. 2013). The child's body had been signalling stress and distress for some time, but these signals had not been heeded. Common signals included the following: a disturbance in sleep (difficulties getting to sleep, waking up in the middle of the night, or waking unrefreshed and fatigued); difficulties eating because food felt like a lump in the child's tummy; increased frequency of abdominal pain, headache, or pain associated with muscle tension elsewhere in the body; a story of viral illnesses that the child found difficult to recover from and that had been followed by prolonged fatigue; and sometimes even the odd panic attack with a racing heart, sweatiness, and difficulty breathing.

The body's signals had not been heeded; the connection between the symptoms and the events in the child's life had not been made; and help for the child to manage her distress, her *dis-ease*, had not been provided (for a discussion of *dis-ease* vs. *disease*, see Online Supplement 1.1). Instead, the child had continued to struggle valiantly onward; she had continued to smile to reassure her parents that she was fine; and when anyone asked, she told them that she was fine. Her symptoms were, in effect, masked, and everyone carried on as always, secure in the belief that the child was resilient, that the child was doing well. But, of course, the child's body was not fine. The child's body told a different story. The body's story suggested that each stress had switched on the child's stress system. With each new stress, the stress system had been activated more and more, and was less and less able to turn itself off. The story that had begun with one functional somatic symptom was now a story of many different symptoms (see, e.g., the story of Paula in Chapter 2).

Translating Clinical Insights into a Research Program

Although the children and their parents typically told me that they were psychologically and emotionally unmarked by the adverse life events that they had experienced, I felt unconvinced. Likewise, although the paediatricians who referred children for treatment of functional somatic symptoms always confirmed that the physical examination was normal, that there was nothing wrong with the children's physical health and no evidence of disease, my impression was that their bodies had activated in response to stress and had not settled back down. It was common for the child's respiratory rate to be elevated—a sign of motor activation, possibly coupled with sympathetic activation. Another such sign was the child's response—with pain—to palpation of their postural muscles, the neck and back muscles that maintain posture and that activate when the body prepares itself for action; this response suggested that those muscles were activated or braced as they would be if the children were readying themselves for self-protective action.

To examine the questions raised by these encounters with patients and families, I was able to use research methodologies developed by two important mentors: the developmental psychologist and attachment researcher Patricia (Pat) Crittenden, and the neuroscientist Leanne (Lea) Williams. For many years (since 1996), alongside other clinicians, I had contributed to Pat's efforts to develop clinical tools to identify patterns of attachment in school-age children and adolescents within her Dynamic-Maturational Model of attachment and adaptation (DMM) (Crittenden 1999; Crittenden et al. 2010; Farnfield et al. 2010). Patterns of attachment—also known as attachment strategies—evolve from infancy through adolescence via one's experience with close others. Attachment strategies function to maximize safety, comfort, and the biological drive for survival and reproduction. Importantly for us, attachment figures also function, across development, as psychobiological regulators. On a daily basis, during playful interactions, attachment figures activate the child's stress system in a moderate way. Likewise, on a daily basis, attachment figures use a range of soothing strategies to help settle the stress system back down again. These repeating interactions with the attachment figure(s) function to regulate, either effectively or ineffectively, the child's developing stress system (see studies listed in Online Supplement 1.3). These early interactions of children are the building blocks of each person's self-regulatory capacities later in life. But when families are stressed—because of commonplace adverse life events, loss events, or trauma—the caregiver's capacity to function as a psychobiological regulator may be compromised.

A key strength of the DMM methodology for assessing attachment is its emphasis on procedural (i.e., memory of past action patterns), affective, and imaged evidence to help coders identify patterns of self-protective organization. For example, in assessing attachment in young children, the focus is on observed behaviour, and in older children, the focus is on the structure of language rather than its content per se. In this way, by going beyond words, the DMM clinical tools allow babies, as well as young children who are not yet verbal or who do not have the cognitive and emotional capacity to articulate their predicaments, to have a voice. And since stress is, for us in this book, embodied, the DMM methodology thus allows the body to *speak*.

I met Lea Williams—now Professor of Psychiatry and Behavioral Sciences at Stanford University and founding director of the Stanford Center for Precision Mental Health and Wellness—in 2005. Lea took me under her wing as my PhD supervisor, and in her lab I was able to do a series of studies that examined biomarkers, or biological markers, (in both the body and brain) of stress-system activation. The cohort included children with FND (and other somatic symptoms) and an equal number of age- and sex-matched healthy controls. Seventy-six children with FND participated in the attachment component of the study, and 57 of those also attended the testing in Lea's lab. Because many of the children were functionally impaired—they could not walk at the time of testing or had non-epileptic seizures (NES)—I made many trips with various wheelchairs to get the children to the lab.

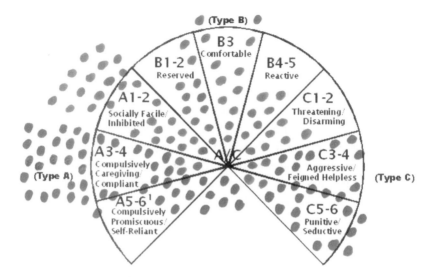

Fig. 4.1 Attachment strategies used by children with functional neurological disorder (vs. healthy controls). The strategies used by children and adolescents with FND are depicted by red dots, and by healthy controls, green dots. The attachment strategies at the top of the circle (A1-2, B1-5, and C1-2) represent the normative attachment strategies. The attachment strategies at the bottom of the circle (A3-4, A5-6, C3-4, and C5-6) represent the at-risk attachment strategies (© Patricia Crittenden. Reprinted with permission)

Identifying Stress and Distress Using Assessments of Attachment

The development of the DMM structured interviews to assess attachment in school-age children and adolescents enabled me to use them in my PhD research program with children presenting with FND (Kozlowska et al. 2011). Blinded coders classified these children with FND as predominantly using at-risk attachment strategies: the Type A+ strategies or the Type C+ strategies (Fig. 4.1). Via linguistic markers, coders also identified unresolved loss or trauma in 75 percent of children with FND versus 12 percent in healthy controls. In a later study, children who had presented to our hospital disabled by chronic/complex pain also predominantly used at-risk strategies (Ratnamohan and Kozlowska 2017). Two large, prospective studies have highlighted the association between the quality of the attachment relationship in early childhood and functional somatic symptoms later in life (Rask et al. 2013; Maunder et al. 2017). For an explanation of the different attachment strategies, see Crittenden (1999) and Online Supplement 4.1.

The overall message from the attachment studies is loud and clear. Children who presented to our hospital for the treatment of functional somatic symptoms—and associated functional impairment—had a long-standing history of relational stress, and they organized self-protectively in ways that maximized safety and comfort in their attachment relationships. For our purposes, given that parents and, more generally, attachment relationships function as the foundation for effective psychobiological regulation, the disruption of attachment relationships evident across studies suggests that these children's stress systems will continue to be more easily and strongly activated in response to any future stress.

Identifying Stress-System Activation Using Biomarkers and Brain Measures

The studies from my PhD research program, which looked at stress-system activation on a group level of analysis, confirmed my clinical impression that children with FND presented in a state of neurophysiological activation/arousal. The group level of analysis—looking at a larger group of children with functional somatic symptoms compared to sex- and age-matched healthy controls—allowed me to identify differences that would not be evident to the paediatrician looking at the test results of a single patient. For references to research articles from my PhD research program, see Online Supplement 1.3.

Autonomic Nervous System

Our studies looking at the autonomic nervous system showed that it was activated too much. Our patients had elevated heart rates (decreased parasympathetic/vagal tone ± sympathetic activation), lower heart rate variability (decreased parasympathetic/vagal tone), and increased skin conductance (sympathetic activation). How dysregulation of the autonomic nervous system contributes to the generation of functional somatic symptoms is discussed in Chapter 6 and in Online Supplement 7.1.

Motor System

Our studies looking at the motor system showed that it was also activated too much. Our patients (with FND) had faster reaction times to emotion faces, reflecting increased vigilance and motor readiness in response to emotional signals. Our patients with NES (a subset of FND) showed that many of these children were also breathing too fast. In other words, they had increased activation of the respiratory motor system, with the consequence that they were hypocapnic at rest: they had lower levels of arterial carbon dioxide because they had exhaled too much carbon dioxide. How hyperventilation and hypocapnia contributes to the generation of functional somatic symptoms is discussed in Chapter 7 and in Online Supplement 7.1.

Immune-Inflammatory System

Our studies looking at the immune-inflammatory system suggested a shift toward a state of low-grade inflammation. What this means is that the children showed a *small* increase in a common marker of inflammation, suggesting that the immune-inflammatory system had been activated by stress—physical or emotional—alongside other components of the stress system. This finding is in contrast to rheumatologic diseases or infections, which show a *large* increase in immune-inflammatory markers. How activation of the immune-inflammatory system contributes to the generation of functional somatic symptoms is discussed in Chapter 9.

Pain

Pain was also documented in all our studies. The term *chronic/complex pain* refers to pain for which available medical explanations either do not explain, or fail to account for the severity of, the child's impairment. In one set of studies, chronic/complex pain was the primary presentation. But when children presented other functional somatic symptoms—for example, FND—pain was also present in 60–84 percent of the children. For more information about chronic/complex pain, see Chapter 9.

Fatigue

Fatigue was also documented in all our studies. Fatigue was present in 33–58 percent of patients even when functional neurological symptoms or chronic complex pain was their primary presenting symptom. For more information about fatigue, see Chapters 9 and 11.

Activation of Brain Systems

We also looked at stress-system activation—and activation of motor-processing regions—on the brain system level. A study looking at cortical arousal using the electroencephalogram (EEG) showed that children with FND showed increased activity in midline regions both in the resting state and in response to an auditory stimulus. These midline regions are involved in salience detection, arousal, pain, and emotional states, and are part of the brain stress systems. Stimuli and body sensations that the brain tags as being *salient* are those that have particular importance for the individual because they signal that the body or the self needs protection from threats to its physical or psychological integrity.

One of the midline regions that we found to be overactivated—the supplementary motor area—is known to have dual role. It functions both as part of the brain stress systems and as a motor-processing region that is involved in motor preparation. Consequently, when the brain stress systems activate, motor function can be affected. How activation of the brain stress systems contributes to the generation of functional somatic symptoms is discussed in Chapter 11.

Brain Structure

Finally, we looked at brain structure using high-resolution MRI to see whether changes in brain function were also associated with subtle changes in brain structure. Importantly, all our patients had clinically normal scans, with no disease or lesions to explain their presentation with functional somatic symptoms. But other structural changes were detected. We found increased grey matter volume—the layers in the brain that contain neuron cell bodies and glial cells—in the supplementary motor area (the same motor area that was overactivated in the EEG study; see above), right superior temporal gyrus (which is involved in face processing), and dorsomedial prefrontal cortex (a region that is part of the brain stress systems). We also found that greater volumes of the supplementary motor area (responsible for motor preparation) correlated with faster reaction times in identifying emotions. These various changes in brain structure (with increased grey matter volume) were likely to reflect experience-dependent plasticity changes that made the children susceptible to the development of functional neurological symptoms (e.g., motor symptoms). For a discussion of plasticity changes, see Chapter 8 and Online Supplement 8.2.

***

To summarize this section: in line with clinical observations suggesting that children with functional somatic symptoms present in a state of stress-related *activation*, our studies looking at attachment patterns, biomarkers of stress-system activation, and brain function and structure showed activation of multiple components of the stress system and concomitant activation of the motor-processing regions and regions involved in pain, salience detection, arousal, and emotion processing. From the stories that the children and their families told, it seemed that the children's stress systems had been previously activated and sensitized (primed) by previous stress, had then been *switched on* by a recent trigger event, but had then somehow failed to *switch off*, the result being the emergence, in these particular children, of functional somatic symptoms.

Embodied Family History

The Family-of-Origin Story

The family-of-origin story—understood as encompassing the lives of previous generations, not all still living—has always held an important place for clinicians who work with children and their families (Kerr and Bowen

1988). In one way or another, stress and perturbations in the lives of previous generations seem to reverberate in each family's problems in the here and now. Many tribal cultures conceptualize healing as involving the healing of the ancestral line (Artlandish Aboriginal Art Gallery 2019).

The importance of the family-of-origin story in children with functional somatic symptoms was first raised by Wencke Seltzer, who worked with families of children presenting with FND (Seltzer 1985). Seltzer noticed that while the families perceived the sick child as 'well-equipped intellectually, well-adjusted socially, and free of psychological or emotional complications' (p. 267), the experiences of the majority of the parents in their own families-of-origin were marked by 'themes of extreme poverty, social humiliation, and family disintegration' (p. 269).

Interest in the effects of family-of-origin history have been rekindled in the last decade as animal and human studies have demonstrated that stress exposure can result in epigenetic alterations that can be transmitted to subsequent generations, increasing the offspring's vulnerability to, among other things, stress-related symptoms, even if these subsequent generations were not exposed to the initial traumatic event (for more, see following section on epigenetics).

Epigenetics: How Stress Weaves Its Way into the Body

Epi comes from the Greek meaning over, above, outer, or around; and *epigenetic* processes are those that influence gene expression without modifying the genetic code itself—typically by increasing or decreasing how the gene is expressed. Epigenetic modifications, the patterns of gene expression that control the body's biological processes, are not themselves static; they are modulated by life experiences and environmental factors in an ongoing way. The epigenetic changes that are the product of adverse life events potentially enhance the responsivity of the child's stress system by changing the expression of genes that are central to stress regulation (e.g., the glucocorticoid receptor gene) (Hyman 2009). The field of epigenetics helps us to understand how stress that occurred in previous generations, during pregnancy, in response to parental stress or poor parental care, or during the child's development 'weaves its way into the neural and biological infrastructure of the child', affecting stress-system function, health, and well-being (Nelson 2013, p. 1098).

In Online Supplement 1.2—Historical Context: The Emerging Science of the Stress System—we discuss how researchers in the 1980s began to recognize that a person's life experiences, especially early-life experiences, actually become biologically embedded in the brain and body.

In Online Supplement 4.2 we list some of the different terms that researchers have used to refer to biological processes through which life experiences alter the function and structure of the brain and body. Many of these terms came into use before we knew anything about epigenetics.

In Online Supplement 4.3 we provide additional information about epigenetic modifications, the biological mechanisms that enable stress-related epigenetic changes to affect health and well-being. We also provide references to the handful of studies that have documented epigenetic changes in patients with functional somatic symptoms, including those with fibromyalgia, irritable bowel syndrome, chronic fatigue syndrome, FND, and chronic/complex pain.

The emerging themes from this body of work is that epigenetic changes—changes in gene expression—are one of the mechanisms by which adverse life experiences weave their way into the brain and body. Although the research in this area is still in its infancy, it appears that changes in gene expression can lead to changes both in stress-system function (e.g., increased activation) and in tissue structure in both brain and body tissues.

The Stress-System Model for Functional Somatic Symptoms

In the final section of this chapter, building on all the information discussed above, we present the stress-system model for functional somatic symptoms. The stress system is made up of multiple interconnected brain-body systems—the autonomic nervous system, hypothalamic-pituitary-adrenal (HPA) axis, immune-inflammatory system, and brain stress systems underpinning salience detection, arousal, pain, and emotional states. These systems form part of a larger, integrated system that protects the individual from a broad range of threats (Chrousos and Gold 1992; Chrousos 2009;

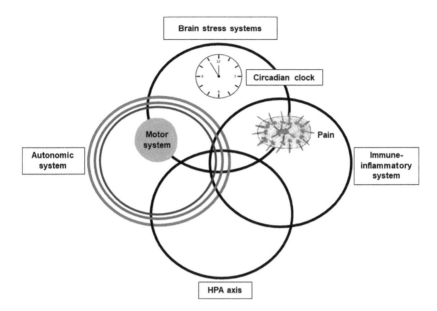

Fig. 4.2 Circles metaphor of the stress-system model for functional somatic symptoms. The overlap between the different components of the stress system—the HPA axis, autonomic nervous system, immune-inflammatory system, and brain stress systems—is presented by the overlap between the circles. The circadian clock is placed within the top circle because the master clock is found in the hypothalamus, a small region located in the base of the brain. The motor system, which includes central and peripheral components, is represented by the pink ball. The placement of the pink ball in the overlap between the brain stress systems and autonomic system reflects that activation of these systems can be accompanied by changes in motor function. The pain system, which also includes central and peripheral components, is represented by the spiky oval. The placement of pain in the overlap between the brain stress systems and immune-inflammatory system reflects that activation of these systems maintains chronic pain. Online Supplement 4.4 includes a version of the circles metaphor that can be printed out (© Kasia Kozlowska 2013)

Kozlowska 2013) (see Fig. 4.2). Activation of any single part of the system, whether by emotional stress, pain, injury, infection, or psychological trauma, can activate or dysregulate other components within the system. When the stress system—or one or more components of the stress system—is activated too much, too little, for too long, or in aberrant ways, or when it fails to return to baseline function, then functional somatic symptoms may arise.

The Stress System in Maintenance and Restorative Mode

In the normal course of events, when the child goes about her daily activities, the brain-body systems that make up the stress system regulate the body: they keep the body functioning within normative physiological limits and ensure that the body has access to sufficient energy resources to face the challenges of daily life. For most children (and most adults), whose lives are full of minor and occasional stress, rapid mobilization and timely termination of stress-system activation occur as the challenges of life are met and addressed, with the body (and stress system) then returning to its baseline function (see Fig. 4.3). When the stress system is functioning in this flexible and healthy way, we refer to it as being in *maintenance and restorative mode—restorative mode*, for short.

Restorative mode is a state of neurophysiological regulation characterized by the easy flow of life processes, an efficient utilization of energy, and the capacity to respond to environmental demands and to the need for tissue regeneration and repair. Restorative mode is associated with what McCraty and colleagues have called *physiological coherence*: the 'degree of order, harmony, stability in', and 'synchronization between', the body's 'various rhythmic activities over any given time period', which in humans involves the near-24-hour period of the human circadian clock (McCraty and Childre 2010, p. 11; McCraty and Zayas 2014). In this way, restorative mode involves *flexibility* in response to environmental needs, *harmony* and *physiological coherence* between its various components, and *efficient energy use*—a flow of life processes that is associated with health, well-being, connectedness, and a subjective sense of comfort or ease.

The Stress System Stuck in Defensive Mode

Unfortunately, when stress is chronic, uncontrollable, unpredictable, cumulative, recurrent, or overwhelming—and the stress system is activated too much, too long, or too frequently—the stress system can get *stuck* in defensive mode (see Fig. 4.3, Frame B). When that happens, the stress system remains activated or, as it were, *switched on*. In this

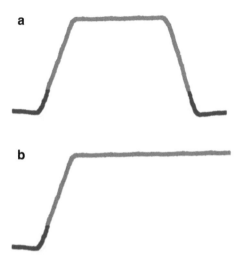

Fig. 4.3   Visual representation of restorative mode and defensive mode. In the normal course of events, the components of the stress system activate to address the challenge presented (denoted in red). They may stay activated for days or even weeks, but then the body returns to *restorative mode* (denoted in blue), its original baseline level of function (see Frame A). The problem is that in the case of many children, the child's body may not return to baseline functioning. In this scenario, even though the challenge or threat has passed, the child remains stuck in *defensive mode* (denoted in red)—and her brain and body may continue to respond as if the threat, whether psychological or physical, were still occurring (see Frame B) (© Kasia Kozlowska 2017)

scenario, biomarkers that mark stress-system activation or dysregulation can be found on a group level of analysis (see earlier section 'Identifying Stress-System Activation Using Biomarkers and Brain Measures').

Not only does the child's body continue to work harder than it needs to, but the body is missing out on the energy renewal, tissue regeneration, and repair functions that take place in restorative mode. *A stress system stuck in defensive mode*—or with one or more of its components stuck in defensive mode—is a system that has lost the ease and flow of life processes, along with the efficient use of energy resources. A stress system stuck in defensive mode is associated with the loss of health, well-being, and connectedness, and with a subjective sense of discomfort or dis-ease. And it can also lead to the production of functional somatic symptoms.

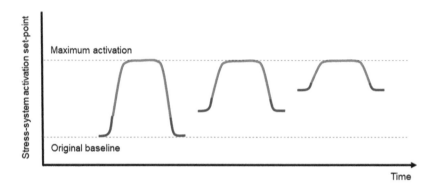

Fig. 4.4 Visual representation of the change in set-points over time in the context of chronic or repeated stress. With repeated stress the set-point—that is, the baseline to which the stress system returns—can change over time. The blue parts of the lines represent the stress system at baseline activation, and the red parts of the lines represent the stress system in an activated state (© Kasia Kozlowska 2017)

Perhaps the most intuitive way of understanding what happens over time—when the stress system is stuck in defensive mode—is that the baseline, or *set-point*, to which the stress system returns, and from which it reacts to new stress, changes over time (see Fig. 4.4). The technical name for the change in set-points is *allostasis*, and the technical term for the long-term biological cost of chronic activation, with a change in set-points, is *allostatic load* (see Online Supplement 1.2). As the set-point moves to higher levels, defensive mode is progressively more engaged even in a 'resting' state, and progressively fewer resources are consequently available, even in that resting state, for repair and maintenance. By the same token, because fewer resources are available for repair and maintenance, the process of restoration is compromised, and recovery from each new stress is difficult and often incomplete.

Visual Metaphors of the Stress-System

Children enjoy looking at pictures, and when we talk to children and their families about the stress system and stress-system activation, we like to draw pictures as we talk. With very young children, we sometimes call the stress system the *danger system*, because the word *danger* is one that even young children understand.

The Circles Metaphor of the Stress System

As discussed above, the circles metaphor provides a simple framework that clinicians can use to organize and make sense of a large—and ever-increasing—body of literature about the way in which the body responds to stress and about the neurobiology of functional somatic symptoms. The model is easily translated into the lay language of daily clinical practice; children and families find it a helpful framework for understanding what is happening to the child's body and why (see case of Paula in Chapter 3).

The overlapping circles highlight the way in which the components are interconnected and interrelated (see Fig. 4.2). In the conversation with the child and family, the overlapping circles help to highlight that when one component of the stress system is activated or dysregulated, other components are also likely to be activated or dysregulated *to some degree*. Very often the child will say something like, 'I see, it is switched on, so now we need to switch it off.'

Online Supplement 4.4 includes a version of the circles metaphor that can be printed out.

The Castle-Fortress Metaphor of the Stress System

The castle-fortress metaphor provides an alternative visual representation of the stress system (see Fig. 4.5). According to this metaphor the stress system is like a castle-fortress. When everything is calm, the castle-fortress (specifically the castle, the place for living) is a calm and welcoming place, with the gates wide open, a place where the tasks of daily life are carried out in a rhythmic and predictable manner (= restorative mode). When the castle-fortress comes under threat, however, the gates of the castle-fortress are shut, the alarm is raised, and the defence towers (specifically those of the fortress) are manned, as needed, to protect the castle-fortress as a whole (= defensive mode). In this metaphor, the stress system, like a castle-fortress, is designed to activate, when necessary, its defence

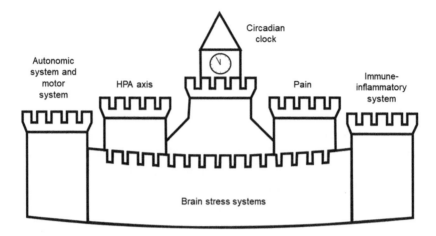

Fig. 4.5 Castle-fortress metaphor of the stress system model for functional somatic symptoms. In this metaphor, each castle tower and the walls surrounding the castle-fortress represent a component of the stress system. Online Supplement 4.4 includes a version of the castle-fortress metaphor that can be printed out (and filled in) (© Kasia Kozlowska 2017)

systems—all of them, if necessary, to maximize protection. Some children, families, and even clinicians find the castle-fortress metaphor of the stress system easier to use than the circles metaphor. In the castle-fortress metaphor, activation of a particular stress-system component can be depicted by shading in the appropriate tower—each of which represents a different component of the stress system. In clinical practice we colour in the towers with red, which, in all the metaphors used in this book, denotes activation into defensive mode (Fig. 4.6).

Online Supplement 4.4 includes a version of the castle-fortress metaphor that can be printed out (and filled in).

The Blue, Red, and Purple Metaphor of the Stress System

The third metaphor used our clinical practice involves colour coding. Blue always represents baseline restorative, healthy mode. Red and purple represent a shift into defensive mode. For example, in the

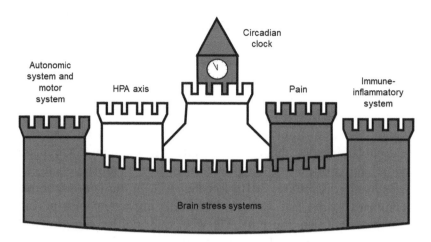

Fig. 4.6 Paula's castle-fortress. Paula—whom we met in Chapters 2 and 3—had a complex history of functional somatic symptoms. In discussions with Paula and the family, we mentioned every component of her stress system as being activated or dysregulated. The symptom of chronic pain began following an injury (colour in the immune-inflammatory tower and pain tower). That injury was followed by sleep disturbance (colour in the clock tower) and functional neurological symptoms (colour in the brain stress systems) in the context of significant bullying. Finally, as Paula became immobile and more and more deconditioned, she developed symptoms related to dysregulation of the autonomic system: panic attacks accompanied by hyperventilation and symptoms of postural orthostatic tachycardia (colour in the autonomic tower [which also includes the respiratory motor system that activates alongside]). Because HPA-axis dysregulation has been documented in studies of women with NES, and because the HPA axis was also likely to be dysregulated due to Paula's reversed sleep pattern, it could also have been coloured in (© Kasia Kozlowska 2017)

autonomic nervous system (see Fig. 4.2), the restorative parasympathetic system is depicted by a light blue line, the sympathetic system by a red line, and the defensive parasympathetic system by a purple line (see also Fig. 6.1). As another example, in the immune-inflammatory system, a macrophage (cell that cleans up debris and is involved in chronic/complex pain) depicted in restorative mode (anti-inflammatory mode) is coloured blue. By contrast, a macrophage depicted in defensive mode (pro-inflammatory mode) is coloured red and purple (see Fig. 9.1).

The Role of Sex Hormones

Stress has a central role in the emergence of functional somatic symptoms in both men and women, but the threshold for developing such symptoms is different for the two sexes. Some female sex hormones—for example, oestrogen—potentiate HPA-axis function and glucocorticoid secretion from the adrenal cortex, accentuate the action of catecholamines in the brain, activate the immune-inflammatory response, and work alongside glucocorticoids to modulate changes in gene expression (Chrousos 2010) (see Fig. 4.7). In this context, chronic or cumulative stress has a more deleterious impact on post-pubertal females than on men and boys. Likewise, this additive engagement of female sex hormones in the stress response, as mediated by the HPA axis, helps to explain why, in civilian settings, women and post-pubertal girls have always been more susceptible to stress-related illnesses and

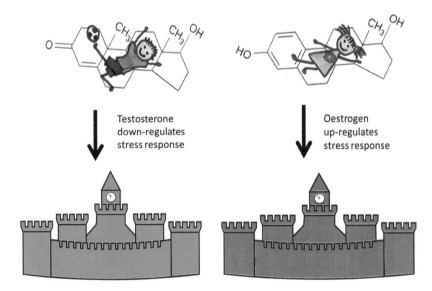

Fig. 4.7 The role of sex hormones in activating the stress response. This figure represents the fact that female hormones (specifically, oestrogen) up-regulate the stress system (see text for description) and that male sex hormones (specifically, testosterone) down-regulate it (© Kasia Kozlowska 2017)

functional somatic symptoms than men and boys. It seems that it takes higher levels of stress—as created, for example, in the context of military combat—to trigger the same symptom presentations in men and boys (see Online Supplement 1.1).

Sex hormones have many diverse roles within the body that are unrelated to their role in reproduction. An emerging body of work looks at the way that sex steroids modulate the expression of immune-inflammatory cells and molecules within the central and peripheral nervous systems, along with the effects of these processes on chronic/complex pain. For example, recent studies suggest that progesterone and testosterone may down-regulate the immune-inflammatory system—shifting it away from an inflammatory state. The implications of these discoveries for the treatment of chronic pain—which involves activation of the immune-inflammatory system on the tissue, spinal, and brain system levels (see Chapter 9)—are the focus of current research (for references see Online Supplement 1.3).

Chapter Summary

In this chapter, and in an effort to make this important scientific material about the stress system a bit more intuitive, we have retraced the first author's steps in developing the stress-system model for functional somatic symptoms. We have also taken time to look at the model itself.

When working with children it is important to be able to explain complex ideas in simple, visual form—and, if possible, in a form that can be drawn in the clinic on a piece of paper and then taken home by the child and her family. The stress-system model for functional somatic symptoms is a simple way of putting together complex information about how the body, brain, mind, and relational environment interact to make a child vulnerable to functional somatic symptoms. In the upcoming chapters we briefly summarize the neurobiology for each component of the stress system in order to provide clinicians who work with children and families a basic understanding of the biology underpinning the stress-system model. In those chapters we try to present the information in a clear, succinct form and to use visual metaphors to summarize large chunks of information. In Chapter 5 we discuss the circadian clock; in Chapter 6, the autonomic nervous system; in Chapter 7, the close coupling between the autonomic and skeletomotor systems; in Chapter 8, the HPA axis; in Chapter 9, the immune/inflammatory system; and in Chapter 10, the important role of the microbiota-gut-brain axis in regulating human health and disease. We complete our discussion of neurobiology in Chapters 11 and 12, which discuss the role of the brain itself and, more broadly, the role of brain systems and the mind in producing functional somatic symptoms.

References

Afari, N., Ahumada, S. M., Wright, L. J., Mostoufi, S., Golnari, G., Reis, V., et al. (2014). Psychological Trauma and Functional Somatic Syndromes: A Systematic Review and Meta-analysis. *Psychosomatic Medicine, 76*, 2–11.

Artlandish Aboriginal Art Gallery. (2019). *Understanding Aboriginal Dreaming.* https://www.aboriginal-art-australia.com/Aboriginal-Art-Library/Understanding-Aboriginal-Dreaming-and-the-Dreamtime/.

Chrousos, G. P. (2009). Stress and Disorders of the Stress System. *Nature Reviews. Endocrinology, 5*, 374–381.

Chrousos, G. P. (2010). Stress and Sex Versus Immunity and Inflammation. *Science Signaling, 3*, pe36.

Chrousos, G. P., & Gold, P. W. (1992). The Concepts of Stress and Stress System Disorders. Overview of Physical and Behavioral Homeostasis. *JAMA, 267*, 1244–1252.

Crittenden, P. M. (1999). Danger and Development: The Organization of Self-Protective Strategies. *Monographs for the Society for Research on Child Development, 64*, 145–171.

Crittenden, P. M., Kozlowska, K., & Landini, A. (2010). Assessing Attachment in School-Age Children. *Clinical Child Psychology and Psychiatry, 15*, 185–208.

Farnfield, S., Hautamaki, A., Nørbech, P., & Sahar, N. (2010). DMM Assessments of Attachment and Adaptation: Procedures, Validity and Utility. *Clinical Child Psychology and Psychiatry, 15*, 313–328.

Felitti, V. J., Anda, R. F., Nordenberg, D., Williamson, D. F., Spitz, A. M., Edwards, V., et al. (1998). Relationship of Childhood Abuse and Household Dysfunction to Many of the Leading Causes of Death in Adults. The Adverse Childhood Experiences (ACE) Study. *American Journal of Preventive Medicine, 14,* 245–258.

Hyman, S. E. (2009). How Adversity Gets Under the Skin. *Nature Neuroscience, 12,* 241–243.

Kerr, M. E., & Bowen, M. (1988). Multigenerational Emotional Process. In M. E. Kerr & M. Bowen (Eds.), *Family Evaluation: An Approach Based on Bowen Theory.* New York: Norton.

Kozlowska, K. (2013). Stress, Distress, and Bodytalk: Co-constructing Formulations with Patients Who Present with Somatic Symptoms. *Harvard Review of Psychiatry, 21,* 314–333.

Kozlowska, K., English, M., & Savage, B. (2013). Connecting Body and Mind: The First Interview with Somatizing Patients and Their Families. *Clinical Child Psychology and Psychiatry, 18,* 223–245.

Kozlowska, K., Scher, S., & Williams, L. M. (2011). Patterns of Emotional-Cognitive Functioning in Pediatric Conversion Patients: Implications for the Conceptualization of Conversion Disorders. *Psychosomatic Medicine, 73,* 775–788.

Maisami, M., & Freeman, J. M. (1987). Conversion Reactions in Children as Body Language: A Combined Child Psychiatry/Neurology Team Approach to the Management of Functional Neurologic Disorders in Children. *Pediatrics, 80,* 46–52.

Maunder, R. G., Hunter, J. J., Atkinson, L., Steiner, M., Wazana, A., Fleming, A. S., et al. (2017). An Attachment-Based Model of the Relationship Between Childhood Adversity and Somatization in Children and Adults. *Psychosomatic Medicine, 79,* 506–513.

McCraty, R., & Childre, D. (2010). Coherence: Bridging Personal, Social, and Global Health. *Alternative Therapies in Health and Medicine, 16,* 10–24.

McCraty, R., & Zayas, M. A. (2014). Cardiac Coherence, Self-Regulation, Autonomic Stability, and Psychosocial Well-Being. *Frontiers in Psychology, 5,* 1090.

McInnis, P. M., Braund, T. A., Chua, Z. K., & Kozlowska, K. (2020). Stress-System Activation in Children with Chronic Pain: A Focus for Clinical Intervention. *Clinical Child Psychology and Psychiatry, 25,* 78–97.

Mollica, R. F., Poole, C., Son, L., Murray, C. C., & Tor, S. (1997). Effects of War Trauma on Cambodian Refugee Adolescents' Functional Health and Mental Health Status. *Journal of the American Academy of Child and Adolescent Psychiatry, 36,* 1098–1106.

Nelson, C. A. (2013). Biological Embedding of Early Life Adversity. *JAMA Pediatrics, 167,* 1098–1100.

Rask, C. U., Ornbol, E., Olsen, E. M., Fink, P., & Skovgaard, A. M. (2013). Infant Behaviors Are Predictive of Functional Somatic Symptoms at Ages 5–7 Years: Results from the Copenhagen Child Cohort CCC2000. *Journal of Pediatrics, 162,* 335–342.

Ratnamohan, L., & Kozlowska, K. (2017). When Things Get Complicated: At-Risk Attachment in Children and Adolescents with Chronic Pain. *Clinical Child Psychology and Psychiatry, 22,* 588–602.

Redding, C. A. (Ed.). (2003). Origins and Essence of the Study. *ACE Reporter, 1,* 1–3. http://thecrimereport.s3.amazonaws.com/2/94/9/3076/acestudy.pdf.

Seltzer, W. J. (1985). Conversion Disorder in Childhood and Adolescence: A Familial/Cultural Approach. Part I. *Family Systems Medicine, 3,* 261–280.

Taylor, D. C. (1986). Hysteria, Play-Acting and Courage. *British Journal of Psychiatry, 149,* 37–41.

5

The Circadian Clock and Functional Somatic Symptoms

Abstract We begin our exploration of the neurobiology of functional somatic symptoms with the circadian clock because every organ, tissue, and cell in our body has a circadian rhythm—and all components of the stress system are regulated by the circadian clock. The integrity of the circadian clock is important in health and dis-ease, and is often Dysregulated in children and adolescents with functional somatic symptoms. We examine the healing functions of sleep and why good sleep is important for subjective well-being, facilitating physiological coherence within the stress system and the body as a whole. We then consider sleep interventions as a good starting place for the treatment of functional somatic symptoms. Improvements in sleep can act as a circuit breaker, the first step in the process of healing, the first step in the process of shifting the body from a dysregulated to a more regulated state.

Electronic supplementary material The online version of this chapter (https://doi.org/10.1007/978-3-030-46184-3_5) contains supplementary material, which is available to authorized users.

97

The Circadian Clock

In our hospital-based Mind-Body Program for functional somatic symptoms, we (the first author [KK] and her clinical team) noticed that many of the children (including adolescents) admitted to the program were bleary-eyed in the morning and that they reported that they had not slept well during the night. The children also reported—and we observed—that after a night of bad sleep, their pain was worse, they felt more nauseous, their fatigue was more pervasive, or they felt more *off* and *ikky* in general. And if the child presented with non-epileptic seizures (NES), we noticed that she was more likely to have one following a night of bad sleep. A bleary-eyed child on ward rounds meant a hard day for everyone. The child would struggle with the Mind-Body Program—to attend the hospital school, to do her physiotherapy, to implement her mind-body strategies to manage arousal and pain—and the multidisciplinary team would struggle to support the ailing child in all these tasks.

Because of these clinical observations, we came to pay the circadian clock a great deal of attention. Regulation of the child's circadian cycle became a priority—the intervention that we implemented first—with all our patients who presented with functional somatic symptoms. As the years went by, we became convinced that regulating the circadian clock made a real difference. It seemed to activate the body's own healing powers, and the patients who slept better in the right phase of the circadian cycle—and not too little or too much—seemed to do better. In the stress-system model for somatic symptoms, the circadian clock is prominently represented within the top circle, which depicts the brain stress systems (see Fig. 4.2). Although the healing powers of sleep have long been recognized (Adam and Oswald 1984), new information about the circadian clock and the restorative functions of sleep have continued to emerge over the last decades. The awarding of the 2017 Nobel Prize in Physiology or Medicine to three scientists—Jeffrey Hall, Michael Rosbash, and Michael Young—for their work on circadian biology has highlighted the overarching role of the circadian rhythm in understanding health and illness (see Fig. 5.1).

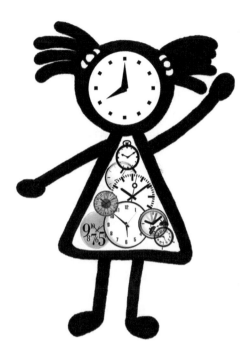

Fig. 5.1   The circadian clock system. The large clock in the brain symbolizes the master clock in the brain's suprachiasmatic nucleus that synchronizes all the secondary clocks in every tissue and every cell of the body (represented by the clocks situated in the body of the figure) (© Kasia Kozlowska 2019)

Evolution

All plants, animals, and humans that live on planet earth have internal biological rhythms that are synchronized with the earth's revolutions as it orbits the sun. From an evolutionary perspective, these inbuilt day and night rhythms—circadian rhythms—have enabled organisms living on our planet to predict when it will be hot and cold, light and dark, and when predators are likely to be out hunting, thereby facilitating adaptations that increase the probability of survival (Smarr 2017). In humans, circadian clocks are genetically inbuilt into all the cells of the body; cells that work together tend to work in harmony and to share a circadian rhythm. In this way, all organs and tissues have their own circadian rhythms.

The central circadian rhythm is generated by the master circadian clock, which lies in the suprachiasmatic nucleus of the hypothalamus (Zelinski et al. 2014). The master clock, along with the genes that drive it, is reset on a daily basis by exposure to morning light via the eyes. The peripheral circadian rhythms present in cells, organs, and organ systems are also regulated by their own gene-based mechanisms. To maintain harmony across and between body systems, the master and peripheral clocks maintain constant communication via a complex system of neuronal and messenger pathways—the autonomic nervous system, neurotransmitters, and neuropeptide and hormone messengers—that are expressed throughout the brain and body (Zelinski et al. 2014). Information from the body is used by the master clock to help synchronize the peripheral circadian clocks (Nader et al. 2010). Synchronization between different clock rhythms facilitates *physiological coherence*. This notion of coherence can be understood as the 'degree of order, harmony, stability' and the 'degree of synchronization' between different body systems in the 'various rhythmic activities' within the body over each near-24-hour period of the human circadian rhythm (McCraty and Childre 2010, p. 11) (see Chapter 4).

The Reciprocal Relationship Between the Circadian Clock and the Stress System

The circadian clock system and the stress system communicate with and regulate each other in many different ways (Nicolaides et al. 2017). Each component of the stress system has its own diurnal rhythm, and synchronization between components facilitates coherence and well-being in a well-regulated body. The master clock regulates the hypothalamic-pituitary-adrenal (HPA) axis, whose end product is cortisol (a glucocorticoid) (see Chapter 8). It activates the axis in the early hours of the morning to facilitate cortisol production and an increase in energy consumption, and deactivates it in the afternoon to decrease cortisol production and energy consumption as the body begins to wind down for the night (see Fig. 5.2). The autonomic system also follows a circadian rhythm (see Chapter 6). Within the autonomic system, the sympathetic system activates in the early hours of the morning—alongside

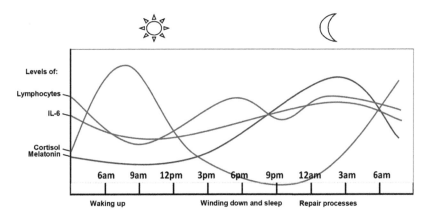

Fig. 5.2 Diurnal rhythms. This figure shows the normal, healthy diurnal rhythms of cortisol, melatonin, lymphocytes (white blood cells), and interleukin-6 (a cytokine) (© Kasia Kozlowska 2019)

the HPA axis—and deactivates at night, when the restorative parasympathetic system activates to support biological processes associated with energy renewal and with healing and repair functions (Buijs et al. 2013). Immune-inflammatory cells, which are found throughout the body and brain, likewise follow a diurnal pattern, regulated by the circadian clock (Labrecque and Cermakian 2015) (see Chapter 9). As noted above, feedback and modulation from all these systems influence circadian clock activity and the setting of diurnal rhythms within the body; these ongoing adjustments to the body's circadian rhythms ensure that the individual is prepared, and at the right times, to respond to challenges, stress, or threat.

Because of the close relationship between the circadian clock and the stress system, dysregulation of one system can lead to dysregulation of the other. Dysregulation of the circadian clock system (e.g., by night shiftwork [in adults] or late-night study routines [in children] or internet surfing throughout the night) can lead to activation of the HPA axis and elevated levels of cortisol (a glucocorticoid). These processes can, in turn, reset the expression of peripheral clock genes and induce additional epigenetic modifications in other body systems. Moving from the opposite direction, when stress leads to activation of the HPA axis and, in turn, to elevated levels of cortisol, the rhythm of the master circadian clock is disrupted, and as described above, peripheral clocks are reset, in this case in order to promote a state of wakefulness and high energy consumption. While this resetting of the peripheral clocks is adaptive in the short term—during periods of stress—because it enables the child to adjust the circadian rhythm–linked activity of her brain and body to properly respond to stress, it is maladaptive in the long term because it adversely affects sleep. Likewise, because of the close relationship between the circadian clock and the autonomic system, dysregulation of one system can lead to dysregulation of the other. For additional references about these interactions, see Online Supplement 1.3.

We can see many of the above processes at work in the following vignette:

> David was a 15-year-old boy who lived with his mother and older brothers. As a baby and toddler, David had lived in a household dominated by strain, conflict, and domestic violence. During primary school David often missed school because of asthma, recurrent abdominal pain, and frequent viral illnesses. After his parents separated (at the beginning of high school), he became depressed. He was treated with a selective serotonin reuptake inhibitor (SSRI) by his family doctor, which helped regulate his mood, but he then stopped taking it. His relationship with his father continued to be strained. As he got older and wanted to spend more time with his friends, his father became jealous of them and complained that David should prioritize time with him. His father's demands were a source of ongoing stress. In high school, David began to suffer from pain that started in his head but then migrated around his body, with an especially painful locus in his lower back. Because of this back pain, David exercised less and less, became physically deconditioned, and missed progressively more school. He began to feel lightheaded on standing up due to an exaggerated heart rate response (orthostatic intolerance, see Chapter 6). At night the pain in his back was at its worst, and David reported that his spine moved and shifted, causing bulging and pain. Unable to sleep at night, David went to bed later and later, and slept into the day. He stopped going to school, stopped seeing the physiotherapist, and became housebound. His mood dropped; he was constantly fatigued; and he began to suffer from suicidal ideation. He then developed functional

neurological symptoms—weakness in the right leg, a turned-in right foot, loss of sensation in the right leg, and an abnormal gait in which he dragged his right leg behind him—and became very depressed. By this time his sleep cycle was entirely reversed.

The above vignette is typical of children with functional somatic symptoms in one crucially important way: children with such symptoms typically present at a point that multiple systems are dysregulated, often with the problems of one exacerbating the problems with another. Another element worth emphasizing is that problems with sleep are typically intertwined with the expression—and exacerbation—of functional somatic symptoms. The first intervention with David was, indeed, to regulate his sleep cycle, thereby correcting his problem of *circadian misalignment*, to which we now turn.

The Health Consequences of Circadian Misalignment

The term *circadian misalignment* refers to a disruption in any of the body's near-24-hour circadian rhythms, including 'inappropriately timed sleep and wake, misalignment of sleep/wake with feeding rhythms, or misaligned central and peripheral rhythms' (Baron and Reid 2014, p. 139). The health consequences of circadian misalignment are substantial.

Jet lag, the misalignment of the circadian clock due to travel across multiple time zones, is probably the commonest example of circadian clock misalignment. It is associated with diverse, but transient, functional somatic symptoms. In addition to daytime sleepiness, fatigue, and a general feeling of not being well and difficulty concentrating, jet lag commonly involves symptoms that reflect disruption of the gut's circadian rhythms: indigestion, nausea, constipation, diarrhoea, and off-schedule defecation.

Shiftwork likewise disrupts light/dark exposure, sleep/wakefulness, rest/activity, or feeding/fasting cycles, all of which are important in maintaining healthy circadian rhythms. After three days of a shiftwork schedule, many metabolites—products of cell metabolism that mark body-system function—show a change in their circadian rhythms and a loss of synchrony with the master circadian clock (Skene et al. 2018). The gut's circadian clock shows circadian rhythm reversal. The body experiences shiftwork as a chronic stress. The chronic circadian misalignment leads to activation and dysregulation of the stress system—autonomic dysregulation and activation of the immune-inflammatory system—along with changes in eating patterns, appetite regulation, glucose regulation, and mood. Chronic dysregulation contributes to an increased risk of medical disorders (e.g., cardiovascular disease), mental health disorders (e.g., depression), and functional somatic symptoms and disorders (e.g., irritable bowel syndrome) (for references see Online Supplement 1.3).

Patterns of Circadian Clock Dysregulation in Children with Functional Somatic Symptoms

Patterns of circadian clock dysregulation can be identified in children with functional somatic symptoms by taking a careful clinical history. As we saw with David, functional somatic symptoms will often result, over time, in difficulties with sleep, but the direction of causality can also go the other way. Difficulties with sleep or disturbed sleep—whether the result of illness, anxiety, depression, academic demands, or lifestyle factors—may contribute to the factors that trigger or maintain the child's functional somatic symptoms.

Kim was a 14-year-old girl who lived with her parents and an older sister. Because Kim's parents were immigrants, they wanted Kim to do well at school and go to university to become a lawyer or a doctor. They had provided Kim—then 12 years old—with tutoring to help her pass exams for a selective school, and the pressure to keep up good grades was relentless. When Kim failed to perform up to expectations, her mother would lose her temper and yell at Kim. Her father said nothing, but Kim could see the disappointment and anger in his face. During the first year of high school, Kim—now 13 years old—had begun to study late into the night. During the school day she was fatigued, and she started to suffer from headaches and bouts of abdominal pain. Whenever Kim's friends suffered from a cold, Kim seemed to catch it and become sick. By the second year of high school, Kim's sleep was very disturbed. She found it difficult to get to sleep; she woke during the night; and she never felt refreshed. She began to experience fainting episodes and had frequent visits to the school nurse. When she began to experience non-epileptic seizures, or NES, the neurology team involved in her care referred her and the family for an assessment with the mind-body team. A subsequent cognitive assessment suggested that Kim was an average student and that the expectations that her parents had from her were way above her capacity.

Sleep problems often interact with other functional somatic symptoms, leading to the following sort of clinical presentation.

Abigail, a 17-year-old girl in the final year of high school, presented following the sudden onset of functional neurological symptoms (functional tremor, gait disturbance, and fluctuating visual disturbances). Her history included the following: four years of unrefreshing sleep, fatigue, and gut symptoms (nausea, plus diarrhoea alternating with constipation), all in the wake of a hospital admission for severe gastritis; and two years of mixed anxiety and low mood. She reported that, after the hospital admission for gastritis, her gut function had never returned to normal, that her sleep had lost the sense of rejuvenation and renewal associated with a good night's sleep, and that, as a consequence, her energy levels had never been the same. For a period of four years she had woken unrefreshed and had struggled, day to day, to meet the challenges of daily living. The additional demands of the final year of high school had proved too much for Abigail. In addition to the symptoms described above, her body had responded to the academic stress with new symptoms of chronic pain in her head and back (of six months duration) along with the functional neurological symptoms that triggered her presentation to hospital.

What is important from the perspective of the stress-system model is the idea of a vicious cycle in which the dysregulated stress system affects the functioning of the circadian clock, and the dysregulated circadian clock affects the functioning of the stress system. As time passes, if the systems are unable to reset themselves back to a healthy pattern, the dysregulation within the body can become self-reinforcing: stress-system activation will continue to disrupt sleep and the physiological coherence of the circadian clock, and disrupted sleep and dysregulation of the circadian clock will maintain dysregulation within the stress system.

The Restorative Functions of Sleep

A dysregulated circadian clock manifesting as a disrupted sleep rhythm is important because it powerfully influences the child's sense of well-being and of physical ease or *dis-ease* (for a discussion of disease vs. dis-ease, see Online Supplement 1.1). When sleep is disrupted, so are the vital restorative functions that occur at night—cleaning up, resetting the homeostatic system, and regeneration and repair—resulting in a loss of well-being. We list some of the restorative functions of sleep below. Clinicians can use this information to engage families in sleep interventions and in the treatment process more generally. For references about each of these processes, see Online Supplement 1.3.

Restorative System 1: Sleep Cleaning by the Glymphatic System

The *glymphatic system* is like a layer of piping that exists in the space between the brain's blood vessels and the feet of glial cells—the brain's immune-inflammatory cells—and that allows waste products from brain cell metabolism to drain out into cerebrospinal fluid. During sleep, when the brain stress systems are switched off (sympathetic tone and catecholamine levels are low), the glymphatic system expands and works at maximum efficiency. In this way, each night as we sleep, the glymphatic system gives the brain a sleep clean.

Restorative System 2: Brain Reboot by Synaptic Shrinking and Resetting

Nerve cells within the brain reboot and reset during sleep. In the sleeping brain the synapses between neurons shrink, which allows new synapses to be made the next day. The nightly process of *synapse shrinking* and *resetting* may facilitate brain health and physical well-being by resetting homeostatic set-points across brain-body systems. Synapse shrinking and resetting allows new learning to take place the next day and facilitates *'smart forgetting'* (Tononi and Cirelli 2014, p. 24). It may also help in the process of processing, dulling, and putting behind painful memories that follow in the wake of adverse life events.

Restorative System 3: Slow-Wave (Deep) Sleep Switches Off Arousal and Inflammation

Slow-wave sleep occurs during the first half of the night, is greatest in young children, and lessens with age (Harvard Medical School, Division of Sleep Medicine 2007). Among other things, the HPA axis and sympathetic system are generally switched off. In addition, in a process sometimes referred to as the *anti-inflammatory reflex* or *cholinergic anti-inflammatory pathway*, the restorative parasympathetic system (vagal nerve) (see Chapter 6) up-regulates and facilitates restoration and repair. The vagal nerve also dampens the production of inflammatory proteins, including cytokines, in the spleen and other body tissues, and it inhibits macrophage activity throughout the body, effectively shutting down the body's inflammatory processes.

Restorative System 4: Sleep Resets Daytime Pain Thresholds

In animal studies, disturbed sleep has been found to increase *pain sensitivity*—a pattern that is also clinically evident in children with functional somatic symptoms. Pain sensitivity may increase for any of the following reasons: improperly reset pain thresholds (see Restorative System 2); increased inflammation or increased sympathetic activation (which activates inflammatory cells) (see Restorative System 3); psychologically depleted coping resources; or multiple interacting processes.

Restorative System 5: Clean-Up and Repair Molecules

During sleep the body secretes hormones and other molecules—including melatonin and growth hormone—that are involved in cell reproduction, tissue regeneration, DNA repair, and radical scavenging. Melatonin secretion is inhibited with the onset of daylight. Regular sleep and maintenance of synchronized circadian rhythms across and between body systems appear to be critical for fine-tuning cell cycles and sleep-related restorative processes that maximize healing, health, and well-being.

Addressing Sleep as a Therapeutic Intervention

As we saw in the section above, all the mechanisms associated with sleep work together to maintain restoration and repair processes, and they contribute in a substantive way to the child's subjective feeling of refreshment and well-being following a good night's sleep. From a clinical perspective, sleep interventions provide the clinician with a starting point for achieving significant changes within a complicated biological system (see Fig. 4.2). Sleep interventions are, when needed, a vital first step in helping the child's body shift from its current, dysregulated state to a state of better regulation, health, and well-being. Given that most children and families intuitively understand that a good night's sleep is important for health and well-being, the clinician has an opportunity to use a sleep intervention as establishing common ground with the child and family. Moreover, because the circadian clock and stress system are so interrelated, failure to normalize the circadian clock makes it much more difficult for the clinician to treat the child's functional somatic symptoms. A dysregulated circadian clock will continue to drive stress-system activation, and stress-system activation will, in turn, continue to drive the production of functional somatic symptoms. By contrast, a better-regulated circadian clock helps harness the body's intrinsic healing functions (see above). And when sleep is stabilized, some of the child's functional somatic symptoms might become less intense or even just melt away, resulting in a much less complicated clinical picture. In any event, the sleep intervention shifts the brain-body system to a more regulated state and increases the probability that other, more focused interventions will actually help to reduce or even resolve the functional somatic symptoms.

In the following vignettes we provide some clinical examples of the types of sleep issues that are part of our clinical practice with children with functional somatic symptoms. The interventions fall along a spectrum. Simple interventions involving sleep hygiene measures are always implemented first and are appropriate for all patients and all clinical settings (Owens et al. 2019).

When the simple interventions fail (or are reasonably expected to fail) to establish restorative sleep, a more assertive intervention is required. These mixed interventions combine sleep hygiene measures with simple medication regimes that are widely used because of their safe profiles—they are well tolerated—or because they have a reasonable evidence base in paediatric practice. Nonetheless, the use of medication requires ongoing monitoring by a medical professional to ensure that medications are used on an interim, short-term basis and discontinued once a healthy circadian cycle and restorative sleep have been re-established.

Finally, still more assertive interventions are reserved for situations characterized by significant functional impairment, where the risk of chronic illness and disability are key concerns. Such presentations may also be complicated by severe anxiety, depression, pain, or opiate/benzodiazepine addiction. These assertive, complex interventions, which are typically undertaken only after other approaches have been trialled, combine sleep hygiene measures with off-label medications, together with withdrawal from opiates/benzodiazepines and the treatment of anxiety and depression. Complex interventions are sometimes seen as controversial because of concerns pertaining to the potential for adverse side effects from medications and long-term misuse of medications by patients (for references discussing the controversy, see Online Supplement 1.3). Such interventions require careful assessment and monitoring, and they need to be limited to inpatient, tertiary care settings or the equivalent, where the patient's clinical response to the intervention can be monitored closely, and where the risks and benefits of the pharmacotherapeutic intervention can be assessed in an ongoing manner.

Three of the following vignettes involve adolescents whom we met earlier in this chapter. The fourth vignette describes a complex intervention implemented in the first author's inpatient setting.

Fifteen-year-old David was very distressed by his functional somatic symptoms—migrating pain worse in the back, and right leg weakness and loss of sensation—and he was highly motivated to be accepted into the inpatient Mind-Body Program. In establishing a treatment contract with David and his mother, the team explained that the program was hard work and that before beginning the program, David needed to engage in some preliminary interventions. First, he needed to return his sleep cycle to a normal rhythm. He could do this over a two-week period by going to bed two hours later each day, until he got to his previous healthy bedtime of 10 p.m. (see Text Box 5.1). Once he reached that point, the team wanted him to take melatonin, a natural substance that the brain secretes to help with sleep, so that his sleep cycle stayed regulated. They also wanted him to eat breakfast in a sunny spot in the house, making sure he got a good dose of morning light. Second, David needed to eat three healthy meals a day—including sufficient vegetables, fruit, and yogurt—to make sure that he had energy for the program and that he was looking after his microbiome, the bacterial community in his gut, which plays a key role in body regulation (see Chapter 10). Third, David needed to restart the antidepressant (an SSRI) that had helped him previously, because the team would be unable to work with him if his mood remained low. In addition, since antidepressants improve the brain's plasticity, they would help his body reset pain set-points and so on (see references in Online Supplement 1.3). Fourth, he needed to go outside the house every day. At first he could mobilize to the front gate, but he had to increase the distance by a minimum of two metres a day. He also needed to re-engage with his physiotherapist. These pre-program interventions would prepare him for the rigours of the Mind-Body Program. David implemented all the above interventions over a six-week period. Subsequently, after his two-week inpatient admission, he was walking with a normal gait, and his pain had decreased significantly. He maintained his improvements over the summer holidays, after which he returned to school full time and initiated ongoing therapy.

Text Box 5.1: How to shift the circadian clock back to a normal, healthy rhythm

The human sleep cycle, which follows the 24-hour circadian clock, can shift itself only about two hours a day (equivalent to two time zones). When trying to move away from a very disrupted sleep cycle—for example, a reverse sleep cycle of sleeping during the day—some children prefer to reset their clocks gradually by going to bed two hours later each day until the targeted sleep time is reached. Going to bed earlier (e.g., by two hours each day) generally does not work. Alternatively, it is much faster and also potentially easier for the child to accumulate sleep debt by staying up all day, all night, and all of the following day, and to then go to bed at the targeted time.

The situation of 14-year-old Kim, whose academic achievement consistently fell short of her parents' expectations, was more complicated.

First, the team engaged Kim and her parents in an education session about how the body responds when it is pushed too hard, and when it does not get enough sleep. Feedback from the separate cognitive assessment was crucial in highlighting that parental expectations that Kim become a lawyer or a doctor were inappropriately high. To address these issues, a referral was made to see the school counsellor, which would help Kim begin to think about other potential career options. The sleep intervention was implemented only after these issues had been aired and Kim's parents had given their explicit consent that she did not need to study into the wee hours of the morning. At that point, the team told Kim and her parents that the first step in treating the fainting events and NES was to regulate Kim's sleep, and that good sleep would, in turn, help Kim's body to regulate itself. A sleep intervention—a more appropriate bedtime, a going-to-bed relaxation exercise, the addition of regular exercise to Kim's daily routine, and the temporary use of some melatonin (for a three-month period)—was implemented. Kim's sleep settled quickly, and her headaches, fatigue, and abdominal pain settled of their own accord. Kim then began to work on strategies to manage her fainting episodes and NES (see Chapter 14). Because the frequency of these events had also decreased with the sleep intervention, this work took place at a slower, more relaxed pace; the pressure and uncertainty were gone since both Kim and her family could see that she was getting better.

The situation of Abigail was even more complicated—and unfortunate.

In addition to having a long history of functional somatic symptoms, 17-year-old Abigail had strong beliefs that medication was bad for the body, and she disliked psychologists and psychiatrists intensely. These attitudes made it difficult for her to engage with the mind-body team. It was not possible, for example, to determine whether melatonin or treatment of Abigail's untreated depression could help her improve the quality of her sleep. Even if Abigail had agreed to trial melatonin or other medications, her strong belief system that these substances would somehow disagree with her would have potentially overridden any therapeutic effect, known as the *nocebo response* (see Chapter 12). It was also not possible to explore mood issues in other ways, to address Abigail's relentless catastrophizing that intruded into her sleep on a nightly basis, or to teach Abigail strategies for down-regulating her arousal. Nor was it possible to engage her in the physiotherapy component of the Mind-Body Program. Abigail felt ashamed and angry that she had developed functional neurological symptoms, and she rejected any interventions that the team had to offer. She transitioned into the adult medical system, where she continued to seek alternate explanations for her health problems. She was eventually lost to follow-up.

As previously noted, in some children the sleep intervention is especially complicated because it is intertwined with the treatment of anxiety, depression, or pain, and also with the need to discontinue unhelpful medications—such as opiates and benzodiazepines—that the child has been prescribed in an effort to manage pain, distress, sleeplessness, and arousal. In this context, when it is necessary to use off-label medications to stabilize the sleep of a child admitted to the first author's Mind-Body Program, the medications are used on an interim, short-term basis, as one small part of an intensive multidisciplinary program—with its concurrent physical, psychological, occupational, and school interventions. And as Winfried Rief and colleagues note in a recent article, enriched 'social and physical environmental stimulation' of the type we provide in the inpatient setting plays an important role in generating positive effects for medications used in psychiatric practice (Rief et al. 2016, p. 51). Once sleep has been stabilized for a period of time—usually a three- to six-month period—any medications that were used to stabilize sleep are withdrawn. The exception is when medications are used also to treat comorbid depression or anxiety.

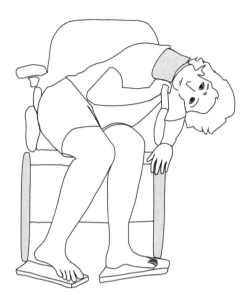

Fig. 5.3 Line drawing of Jai. This line drawing shows Jai dangling over the edge of his wheelchair at the beginning of his admission into the Mind-Body Program (© Kasia Kozlowska 2019)

Jai was a 14-year-old boy presenting with a six-week history of painful fixed dystonia in the neck—which twisted his head to the left—a four-week bilateral leg weakness and difficulties with coordination of his legs, and a two-year history of irritable bowel syndrome. On assessment for the inpatient Mind-Body Program, Jai presented in a wheelchair, his neck supported by a Miami J collar. He was in constant pain and a chronic state of hyper-arousal (manifest by an elevated respiratory rate of roughly 25 breaths per minute). Jai's chronic pain was punctuated by painful neck spasms—brought on by any attempt to change his position—during which he would turn white, shake, and clench his teeth. His body was generally twisted, and he dangled out over the edge of the wheelchair in a C-shape (see Fig. 5.3). He was unable to stand or mobilize independently, and his mother and nursing staff helped him with all activities of daily living. At night, Jai was unable to initiate sleep. He would eventually fall asleep between midnight and 2 a.m., only to wake in pain 3–4 hours later, at which point he begged the nurses to transfer him back to his wheelchair because he was unable to manage the pain in his twisted position in the bed. On presentation he was medicated with high doses of diazepam for the dystonia and oxycodone hydrochloride (an opioid medication) for pain. A month into the admission he disclosed severe and long-standing anxiety and depression.

Jai's sleep intervention began with simple sleep hygiene measures, moved to a combination of sleep hygiene measures and simple medications with a reasonable evidence base, and subsequently moved to a complex intervention using off-label medications. This last, complex intervention, monitored by a child psychiatrist (KK) and a pharmacist specializing in psychopharmacology, was necessary in order to simultaneously manage arousal and sleep, pain and opiate/benzodiazepine withdrawal, and mental health issues. The intervention is described in further detail below. (For the rationale behind our choice of medications and references, see Online Supplement 5.1.)

- *Establishing a regular bedtime/waking schedule.* In addition to setting a reasonable schedule, we banned electronics in the late evening (which would otherwise contribute to keeping Jai awake into the early hours of the morning).
- *Opening of curtains and switching on room lights in the morning to ensure exposure to the bright Australian sunlight.*
- *Melatonin* (3 mg, then 6 mg, then 9 mg) to help Jai with sleep initiation. This helped a little.
- *Decreasing arousal (in this case, by adding nighttime clonidine).* Together with the melatonin, the clonidine enabled Jai to fall asleep at night at his 11 p.m. bedtime, but it failed to keep him asleep. Jai continued to wake with pain and to remain awake in the early hours of the morning.
- *Using quetiapine to improve sleep quality and length* (25 mg titrated to 75 mg). Jai's sleep normalized; he did not awake from pain in the middle of the night; and he stopped experiencing each night as a form of torture (twisted, in pain, and, in terms of mobility, helpless). The improved sleep also increased his capacity to participate in the program.
- *Discontinuing benzodiazepines.* The diazepam was ceased on admission into the program because of its addictive properties.
- *Discontinuing opiates.* Although opiates alleviate pain in the short term, using them to alleviate chronic pain ends up potentiating the pain (for references see Online Supplement 5.1). In this context, the

opiates were slowly withdrawn over a period of months (for details see Khachane et al. [2019]).

- *Trialling botulinum toxin type A (Botox).* The botulinum toxin decreased both the frequency of Jai's debilitating neck spasms and the pain associated with them.
- *Quetiapine* was changed to mirtazapine (7.5 mg titrated to 22.5 mg) when Jai disclosed long-standing severe anxiety and depression. Despite significant sleep disruption during the changeover, Jai's sleep eventually settled at the higher dose. After roughly six weeks on mirtazapine, Jai's mood began to improve, and his pain settled even further.
- *Self-hypnosis* was added to the sleep routine once the team discovered that Jai was highly hypnotizable (see Chapter 15). Jai used self-hypnosis to help him position his body for sleep and to help him fall back to sleep if he awoke.

The entire sleep intervention, as described above, took three months. It was six months into his Mind-Body Program before Jai could sit and sleep in a normal position, and seven months into the program before he started to stand independently and mobilize on crutches, and was discharged. One month after discharge—after more than eight months of illness—he began to walk independently. For a detailed description of Jai's case and all components of the intervention with Jai, see Khachane and colleagues (2019).

Sleep Interventions as the Groundwork for Effective Treatment

In the Mind-Body Program, we celebrate good sleep and highlight it as the child's first therapeutic achievement on the path toward health and well-being. We also ask the child to protect her sleep at all costs— no late nights or sleeping in until things have settled. Unless the child comes from a culture where naps are part of the sleep routine, we avoid naps during the day and replace them with rest times, during which the child implements self-regulation strategies.

The vignettes in this chapter highlight the many different interventions that clinicians can use to help stabilize the child's sleep: education about sleep, circadian alignment, the management of electronic devices, sun exposure on waking, the addition of regular exercise to the daytime routine, relaxation, hypnosis (or other regulation techniques) at bedtime, and prescribing melatonin and other medications.

The use of medication requires that a child psychiatrist or paediatrician be a core member of the multidisciplinary team and that the risks of using medication (because of the potential side effects) and of not using medication (because of the potential for chronic illness and disability) be carefully assessed. While the concerns about inappropriate and long-term use of unnecessary or ineffective medications are important to keep in mind, we know from our clinical experience that—unless and until the child obtains good, restful, restorative sleep—other interventions are much less likely to succeed, and improvement is likely to be minimal or far too long in coming. Failing to treat functional symptoms—including disrupted sleep—efficaciously has its own risks. From a neurobiology perspective one can expect that the neurophysiological dysregulation, brain connectivity changes, and brain plasticity changes that occur in functional somatic disorders may become irreversible—and the presentation chronic—if the patient's neurobiological system is not stabilized in a timely fashion. In this context, we have included multiple vignettes, ranging from clinical scenarios in which the sleep component can be easily managed to ones in which the sleep component is especially difficult or even impossible to treat. Our hope is that this range of cases will help the reader to understand the diversity of presentations for functional somatic symptoms and also to understand the resulting need for flexibly adjusting to the challenges presented by each particular patient.

* * *

In this chapter, we have seen that the circadian clock and the stress system are closely interconnected, that activation of the stress system can adversely affect the circadian clock, and that disruption of the circadian clock can activate or dysregulate the stress system. These interconnections can create a vicious cycle that contributes to the child's lack of well-being—dis-ease—and to the emergence of functional somatic symptoms.

Early goals in any treatment are to shift the child toward better sleep, a healthier circadian rhythm, and coordination of circadian rhythms between body systems. Not only will the child's sense of well-being—of physical and psychological ease—improve, but achieving these preliminary goals will result in a better-regulated stress system and will facilitate the treatment of functional somatic symptoms. In Chapter 6 we discuss the autonomic system and its role in generating functional somatic symptoms.

References

Adam, K., & Oswald, I. (1984). Sleep Helps Healing. *British Medical Journal (Clinical Research Ed.), 289,* 1400–1401.

Baron, K. G., & Reid, K. J. (2014). Circadian Misalignment and Health. *International Review of Psychiatry, 26,* 139–154.

Buijs, R. M., Escobar, C., & Swaab, D. F. (2013). The Circadian System and the Balance of the Autonomic Nervous System. *Handbook of Clinical Neurology, 117,* 173–191.

Harvard Medical School, Division of Sleep Medicine. (2007). *Natural Patterns of Sleep.* http://healthysleep.med.harvard.edu/Healthy/Science/What/Sleep-Patterns-Rem-Nrem.

Khachane, Y., Kozlowska, K., Savage, B., McClure, G., Butler, G., Gray, N., et al. (2019). Twisted in Pain: The Multidisciplinary Treatment Approach to Functional Dystonia. *Harvard Review of Psychiatry, 27,* 359–381. https://pubmed.ncbi.nlm.nih.gov/31714467/.

Labrecque, N., & Cermakian, N. (2015). Circadian Clocks in the Immune System. *Journal of Biological Rhythms, 30,* 277–290.

Mccraty, R., & Childre, D. (2010). Coherence: Bridging Personal, Social, and Global Health. *Alternative Therapies in Health and Medicine, 16,* 10–24.

Nader, N., Chrousos, G. P., & Kino, T. (2010). Interactions of the Circadian CLOCK System and the HPA Axis. *Trends in Endocrinology and Metabolism, 21,* 277–286.

Nicolaides, N. C., Charmandari, E., Kino, T., & Chrousos, G. P. (2017). Stress-Related and Circadian Secretion and Target Tissue Actions of Glucocorticoids: Impact on Health. *Frontiers in Endocrinology, 8,* 70.

Owens, J. A., Chervin, R. D., & Hoppin, A. G. (2019). *Behavioral Sleep Problems in Children.* https://www.uptodate.com/contents/behavioral-sleep-problems-in-children.

Rief, W., Barsky, A. J., Bingel, U., Doering, B. K., Schwarting, R., Wohr, M., & Schweiger, U. (2016). 'Rethinking Psychopharmacotherapy: The Role of Treatment Context and Brain Plasticity in Antidepressant and Antipsychotic Interventions'. *Neuroscience and Biobehavioral Reviews, 60,* 51–64.

Skene, D. J., Skornyakov, E., Chowdhury, N. R., Gajula, R. P., Middleton, B., Satterfield, B. C., et al. (2018). Separation of Circadian- and Behavior-Driven Metabolite Rhythms in Humans Provides a Window on Peripheral Oscillators and Metabolism. *Proceedings of the National Academy of Sciences of the United States of America, 115,* 7825–7830.

Smarr, B. (2017, October 3). Circadian Rhythm: This Year's Nobel Prize Winners Are Changing Everything We Know About Medicine and Biology. *Quartz.* https://qz.com/1092753/circadian-rhythm-this-years-nobel-prize-winners-are-changing-everything-we-know-about-medicine-and-biology/.

Tononi, G., & Cirelli, C. (2014). Sleep and the Price of Plasticity: From Synaptic and Cellular Homeostasis to Memory Consolidation and Integration. *Neuron, 81,* 12–34.

Zelinski, E. L., Deibel, S. H., & McDonald, R. J. (2014). The Trouble with Circadian Clock Dysfunction: Multiple Deleterious Effects on the Brain and Body. *Neuroscience and Biobehavioral Reviews, 40,* 80–101.

6

The Autonomic Nervous System and Functional Somatic Symptoms

Abstract In this chapter we continue our exploration of the neurobiology of functional somatic symptoms by considering the autonomic nervous system. In response to stress, the autonomic system activates into defensive mode to prepare the body for protective action. And when protective action is no longer necessary, the system typically deactivates. But if the child has faced stress that is chronic, uncontrollable, unpredictable, cumulative, recurrent, or overwhelming, the autonomic system may remain activated and represent an ongoing burden on the body. In this chapter we discuss functional somatic symptoms that are the direct expression of the activation or dysregulation of the autonomic system.

We have chosen to discuss the autonomic nervous system next because the functional somatic symptoms related to the stress-related activation of this system are common both in daily life and in clinical practice. Activation and dysregulation of the autonomic system in

Electronic supplementary material The online version of this chapter (https://doi.org/10.1007/978-3-030-46184-3_6) contains supplementary material, which is available to authorized users.

children (including adolescents) has been documented across the full spectrum of functional disorders (see table in Online Supplement 6.1). Therapeutic approaches that target the autonomic system are therefore a cornerstone of treatment (see Chapter 14). More broadly, some approaches to psychotherapy—for example, Peter Levine's Somatic Experiencing, Patricia Ogden's Sensorimotor Psychotherapy, or Kathy Kain's use of therapeutic touch—use tracking and settling/release of autonomic activation patterns as their primary therapeutic tools (Levine 1997; Payne et al. 2015; Ogden and Fisher 2015; Kain and Terrell 2018). And these activation patterns are so important and, to the trained therapist, so tangible that some therapists from the bodywork tradition 'listen' only to the story told by the body and *never* ask for the body's story to be told in words. Understanding the autonomic system and its patterns of activation also enables clinicians to devise therapeutic approaches for infants and preverbal children (Porges et al. 2019).

What that all means for us in clinical practice is that we need to identify and understand the relevant patterns of autonomic activation if we are to make good progress is treating our patients. While this chapter focuses on the body expression of symptoms associated with the autonomic nervous system, it is important to keep in mind that the autonomic system is regulated by the brain (Craig 2005) and that changes in autonomic activation also involve changes in the brain stress systems (see Chapter 11). In the stress-system model, the interdependence between the autonomic system and brain stress systems is represented by the overlapping circles in Fig. 4.2.

On a final note, we hope that as readers make their way through this chapter, they will bring to mind the patterns of activation that their own bodies experience in the face of stress. Understanding their own patterns of activation will enable psychotherapists to be more effective in recognizing them in the children they work with.

The Autonomic Nervous System and Body Regulation

The *autonomic nervous system* relies on electrical signalling by neurons to fine-tune body state second-by-second. Its *afferent*, interoceptive nerves (from the body to the brain) carry information to the brain about the body's physiological condition (Craig 2003). The autonomic system's *efferent* nerves (from the brain to the body) innervate all the internal organs and tissues of the body, such as the heart, liver, bladder, gut, white and brown fat, immune cells, and connective and other tissues, including the fascia and the smooth muscle within the blood vessels and body organs. All the organs and tissues from inside the body are called the *viscera*. Because the efferent nerves innervate the viscera, including heart muscles and constriction or relaxation of smooth muscle, they are sometimes referred to *visceromotor nerves*.

The autonomic nervous system has two main components: the *sympathetic system* and *parasympathetic system*. The latter includes both a *restorative* and a *defensive* component. The differentiation between the restorative and defensive components of the parasympathetic system is the work of Stephen Porges (2011) (see Online Supplements 1.2 and 6.1). The main nerve containing parasympathetic nerve fibres, both restorative and defensive, is the *vagal nerve*, and for this reason the terms referring to that nerve, including *vagal* and *vasovagal*, are often used to refer to parasympathetic activation. See Fig. 6.1 and following sections for further details.

The Autonomic Nervous System and Attachment Figures

The baseline balance between these three components of the autonomic nervous system is substantially influenced by attachment figures, who function as biopsychosocial regulators (for references see Online Supplement 1.3). In this capacity, sensitive attachment figures help children develop good autonomic regulation characterized by higher restorative parasympathetic activation and lower sympathetic activation. By contrast, attachment figures who are themselves dysregulated are unable to help their children regulate. Stress—whether physical (illness or injury) or psychological (worry, fear, conflict in interpersonal relationships)—has an adverse effect on the autonomic system balance in both attachment figures and their children. Interventions that promote

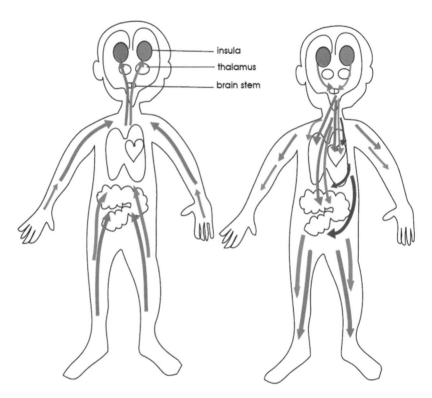

insula
thalamus
brain stem

Fig. 6.1 A simplified functional visual representation of the autonomic nervous system. Afferent signals from the body to the brain provide the brain with interoceptive information about the state of the body (figure on the left). Efferent signals from the brain to the body—involving both the *sympathetic* and *restorative parasympathetic systems*—provide second-by-second fine-tuning of body state (figure on the right). In addition, when needed (as in response to threat), the *sympathetic nerves* (depicted in red) *up* body arousal by increasing heart rate, activating the secretion of adrenalin (from the adrenal glands), adjusting vascular tone, and so on. Likewise, *restorative parasympathetic nerves* (depicted in blue) *down* body arousal (e.g., by decreasing heart rate). The *defensive parasympathetic* nerves (depicted in purple) work alongside the sympathetic system in response to threat by activating defensive programs in the gut and in the heart. Online Supplement 4.4 includes a version of the functional visual representation of the autonomic nervous system that can be printed out (© Kasia Kozlowska 2013)

restorative parasympathetic activation via touch, vocal connection, eye-to-eye contact, and emotional communicating serve to support autonomic regulation in young children (Porges et al. 2019) (Fig. 6.2).

The Autonomic Nervous System Under Conditions of Low Stress and Safety

Under conditions of safety and low stress, the sympathetic and parasympathetic systems work together continually, and in a complementary manner, to regulate body state. For example, in the heart the sympathetic system functions like an accelerator (increasing heart rate when needed), and the parasympathetic system functions like a brake (decreasing heart rate). Similarly, in most situations the sympathetic nerves activate immune-inflammatory cells into defensive mode (when needed), and parasympathetic nerves down-regulate immune-inflammatory cells into restorative mode.

Sympathetic efferent nerves to body organs and tissues innervate, and with the exception of the gut and bladder, usually activate those organs on a second-by-second basis to maintain ongoing bodily functions. Via activation of the adrenal medulla, the sympathetic system also facilitates the release of adrenaline and noradrenaline, thereby enabling the catabolic, energy-expending responses that are needed to maintain body functions.

Restorative parasympathetic efferent nerves also innervate body organs and tissues to regulate body state, but in a manner that complements, and sometimes counteracts, the sympathetic system. Their priority, however, is to efficiently manage key life processes such as digestion (to appropriate energy from food), elimination of waste products, energy conservation, and tissue regeneration and repair, as well as to maintain a body state that facilitates close emotional connection with significant others (Porges 2011; Porges and Carter 2011). For a detailed account of specifically which nerves innervate which organs and tissues, see Wehrwein and colleagues (2016).

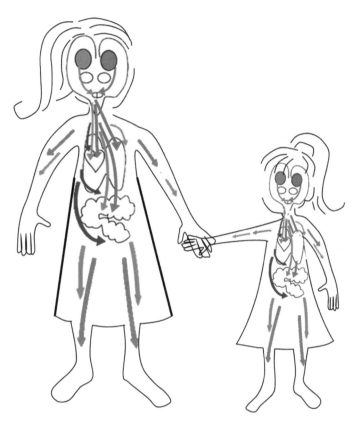

Fig. 6.2 Mother and child co-regulating. This figure depicts a mother figure (and her autonomic nervous system), a child figure (and her autonomic nervous system), and the co-regulation between them (© Kasia Kozlowska 2019)

With the exception of an ongoing role in *orienting* to sudden changes in the environment that may represent potential danger—which results in a decreased heart rate—*defensive* parasympathetic efferents are largely offline, waiting in the background to activate in response to threat.

Thus, overall—under conditions of safety and low stress—the sympathetic system has a catabolic effect, causes the release of energy, and is associated with arousal, whereas the parasympathetic system has an anabolic effect, increases saving and storing of energy, and is associated with rest and restoration. Under such conditions, the child is rarely aware of body changes mediated by the autonomic nervous system. She may notice when her stomach rumbles with hunger, or when her heart thumps and skin sweats after she has been running, or when she blushes and her face heats up. But most of the time the autonomic system just chugs along in the background.

The Autonomic System Under Conditions of Acute Stress, and Episodic Functional Somatic Symptoms

Under conditions of stress or in response to signals of danger, the sympathetic and parasympathetic systems shift into their respective defensive modes:

Sympathetic system (see Fig. 6.3). In response to threat or danger—whether physical, psychological, or both—the sympathetic system revs up. In the body as a whole, increased sympathetic activation raises energy consumption, heart rate, and vascular resistance, all in order to prepare the body for defensive action. Children may consequently experience what they describe as a thumping heart (a high heart rate), sweatiness (activation of sweat glands), and sudden changes in body temperature (changes in dilation and constriction of blood vessels near the skin). In the mouth and gut—as a means of making energy available for more urgent purposes—sympathetic activation disrupts, and potentially entirely shuts down, salivary gland, gastric, and colonic function. Because salivary glands are affected, dry mouth is a common symptom of sympathetic arousal. In some cases of chronic sympathetic arousal, the child feels that the food she swallows is just sitting in the stomach (sometimes described as having what feels to be a rock in the stomach) or that she 'just can't eat'. In other cases the child experiences symptoms of constipation. Increased sympathetic activation also affects sleep, with children describing difficulties with sleep initiation and increased arousals in the early hours of the morning (see also Chapter 5).

Parasympathetic system. Stress triggers a response in both the restorative and defensive parasympathetic systems.

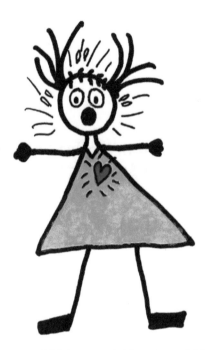

Fig. 6.3 A girl in a state of high arousal. The state of high arousal, in which sympathetic activation, including that of the sweat glands in the skin and smooth muscles of the pupils and eyelids, is coupled with skeletomotor activation. The child often describes a thumping heart, sweatiness, feelings of heat on the inside, tightness in the muscles of the body, and an increased breathing rate or a sensation of not getting enough air. The observer may be aware of dilated pupils and a widening of the eyes (© Kasia Kozlowska 2019)

The activity of the *restorative parasympathetic system* decreases. Most importantly, withdrawing the parasympathetic break on the heart increases the heart rate immediately and also frees the sympathetic system to increase the heart rate, if necessary, even more. In addition, withdrawal of restorative parasympathetic activity and activation of the sympathetic activity is associated with lower pain threshold in the gut (i.e., more susceptibility to pain), which creates a risk for developing hyperalgesia (pain responses to stimuli that do not trigger pain in healthy controls) (see Online Supplement 1.3). This is probably why abdominal pain is such a common symptom in young children who experience significant stress and also why adults experiencing severe stress or anxiety sometimes report that something makes them 'feel sick to the stomach'.

Altan was a 10-year-old boy in year 4 of primary school. His family had moved house in the middle of the academic year, and he was now attending a new school, where he was the target of teasing from boys in the year above him. Altan began to worry about going to school. In particular, he was worried about being waylaid by the boys at the front gate and teased. At night he had trouble falling asleep (decreased restorative parasympathetic [vagal] activation, increased sympathetic activation, and increased hypothalamic-pituitary-adrenal [HPA] axis activation [see Chapter 8]). In the mornings he was unable to eat and complained of abdominal pain and nausea, and sometimes he vomited (decreased restorative parasympathetic [vagal] activity and activation of defensive parasympathetic [vagal] programs to the gut). Altan's symptoms melted away when a neighbour suggested that Altan walk to school with her twin boys, who were in year 6. Altan now happily went to go to school feeling safe—and with a settled autonomic nervous system—in the presence of his new buddies.

Alongside the withdrawal of the restorative parasympathetic system, the *defensive parasympathetic system* lowers its set-point, which enables this system to activate its defensive programs for the heart and for the gut and bladder more readily, thereby working in tandem with the sympathetic system to defend the child's body from threat or danger. Again, it is important to note that these defensive parasympathetic programs are usually offline; they are activated only when the sympathetic system reaches a certain threshold involving severe or imminent threats or danger or when defensive parasympathetic fibres are (reflexly) activated by threat stimuli.

In response to a threat or danger that arises suddenly (including sudden pain or shock), activation of defensive parasympathetic (vagal) nerve fibres to the heart (see Fig. 6.4) can suddenly slow it down (bradycardia) or briefly stop it (resulting in asystole)—which is, in extreme circumstances, itself a defence response (Roelofs et al. 2010). Possible manifestations include dizziness and giddiness (symptoms that occur before a faint) or actual fainting. The most well-recognized expression of this response is blood phobia—that is, fainting in response to the sight of blood (Ost et al. 1984).

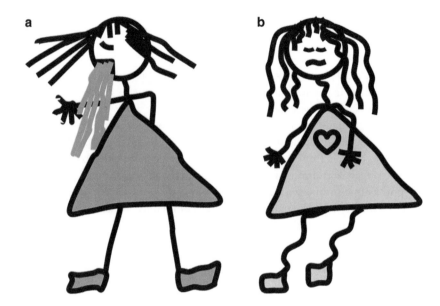

Fig. 6.4 Activation of defensive parasympathetic programs to the gut and heart. *Frame A*. Activation of defensive parasympathetic programs to the gut causes activation of nausea and vomiting programs in this child. *Frame B*. Activation of defensive parasympathetic programs (vagal nerve fibres) to the heart causes threat-induced fainting in this child (© Kasia Kozlowska 2018)

In the following vignette of Jean-Luc, we see a man whose fainting episodes started as a child and recurred well into middle age (with potentially still more to come). Jean-Luc, like his mother, suffered from fainting events mediated by activation of the defensive parasympathetic (vagal) nerve fibres to the heart—an activation that was usually, but not always, induced by acute pain.

At 12 years of age, after his mother tapped him on the elbow—on the ulnar nerve—as a reminder of good table manners, Jean-Luc's eyes rolled back, and he fell off his chair to the floor. At 20, in a science lab, he fainted when his procedure on a live frog (in preparation for dissection) went badly amiss. At 44, he fainted in response to an intense stomach pain in a pub, hitting his head on the counter. Because he was bleeding, and because the pub's bouncers assumed that he had been causing trouble, he was thrown out onto the street with a warning. At 54, he twisted his leg and fractured his fibula while playing ball with a group of children at a party. During the sudden sharp intense pain, he fell to the ground, aware that he was losing consciousness. At 55, Jean-Luc was asleep in a hotel in Europe. In the middle of the night he woke up with a growing pain in his stomach from food poisoning or a gastrointestinal bug. As the pain got worse, he got up to go the bathroom to vomit (defensive parasympathetic program). The next part of the story is given in Jean-Luc's own voice: 'I vomit all my guts in the toilet, and it seems to get better. Then a second wave comes, very sharp and intense, and I lean again over the toilet bowl. I don't remember passing out. Next I wake up. My body is stuck between the toilet and the wall in a weird position. Luckily, I did not fall from high and did not hit anything. I don't know how long I have been there, but most probably not more than a few minutes.'

Activation of defensive parasympathetic programs for the gut and bladder manifest as nausea and vomiting (see Fig. 6.4) and as fear-induced faecal or urinary incontinence or simply as an increase in (sudden) bowel motions or urinary frequency, with the consequence that the child complains that she repeatedly needs to run urgently to the toilet to defecate or urinate. Common examples of this mechanism—which many readers will be familiar with—include the feeling of nausea in response to an aversive stimulus/memory or the need to run to the toilet to empty the bladder before public speaking. These defensive programs were developed (via evolution) to empty the gut in case of poisoning or infection, or to rid the body of unnecessary weight when flight was required. The defensive parasympathetic programs to empty the gut can operate at the same time as the sympathetic programs that tend to shut down the gut, so that the child can experience alternating bouts of diarrhoea and constipation.

Chronic Activation or Dysregulation of the Autonomic Nervous System in Children with Functional Somatic Symptoms

Chronic activation or dysregulation of autonomic function is a pervasive feature of functional presentations. It contributes to, and helps maintain, dysregulation of the stress system as a whole and the associated, nonspecific symptoms of fatigue, nausea, disrupted sleep, sensation of a beating heart, and so on. But in some cases this chronic activation/dysregulation of autonomic function expresses itself in stable, repeating symptom patterns in one or more body systems. Because these symptom patterns are both recognizable and common, they have been given medical names such as irritable bowel syndrome, irritable bladder, and orthostatic intolerance (also known as postural orthostatic tachycardia syndrome [POTS]). For historical terminologies pertaining to autonomic dysregulation—for example, in soldiers from the American Civil War—see Online Supplement 1.1.

The following vignette of Barbara highlights how the concomitant increase in sympathetic activity, decrease in restorative parasympathetic activity, and increase in defensive parasympathetic activity can manifest in chronic gut symptoms.

Barbara was a 13-year-old girl with a two-year history of chronic abdominal pain and nausea, punctuated by episodes of recurrent vomiting that led to dehydration and that brought her repeatedly to hospital. Barbara and her family were refugees. Many of Barbara's relatives in her home village—including her father and older brother—had been threatened by armed militia, sometimes at gun point. Barbara's immediate family fled the village, but the rest of her relatives stayed behind. On arrival to Australia, Barbara had nightmares about the well-being of her aunt, who had helped raise Barbara and her siblings. At night Barbara often woke from her nightmares sweaty and with her heart racing (sympathetic activation). She also began to suffer from recurrent episodes of abdominal pain (changed pain thresholds associated with increased sympathetic, and decreased restorative parasympathetic, activity), leading to frequent visits to the local hospital's emergency department. A year after arrival, she and other members of her family experienced a bout of gastritis that required, in her case, admission to hospital. After the gastritis resolved, she continued to feel nauseous, had trouble eating, and suffered from vomiting episodes (activation of defensive gut programs mediated by the defensive parasympathetic system). Her abdominal pain also spread: she now also suffered from headache and pain in the hip (central pain sensitization/activation of pain maps; see Chapter 11). Her nausea and retching were triggered on a daily basis, whenever it was time to eat a meal (activation of defensive parasympathetic system and defensive gut programs). She had difficulty maintaining her weight. She missed a lot of school. When Barbara experienced any emotional stress or distress—for example, when she had a falling out with a friend, when her father was unwell, or when there was conflict with a teacher—her symptoms (pain, nausea, and vomiting) would be triggered, and she would present to the emergency department in a dehydrated state. (For other factors that could have contributed to Barbara's presentation, see Chapter 10 about the microbiota-gut-brain axis.)

The following vignette of Carmen highlights how the loss of a parent can lead to chronic autonomic dysregulation presenting as fainting episodes. We can hypothesize that the sudden death of Carmen's father led to significant distress and concomitant autonomic activation—a withdrawal of restorative vagal activity, plus sympathetic arousal—as well as a changed set-point for activation of the defensive parasympathetic system (defensive vagus), resulting in more frequent activation of the defensive parasympathetic system (defensive vagus) and frequent fainting (vasovagal) events. Previously for Carmen, such events had been episodic—for example, in response to the sight of blood.

Carmen was a 14-year-old girl from a middle-class family. Prior to the death of her father in a motor vehicle accident, Carmen had occasionally fainted when standing in the heat. Having her blood taken or seeing the needles used for vaccination also made her queasy, and in a few instances she had fainted. Following her father's death, Carmen's distress was extreme, and she thought of her father frequently. At school she began to have almost daily episodes of fainting (activation of the defensive parasympathetic fibres [defensive vagus] to the heart). Her friends reported that she would turn white, drop to the ground, and recover herself soon after. On several occasions she sustained significant injuries to her arms and head. Carmen has no memory of the faints.

Autonomic dysregulation manifesting as orthostatic intolerance (or POTS) expresses itself via physical symptoms of dizziness, giddiness, palpitations, lightheadedness, near-fainting, and fainting on standing up from a reclined or sitting position. It involves too little restorative parasympathetic (vagal) activity (allowing heart rate to increase), too much sympathetic activity (through which heart rate increases even more), and no change in blood pressure (Stewart 2012; Wells et al. 2018) (for details about POTS and additional references, see Online Supplement 6.1). Orthostatic intolerance is often accompanied by nausea—or even abdominal pain or vomiting—reflecting concomitant activation of defensive gut programs by the defensive parasympathetic system. It is frequently comorbid with other functional somatic symptoms or syndromes. Because the autonomic nervous system is very sensitive to stress, orthostatic intolerance is a common consequence of physical or psychological stress, such as surgery, a viral illness, gravitational deconditioning (too much bed rest), puberty (growth spurt or, for girls, the onset of menstruation), a traumatic event, cumulative adverse life events, or ongoing distress in the context of family conflict.

In the following vignette of Ines, we see orthostatic intolerance in a young girl with non-epileptic seizures and social anxiety. The standing test mentioned as part of the vignette is done on waking. The child stands for ten minutes with heart rate and blood pressure being taken at one-minute intervals. A heart rate increase of ≥ 40 beats per minute (accompanied by symptoms) without a significant lowering of blood pressure gives a good indication of orthostatic intolerance.

Ines was a 13-year-old girl living with her parents and her older sister. Ines was bullied throughout primary school, which she had managed by avoiding close friendships. She also had a history of fainting if she stood too long in the heat. When Ines was in high school, her sister was assaulted. In the aftermath of the assault, the sister became depressed and began to self-harm. Ines worried about her sister: her mind produced vivid images of her sister being assaulted, being carved up with a knife, and dying from suicide. Ines presented with non-epileptic seizures—zoning-out events lasting minutes, plus periods of collapse and unresponsiveness lasting minutes to hours. She also reported nausea, wobbliness, fatigue, and dizziness. The latter cluster of symptoms typically manifested on standing. Sometimes she also had diarrhoea. During a ten-minute standing test, Ines was found to have a high baseline heart rate of 90 (>75th percentile) that increased to 160 during the test, with no drop in blood pressure, all consistent with orthostatic intolerance and a diagnosis of POTS.

Orthostatic intolerance is also frequently encountered in chronic pain patients secondary to a loss of physical conditioning that has resulted from a lack of exercise:

> Orthostatic intolerance was confirmed in Paula, the bed-bound 15-year-old girl with chronic pain and recent onset of functional neurological symptoms (leg weakness and functional blindness), whom we met in Chapters 2 and 3. Immediately upon waking in her hospital bed, Paula would begin catastrophizing about her pain, about feeling sick, and about going to the hospital school. Her heart rate would range around 85, and her respiratory rate around 25. On a standing test, Paula's heart rate rose from 84 beats per minute to 146 beats over six minutes, with no significant drop in blood pressure (see Table 3.1). Paula felt sick and lightheaded; her respiratory rate increased; and her panic increased. It increased again when she was taken to school, culminating in a panic attack.

Another pattern of autonomic dysregulation is overactive bladder, manifesting as urinary frequency or urgency, which is thought to involve too much (defensive) parasympathetic activity coupled with too little sympathetic activity (Aydogmus et al. 2017). (For a discussion of urinary retention, see Chapter 7.)

> Ghani was a 12-year-old girl who spent one month in hospital, confined to her bed with pneumonia. When Ghani was discharged home, she continued to experience symptoms of fatigue, dizziness, and intermittent headaches, and she had difficulties concentrating on her schoolwork and could manage only half days at school. She also developed urinary frequency and felt like she needed to go to the toilet all the time. All urology tests were normal. A standing test showed that when Ghani stood up from a resting position, her blood pressure was stable, but her heart rate increased by 69 (90 to 159) beats per minute (reflecting significant sympathetic activation on standing). A hyperventilation challenge showed chronic hyperventilation (see Chapter 7). The diagram of the autonomic nervous system (see Fig. 6.1) was used to explain that the long period in bed—because of the pneumonia—had contributed to dysregulation of the autonomic system, that this dysregulation was causing Ghani's irritable bladder symptoms and her dizziness on standing, and that it was

contributing to her symptom of fatigue. To help regulate her autonomic nervous system and switch down her respiratory motor system, Ghani added breath training to her home rehabilitation/recovery program.

As noted earlier, Online Supplement 6.1 presents a table summarizing paediatric studies showing autonomic dysregulation in relation to wide-ranging functional problems, including chronic pain/chronic abdominal pain, irritable bowel, chronic fatigue, functional neurological disorder, and disturbed sleep.

* * *

We hope that after reading this chapter, the mental health clinician working with children will be better able to identify and track patterns of activation in the body—both by asking the child and family better questions, and by observing activation patterns in the body itself. We are confident that the clinician will discover that a large number of child patients suffer from symptoms that pertain to activation or dysregulation of the autonomic nervous system (see vignettes scattered through this chapter). The child, in turn, will find it very reassuring to know that the clinician understands the language spoken by the body, understands the manner in which the body is causing the symptoms, and knows how to implement strategies that can help the child settle her body and, as in Chapter 3's vignette of Paula, enable the symptoms to melt away.

References

Aydogmus, Y., Uzun, S., Gundogan, F. C., Ulas, U. H., Ebiloglu, T., & Goktas, M. T. (2017). Is Overactive Bladder a Nervous or Bladder Disorder? Autonomic Imaging in Patients with Overactive Bladder via Dynamic Pupillometry. *World Journal of Urology, 35*, 467–472.

Craig, A. D. (2003). Interoception: The Sense of the Physiological Condition of the Body. *Current Opinion in Neurobiology, 13*, 500–505.

Craig, A. D. (2005). Forebrain Emotional Asymmetry: A Neuroanatomical Basis? *Trends in Cognitive Sciences, 9*, 566–571.

Kain, K. L., & Terrell, S. J. (2018). *Nurturing Resilience: Helping Clients Move Forward from Developmental Trauma: An Integrative Somatic Approach.* Berkeley, CA: North Atlantic Books.

Levine, P. (1997). *Waking the Tiger: Healing Trauma.* Berkeley, CA: North Atlantic Books.

Ogden, P., & Fisher, J. (2015). *Sensorimotor Psychotherapy: Interventions for Trauma and Attachment.* New York: Norton.

Ost, L. G., Sterner, U., & Lindahl, I. L. (1984). Physiological Responses in Blood Phobics. *Behaviour Research and Therapy, 22,* 109–117.

Payne, P., Levine, P. A., & Crane-Godreau, M. A. (2015). Somatic Experiencing: Using Interoception and Proprioception as Core Elements of Trauma Therapy. *Frontiers in Psychology, 6,* 93.

Porges, S. W. (2011). *The Polyvagal Theory: Neurophysiological Foundations of Emotions, Attachment, Communication, and Self-Regulation.* New York: Norton.

Porges, S. W., & Carter, S. (2011, October). *Polyvagal Theory, Oxytocin and the Neurobiology of Love and Attachment: Using the Body's Social Engagement System to Promote Recovery from Experiences of Threat, Stress and Trauma.* Seminar, Sydney, Australia.

Porges, S. W., Davila, M. I., Lewis, G. F., Kolacz, J., Okonmah-Obazee, S., Hane, A. A., et al. (2019). Autonomic Regulation of Preterm Infants Is Enhanced by Family Nurture Intervention. *Developmental Psychobiology, 61,* 942–952.

Roelofs, K., Hagenaars, M. A., & Stins, J. (2010). Facing Freeze: Social Threat Induces Bodily Freeze in Humans. *Psychological Science, 21,* 1575–1581.

Stewart, J. M. (2012). Update on the Theory and Management of Orthostatic Intolerance and Related Syndromes in Adolescents and Children. *Expert Review of Cardiovascular Therapy, 10,* 1387–1399.

Wehrwein, E. A., Orer, H. S., & Barman, S. M. (2016). Overview of the Anatomy, Physiology, and Pharmacology of the Autonomic Nervous System. *Comprehensive Physiology, 6,* 1239–1278.

Wells, R., Spurrier, A. J., Linz, D., Gallagher, C., Mahajan, R., Sanders, P., et al. (2018). Postural Tachycardia Syndrome: Current Perspectives. *Vascular Health and Risk Management, 14,* 1–11.

7

The Skeletomotor System and Functional Somatic Symptoms

Abstract In this chapter we continue our exploration of the neurobiology of functional somatic symptoms by considering the skeletomotor system. When the stress system activates, the skeletomotor system activates in tandem, to prepare the body for protective action. And when protective action is no longer necessary, the skeletomotor system typically deactivates. But if the child has faced severe stress of one kind or another, with the consequence that stress-system activation is maintained, activation of the skeletomotor system may also be maintained even though there is no immediate need. This maladaptive activation of the skeletomotor system may express itself in aberrant motor patterns. Some of these patterns are easily recognizable as body responses to threat that have somehow remained activated even in the absence of current threat. Other motor patterns mimic neurological conditions and result in significant functional impairment. In this chapter we also

Electronic supplementary material The online version of this chapter (https://doi.org/10.1007/978-3-030-46184-3_7) contains supplementary material, which is available to authorized users.

introduce the reader to the fascia system. The fascia envelops and supports skeletal muscle (and other organs and tissues) and plays an important role in symptoms involving the skeletomotor system.

The skeletomotor system includes skeletal muscles, the motor nerves that innervate these muscles, and the motor-processing regions in the brain that control all aspects of motor function. *Skeletal muscles* are made up of *striated* muscle fibres (cells) that attach to the *bones of the body*. These muscles enable the body to move and to address, through action, the challenges of daily life. Anatomists refer to the motor nerves that innervate these muscles as *somatomotor nerves*. The word *soma* comes from the Greek and means *body* (or *body proper*). The skeletomotor system manages motor activation of the body (soma) as a whole. By contrast, as we saw in Chapter 6, the efferent nerves of the autonomic nervous system, known as *visceromotor nerves*, innervate heart muscle and smooth muscle—which is found in body organs and tissues (e.g., blood vessels and glands)—and also control increases in body arousal. For the origins and anatomy of different types of muscles, see Online Supplement 7.1.

Because functional symptoms pertaining to the skeletomotor system frequently involve pain, we must also mention the afferent nerves—which are part of the interoceptive system—that carry information about body state (including pain) from skeletal muscle to the spinal cord and then to the brain. These afferent interoceptive nerves play a key role in chronic musculoskeletal pain. Locally, in chronic pain the endings of these nerves may release pro-inflammatory molecules in skeletal muscle (called neurogenic inflammation). The nerves themselves (separate from the activity at their endings) carry interoceptive and pain information from muscle to the spinal cord. In the spinal cord—which is part of the central nervous system—these same nerves release pro-inflammatory molecules, resulting in *central sensitization*, a state in which pain signals are maintained and amplified. In turn, this central sensitization (in the spinal cord) activates nerves carrying pain signals through the spinal cord to the brain, where they help maintain activation of pain maps and the subjective experience of pain. For further discussion of pain and pain maps, see Chapters 9 and 11.

Functional somatic symptoms associated with the skeletomotor system are wide ranging. Individual children (including adolescents) have their own characteristic patterns of skeletomotor response to stress. One simple way of conceptualizing this idea, which is used to organize the present chapter, is to borrow a notion introduced by Leah Helou and colleagues (2018), who refer to 'laryngeal muscle responders': individuals who respond to stress by tightening up the laryngeal muscles that make up the voice box. By the same token, and as discussed in this chapter, some children respond to stress by activating their postural muscles; others activate their respiratory muscles; others the muscle groups involved in actions such as coughing; and so on. Importantly for our purposes, each of these different patterns, when excessive, maladaptive, or aberrant, can present as functional somatic symptoms. But just how any particular pattern of symptoms is classified or described will depend upon the medical professional initially consulted. For example, excessive activation of laryngeal muscles may be called *functional/habit/psychogenic cough* (if presenting with a cough to a respiratory physician), *muscle tension dysphonia* (if presenting with loss of voice to a speech pathologist), *functional dysphagia* (if presenting with *concurrent* difficulties in swallowing to a gastroenterologist), *muscle tension dysphagia* (if presenting with difficulties in swallowing to an otorhinolaryngologist), or *functional tic disorder/functional neurological disorder* (FND) (if presenting with vocal noises to a neurologist). For references see Online Supplement 1.3.

The Skeletomotor System Works Together with the Autonomic Nervous (Visceromotor) System

Activation of the skeletomotor system and activation of the autonomic nervous system occur hand in hand. The two systems function as *coupled* systems (Koizumi and Brooks 1972; Dum et al. 2016; Jafari et al. 2017) (see Fig. 7.1). They work together as an integrated whole. This collaboration begins on the brain system level and flows through to the body system level. Activation of the autonomic system—in particular, an increase

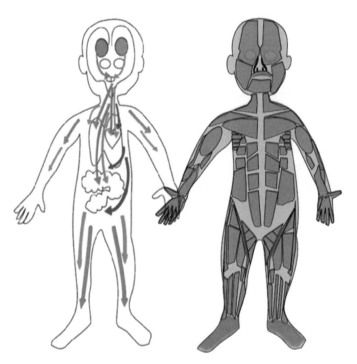

Fig. 7.1 The autonomic and skeletomotor systems as coupled systems. The figure on the left represents the efferent (motor) component of the autonomic system. The *sympathetic* nerves are depicted in red. The *restorative* parasympathetic nerves are depicted in blue. The *defensive parasympathetic* nerves are depicted in purple. The figure on the right represents the skeletomotor system. The holding of hands represents the coupling between the two systems. The autonomic system—also known as the visceromotor system—activates to mediate increases in body arousal and motor changes in the organs and tissues. The skeletomotor system activates to mediate an increase in breathing rate (to keep up with the body's increased need for oxygen for producing energy), to increase tone in skeletal muscles to prepare the body for action, and to generate movement. The systems work together as an integrated whole (© Kasia Kozlowska 2017)

in sympathetic arousal—is typically accompanied by activation of the skeletomotor system, and vice versa. Likewise, when one of these systems becomes excessively activated or dysregulated, the other does so, too.

Because of this coupling between systems, some therapists refer to coupled activation of the autonomic nervous system and skeletal muscle as *tension patterns* (Baker 2017) or as *stress-related bracing* or *patterns of constriction* or *contraction* (see Online Supplement 7.1). Body-oriented psychotherapists—such as those working from Peter Levine's Somatic Experiencing, Patricia Ogden's Sensorimotor Psychotherapy, or Kathy Kain's use of therapeutic touch—use tracking and settling/release of autonomic/skeletal muscle/fascia activation patterns as their primary therapeutic tools (Levine 1997; Payne et al. 2015; Ogden and Fisher 2015; Kain and Terrell 2018).

Brain Stress Systems and Skeletomotor Function

While this chapter focuses on the body expression of aberrant motor symptom patterns, it is important to highlight that all of the symptom patterns described below also involve, and are the result of, excessive activation of the brain stress systems (for further discussion see Chapter 11). That is, excessive activation of the brain stress systems appears either (1) to maintain activation of motor-processing regions that are associated with and generate specific aberrant motor patterns or (2) to disrupt motor processing in the brain, generating unusual motor patterns that mimic neurological diseases (and are diagnosed as FND).

Symptoms Associated with Muscles That Stabilize Body Posture

Sympathetic activation and its state of high arousal are typically coupled with increased tone in postural muscles, which stabilize body posture and ensure that the body is prepared for action. Increases in tone involve activation of both skeletal motor units (detectable on electromyogram) and muscle spindles (detectable with needle microelectrodes) (for muscle spindles and pain, see Online Supplement 7.1). Increased tone in postural muscles also occurs in stressful situations for which actions either are not required or cannot actually be taken effectively. Such situations include those whose origins are psychological (e.g., anticipatory anxiety, catastrophizing, traumatic memories), interpersonal (e.g., conflicts within relationships), or even intellectual (e.g., difficult cognitive tasks). For example, a child may have an urge to punch a bully in the face, but this type of physical, protective action is generally deemed inappropriate in the current cultural context, and is typically inhibited. The upshot is that the body will still activate the motor action pattern (the skeletal muscles preparing for action, including the punch) but without the follow-up action—the punch itself—taking place.

Mild increases in muscle tone involving particular action patterns in response to psychological, interpersonal, or intellectual stress are common and will generally abate relatively quickly. But persistent or recurring increases in tone can be maladaptive (Westgaard et al. 2013) and may result in pain or sensations of tension in the head, neck, back, hamstring, and calf muscles. In children, this sort of excessive musculoskeletal tension can usually be identified as tenderness, trigger points, and increased muscle tension on palpation (Simons et al. 1999). Such increases in tone—the patterned activation of muscles—will typically contribute to symptoms of fatigue. And if the activation of these muscles is recurrent and ongoing, all the factors that are associated with, and that maintain, chronic pain potentially come into play (see above and Chapters 9 and 11).

Greta, a 17-year-old girl in the final year of high school, was hoping to become a doctor; her study schedule was often gruelling. After any protracted period of studying, Greta suffered from tension and pain in the muscles that support posture: the muscles of her neck, shoulders, and legs (hamstrings and calves). At night the hamstring muscle on the right throbbed with pain.

Symptoms Arising in Connection with Muscles of the Respiratory Motor System: Hyperventilation

'Hyperventilation is a respiratory stress response that occurs most typically in situations of uncontrollable stress, fear, and pain' (Jafari et al. 2017, p. 997). In states of arousal, sympathetic activation is coupled with increases in respiratory rate to ensure an increase in the oxygen (O_2) supply to cells for the production of energy—a process known as cellular respiration (see section on cellular respiration in Online Supplement 7.1). Carbon dioxide (CO_2), the waste product of cellular respiration, diffuses into the blood and is then eliminated by the lungs. The homeostatic range for arterial CO_2 is 36–52 mm Hg (up to 52 mm Hg in sleep). If the arterial CO_2 is below the homeostatic range—the gold-standard test for hyperventilation—then the child is, by definition, hyperventilating. That is, the child is breathing faster than needed by metabolic demand, faster than required to eliminate the CO_2 produced by cellular respiration. In such circumstances—with activation of the respiratory motor system (skeletal muscles that mediate respiration) exceeding the body's actual oxygen need—functional somatic symptoms may arise.

Transcutaneous monitors—a small probe placed on the finger—now enable researchers to measure arterial CO_2 noninvasively by its diffusion across the skin. Arterial CO_2 is denoted as pCO_2: the p refers to the partial pressure of carbon dioxide in the arterial blood when measured by a transcutaneous monitor.

In clinical practice, where transcutaneous monitors are not usually available, respiratory rate—with the guidance from reference ranges (Fleming et al. 2011, p. 3636)—is used as an approximate measure of hyperventilation. Very high resting-state respiratory rates (>25 breaths per minute in children 9 years and older; see following vignette) fall above the 99th percentile and are a clear indictor of an overactivated respiratory motor system—and hyperventilation. High breathing rates ($\geq$21 breaths per minute for children 8–11 years and $\geq$19 breaths per minute for adolescents 12–15 years) fall above the 75th percentile and are highly suggestive of an overactivated respiratory motor system and hyperventilation (Kozlowska et al. 2017; Chudleigh et al. 2019).

Twelve-year-old Bella presented to the emergency department with a recurrence of non-epileptic seizures (NES) and an increase in the frequency of her fainting episodes in the context of long-term diagnoses of postural orthostatic tachycardia syndrome (POTS) and irritable bowel syndrome. The emergency doctor observed hyperventilation before and during the NES, with respiratory rates of over 40 breaths per minute. The video electroencephalogram (EEG) tracing was normal. The transcutaneous probe that measured arterial CO_2 showed that Bella was already hyperventilating in the resting state (pCO_2 of 34 mm Hg, before Bella was instructed to hyperventilate as part of the hyperventilation challenge). During the hyperventilation component itself—when the technician used a pinwheel to help Bella hyperventilate—Bella's head dropped, and she became unresponsive, dropping the pinwheel at 25 mm Hg (a pattern that replicated some of her NES). During the 15-minute recovery period, Bella failed to return to homeostasis (see Fig. 7.2). Her resting-state heart rate was frequently ≥90 beats per minute (above the 75th percentile), and her resting heart rate variability (a measure of calmness) on the biofeedback device used by the team was low (reflecting low restorative parasympathetic activity). Taken together, the biomarkers suggested overactivation of the respiratory motor system coupled with overactivation of the autonomic nervous system.

Hyperventilation and low pCO_2 are associated with a cascade of neurophysiological changes (for the neurophysiology of hyperventilation, see Online Supplement 7.1). As with other biological responses, the pattern of each child's individual response to hyperventilation varies from one child to another (see Fig. 7.3 picturing children with different responses). What this means clinically is that some children experience, for example, florid symptoms in response to hyperventilation, whereas some children do not. It also means that many patterns of presentation can be encountered clinically, with different children presenting with different symptom patterns involving different body systems. Clinicians therefore need to keep in mind the entire spectrum of hyperventilation-related symptoms and to be able to identify these symptoms in any particular child, whether the symptoms occur in isolation (e.g., hyperventilation-induced chest pain) or alongside other hyperventilation-induced symptoms (e.g., hyperventilation-induced chest pain plus changes in consciousness). In addition, children can present with chronic hyperventilation combined with sudden, time-limited periods of hyperventilation (like Bella), or they can present with such time-limited increases alone, in which case their respiratory rates (and arterial CO_2) in the relaxed, resting state may be normal.

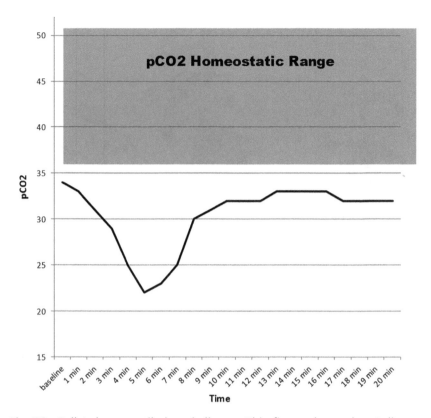

Fig. 7.2 Bella's hyperventilation challenge. This figure shows that Bella was hyperventilating at baseline, even before the EEG technician asked her to hyperventilate. She then dropped her pCO_2 further (as expected) but was unable to reach the homeostatic range—or even her baseline level—after a 15-minute recovery period (© Kasia Kozlowska 2017)

Hyperventilation is associated with major changes in both the body generally (not just the respiratory system) and the brain.

In the Body

Hyperventilation causes sensory and motor nerves to become activated. Excessive activation of nerves may cause pins and needles in the hands and feet, twitchy muscles, or even spasms in the hands or feet

When I hyperventilate ....

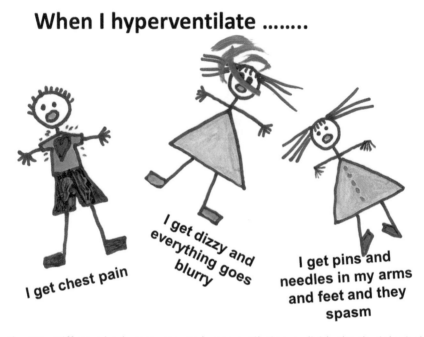

I get dizzy and everything goes blurry

I get chest pain

I get pins and needles in my arms and feet and they spasm

Fig. 7.3 Different body responses to hyperventilation. Individuals' physiological responses to hyperventilation vary widely, as these three examples of hyperventilation indicate. The boy on the left experiences chest pain due to constriction of cardiac arteries. The girl in the middle experiences dizziness and blurry vision due to constriction of cerebral arteries. The girl on the right experiences pins and needles (paraesthesias) and painful cramps of muscles in hands and feet (carpopaedal spasms) due to increased excitability of sensory and motor axons in the peripheral nervous system (© Kasia Kozlowska 2017)

(carpopedal spasms). Hyperventilation also causes vasoconstriction of arteries supplying blood and oxygen to the heart. Excessive vasoconstriction decreases blood flow and delivery of oxygen, and may cause hyperventilation-induced chest pain. Sustained increases in respiratory rate over time—which increase the body's demand for energy—will contribute to symptoms of fatigue. When talking with the family, the clinician can point out that the child's respiratory motor system is working very hard and that it is not surprising that the child feels fatigued and exhausted.

In the Brain

Hyperventilation initially causes cortical excitation; that is, it increases brain arousal and neuron excitability. High levels of cortical arousal can impair prefrontal cortex function, shift the brain to a defensive mode of organization, and increase the probability that evolutionarily more primitive modes of neurological function will emerge (Arnsten 2015).

If hyperventilation continues beyond the short term, it causes (to an extent that varies from individual to individual) vasoconstriction of arteries supplying blood and oxygen to the brain, resulting in decreased blood flow and delivery of oxygen, and in some degree of cerebral hypoxia. Symptoms of cerebral hypoxia include dizziness, changes in vision (ranging from changes in colour to complete blackout), decreasing levels of consciousness (to loss of consciousness), loss of muscle tone (potentially culminating in falling), and so on. The prefrontal cortex is particularly sensitive both to cortical arousal and to hypoxia.

What this means clinically is that some children will have changes in consciousness with hyperventilation. In some cases, their heads will drop, and they will be 'out of it' for a few seconds; other children may faint; others may have episodes of crying and distress (loss of top-down inhibition); and still others will go into an altered, dissociated state. In extreme cases, the child may even experience an NES, with spasmodic movements (Kozlowska et al. 2017). The stressed brain undergoes a cascade of neurobiological changes that we are only just beginning to understand. Hyperventilation contributes to these changes in a major way. Importantly, interventions that target breathing and that improve regulation of the respiratory motor system provide powerful tools to help the child regulate her brain and body (see vignette of Bella, below).

> Twelve-year-old Bella, whom we meet earlier in the chapter, learnt to identify body symptoms that signalled that she was beginning to hyperventilate, including not feeling real and a sense of 'spacing out', a change in the quality of auditory and visual stimuli, a cold feeling in the chest and stomach, and feeling dizzy. Bella learnt to implement a slow-breathing strategy—at the point that she first noticed the warning signs—to avert the pending NES.

Symptoms Associated with Increased Tone in Laryngeal Muscles and the Vocal Folds

The intrinsic laryngeal muscles that are involved in voice production are striated muscles attached to cartilage (for details about striated muscles, see Online Supplement 7.1). The *vocal folds*—also popularly known as *vocal cords*—are made up of mucous membrane and intrinsic laryngeal muscle. Sound is produced when the vocal folds vibrate. In states of high arousal, sympathetic activation is coupled with increased tone in the laryngeal muscles, together with increased tone in the postural muscles of the neck, back, and legs (Helou et al. 2013, 2018; Kozlowska et al. 2015) (see also Online Supplement 7.1). This increase in laryngeal muscle tone causes an increase in the pitch of the voice, with the consequence that the vocalizations of stressed children are high in pitch. The same things happen in other mammals, for example, rat pups emit high-pitched—actually, ultrasonic—vocalizations on separation from their mothers, which the rat pups find to be very stressful (for references see Online Supplement 1.3).

Functional presentations involving the laryngeal muscles/vocal folds include functional aphonia (total loss of voice), functional dysphonia (high-pitched baby voice, whispered phonation, falsetto voice, vocal fatigue, voice instability [including a breathy, hoarse, or rough voice]), diplophonia (with two tones concurrently), and a voice that breaks uncontrollably or has a tight, strained, or strangled quality (Baker 2017).

Akin to other functional neurological symptoms, symptoms involving the laryngeal muscles/vocal folds are associated with aberrant patterns of motor activation in the brain and with aberrant activation of the brain stress systems (Dietrich et al. 2012; Roy et al. 2019) (see Chapter 10). Likewise, patients with functional voice disorders, like others with functional somatic symptoms, typically present to the health care system with a single set of functional symptoms, but, if asked, they also report other symptoms pertaining to activation of the stress system more generally (Demmink-Geertman and Dejonckere 2002; Helou et al. 2018) (see Online Supplement 7.1).

The case of Brian is an amalgam kindly put together by our colleague Jan Baker, a speech pathologist who has particular expertise with functional voice disorders (Baker 2017).

Brian, a 15-year-old boy, presented for speech therapy assessment with a functional dysphonia of four years' duration. Even though Brian was post-pubertal—puberty had started at age 11 years—his voice pitch remained abnormally high, with marked vocal instability in the form of uncontrollable pitch breaks from falsetto phonation to a rough, diplophonic voice. Other names for this type of functional dysphonia are *puberphonia* and *mutational falsetto*. Brian had seen many speech therapists and ear, nose, and throat specialists. Repeated laryngoscopic assessments had confirmed the following: normal laryngeal and vocal-fold structures; extreme tension in the extrinsic and intrinsic laryngeal muscles; and tight sphincteric constriction of the false vocal folds, often obliterating the view and interfering with the function of his true vocal folds. A trial of botulinum toxin injection into Brian's false vocal folds had been administered on one occasion in order to elicit relaxation of this extreme pattern of supraglottic constriction, but the intervention was not effective.

On presentation, Brian appeared to be physically tense, with raised shoulders, high clavicular breathing, and a tight jaw. He appeared anxious and shy, found it difficult to make eye contact, and noted that he found his high-pitched voice both embarrassing and debilitating. He acknowledged that his parents and school teachers were concerned about the effect that his voice was having on his school attendance and also about his reticence to join in activities with other young people. His developmental history, carefully put together by the therapist, disclosed no severely stressful life events or difficulties either at the onset of puberty or over the four-year period of his dysphonia.

In the ordinary course of events, a brief, one- or two-session intervention by a speech pathologist is effective in restoring normal phonation in adolescents such as Brian. For Brian, however—because he had not disclosed the psychological stress that was driving the functional dysphonia (see below)—the intervention took months of coordinated effort involving Brian, his family, his school teachers, and two close friends. Standard behavioural techniques to facilitate normal phonation proved ineffective. The breakthrough came when Brian was able to experience his normal voice in association with a strongly felt emotion—in Brian's case, his laughter while watching television in the privacy of his bedroom. A strategy was devised to record Brian's voice during a particular program that he enjoyed. In the recording of Brian's free, uninhibited emotional laughter, Brian heard and recognized his normal voice at a pitch and quality appropriate to his age and maturity. The essence of this intervention was to build upon his spontaneous motor functioning (in the form of laughter), thereby changing the focus of attention and releasing his voice from cortical, or 'top-down', control and interference. It was only after many months of therapy—with Brian being held in both a trusting therapeutic relationship and trusting relational network (family, teachers, and friends) while searching for his true voice—that he was able to raise and address issues that had been troubling him since the age of 12. Ever since his voice started to break (at puberty), Brian had held fears that he might be gay—which he now felt able to discuss.

In rare cases, an overly robust motor response in the larynx can cause complete adduction of the vocal folds, ventricular bands, and supraglottic structures, thereby closing the airway, cutting off or reducing oxygen supply, and causing hypoxia. Potential sequelae include a change in consciousness, fainting, or fainting followed by a hypoxia-related NES. In some cases, this sphincteric vocal fold adduction is misdiagnosed as asthma. For clinical vignettes detailing atypical, stress-related motor responses in the larynx, see Kozlowska and colleagues (2018a, b).

Mika was a 9-year-old boy with a history of chronic, treatment-resistant asthma and weekly presentations to hospital. He was very anxious about his asthma attacks. Sometimes when Mika thought that he was having an asthma attack, he would begin to panic, his heart would race, and he would begin to breath quickly, coughing intermittently and taking in huge, noisy gulps of air. In this state of high arousal, his vocal folds would adduct, thereby closing his air passage. During one such event, the respiratory specialist visualized the adduction of the vocal folds using a laryngoscope. Mika's noisy breathing would suddenly stop, his eyes would roll back—a blue tinge around his lips signalling hypoxia—and he would slump to the side. Sometimes Mika would be incontinent of urine, and sometimes his body would jerk and shake (a hypoxia-related NES). (This vignette was first presented in Kozlowska et al. 2018a.)

Symptoms Associated with Muscles of the Inner Ear

The muscles of the inner ear—the tensor tympani and stapedius—are the smallest striated muscles in the body. Contracting in response to noise, they inhibit, through what is known as the *acoustic reflex*, the vibrations of the small bones in the middle ear and thereby inhibit, in turn, the transmission of sound. In children, persisting tinnitus or sound sensitivity is often triggered by physical stress (e.g., attendance at a loud concert) or infection (e.g., a viral infection). Akin to other functional somatic symptoms, aberrant motor patterns that maintain tinnitus appear to be maintained by ongoing activation of the brain stress systems (Chen et al. 2017; Leaver et al. 2011) (see Chapter 11). For vignettes see Louisa in Chapter 2 and Bellynda in Chapter 8.

Symptoms Associated with Muscles Involved in Coughing

Coughing is a motor pattern that involves muscles of the larynx, pharynx, chest, and diaphragm. Cough is a defensive reflex that 'preserves the gas-exchanging functions of the lung by facilitating clearance of aspirate, inhaled particulate matter, accumulated secretions, and irritants that are either inhaled or formed at sites of mucosal inflammation' (Canning et al. 2014, p. 1633). The cough reflex can be triggered by activation of parasympathetic (vagal) afferents from the larynx, trachea, and bronchi, as well as by irritation of the lower oesophagus (in a subgroup of individuals) or by mechanical stimulation of the ear (mechanical stimulation of afferent vagal fibres in the external auditory canal can activate the cough reflex in another subgroup of individuals). Functional cough (also known as *habit* or *psychogenic* cough) or throat clearing usually develops in the wake of an infection involving the pharynx or the bronchi. Like other functional disorders, functional cough is an aberrant motor pattern that is presumably maintained by ongoing activation of the brain stress systems (Canning et al. 2014). The symptoms of functional cough may range from mild coughing to intense, almost constant coughing that resembles a goose honking or a dog or seal barking. The third author (HH) had a patient who had been 'barking' almost continuously for more than a year.

Symptoms Associated with Muscles Involved in Swallowing, Belching, and Rumination

Functional somatic symptoms can also occur in connection with motor patterns that involve the striated (skeletal) muscles in the throat, neck, and chest (innervated by somatomotor nerves) and smooth muscle in the upper gastrointestinal tract (innervated by the autonomic nervous system). These muscles work together to enable swallowing, belching, and rumination. Gastroenterologists commonly refer to the functional somatic symptoms associated with these processes as (aberrant) *behaviours*, *habits*, or *reflex responses* that develop as reactions to stimuli such as food, infection, strong emotions, or even acute work pressure. Functional disorders associated with swallowing and belching (and unrelated to any organic pathology) include globus sensation (the feeling of having a lump in the throat), excessive belching (bringing up air), rumination/regurgitation (bringing up food, in a process similar to belching), and other unwanted action patterns mediated by this group of muscles. Akin to other functional somatic symptoms, these motor patterns appear to be maintained by ongoing activation of the brain stress systems (Tornblom and Drossman 2018) (see Chapter 11).

For more information—and references—about the mechanics (muscle patterns) in belching, rumination/regurgitation, and globus sensation, see Online Supplement 7.1.

Functional symptoms involving muscles of breathing and swallowing can present as lone symptoms (see case of Fiona in Kozlowska [2013]), as a cluster of symptoms involving breathing or swallowing functions, or, as in the following case of Maddie, alongside other functional neurological symptoms.

Maddie, a 15-year-old girl—the youngest of six children—attended a special school for the intellectually impaired. Maddie's family split their time between the farm (run by the family, and now her father, for generations) and the city (where Maddie lived with her mother, whose chronic medical condition required her close proximity to the hospital). Despite her intellectual disability, Maddie had done well because she had always been supported by her siblings. But when Maddie turned 15, her sister—the last sibling living in her mother's house—left home to get married, leaving Maddie responsible, all on her own, for managing the house, the physical and emotional needs of her ill mother, and the continuing demands of her own schooling. Three months into this new arrangement, Maddie experienced a fall, knocking her head and hurting her right knee. In the very short term, she suffered from a loss of memory—she no longer remembered that her sister had left home—and also from pain in her right knee. Over the next month, the memory loss did not resolve, and the pain spread to involve Maddie's whole leg. After seeing many doctors, who could find no medical explanation for her problems, Maddie was referred to the complex pain clinic.

Because the farm work was at its peak in and around this time period, the visits from those living on the farm—Maddie's father and some of her siblings—were brief, and Maddie became more and more distressed. Three months after her fall, she began to complain of a lump in the throat that fluctuated in intensity, that came and went, and that, when present, made it difficult to swallow food. Maddie also began to experience episodes of panic: breathlessness, dizziness, blurred vision, sweatiness, a pounding heart, and tingling in the fingers, feet, neck, back, shoulders, and left side of the face. During these episodes, Maddie's respiratory rate would reach 40 breaths per minute, which she was unable to lower. The panic attacks soon morphed into NES, which sometimes lasted over an hour (Kozlowska et al. 2018a). During the NES, Maddie was unresponsive, and her body shook and jerked. Sometimes she was aware of what people said around her, and sometimes not. Following one prolonged NES, Maddie experienced a range of other functional neurological symptoms that took weeks to resolve: she lost power in her legs and could no longer feel them, was unable to void her bladder, lost her capacity to talk, and had difficulty swallowing, with the consequence that saliva dribbled from the corner of her mouth. After substantial work regarding regulation strategies and some changes in the family situation, Maddie regained use of her legs, bladder, voice, and swallowing, and joined her father and siblings on the farm. Because her NES had not yet resolved, she initially wore a bike helmet when mobilizing around the property. Twelve months later, all her symptoms had fully resolved, and Maddie was happily contributing to the running of the family farm, with intermittent visits to her mother in the city.

Symptoms Associated with Muscles in the Bladder Sphincter

The skeletal muscle in the bladder sphincter is innervated by somato-motor nerves. The smooth muscle in the bladder sphincter is innervated by sympathetic (visceromotor) nerves, and the smooth muscle in the bladder wall is innervated by parasympathetic (visceromotor) nerves. Urination is a coordinated response involving (1) inhibition of sympathetic efferents and relaxation of smooth muscle fibres in the urethral sphincter, (2) inhibition of somatic efferents and relaxation of striated muscle fibres in the urethral sphincter, and (3) activation of efferent parasympathetic fibres and concomitant contraction of the bladder wall. Because the skeletomotor and autonomic (sympathetic) systems are coupled, stress-related activation of the sympathetic efferents coupled with activation of somatomotor efferents to the sphincter may be responsible for stress-related (functional) bladder retention. For brain regions involved in urination, see references in Online Supplement 1.3.

Symptoms That Mimic Neurological Diseases

For completeness, we mention symptoms that mimic neurological conditions such as stroke, epilepsy, or infections of the brain. Common symptoms include weakness or paralysis of the legs or arms, loss of coordination of the legs, and contraction of muscles, causing abnormal posture of the limbs (dystonia). We discuss these presentations in more detail in Chapter 11. Neurologists consider these symptoms under the umbrella of FND. Some presentations associated with increased tone in laryngeal muscles and the vocal folds are also included under FND.

Likewise, bladder retention sometimes occurs alongside other FND symptoms and may be included under FND because it mimics neurological conditions involving the spinal cord.

The Fascia

Fascia—connective tissue—is present throughout the body (Stecco 2015). *Superficial fascia* refers to a fibrous layer that lies within the skin and that covers the body. This fascia protects the body as a whole. *Deep* (muscular) *fascia* 'refers to all of the well-organized, dense, fibrous layers that interpenetrate and surround muscles, bones, nerves and blood vessels, binding all of these structures together into a firm, compact, continuous mass' (Stecco et al. 2016, p. 162). This fascia helps maintain posture and supports body movements. *Visceral fascia* refers to the layers of connective tissue that surround, wrap, and help suspend the organs and tissues. This fascia plays a role in maintaining homeostasis—the internal environment of the body.

The fluidity or rigidity of the fascia system is linked to the child's sense of health and well-being. Healthy interactions between the child and the attachment figure, including physical contact that modifies the fascia system—for example, soothing touch such as holding the child tight or stroking the child's body—will simultaneously settle the autonomic system, deactivate the skeletomotor system, and modify both the pliability and texture of the fascia, contributing to the child's sense of physical and emotional well-being (Schleip 2003; Schleip and Klingler 2019). Likewise, many of us find that therapeutic touch or physical palpation techniques help release tension patterns in our own bodies.

By contrast, activation of the autonomic system, with an increase in sympathetic arousal, is typically accompanied by increased activity of skeletal muscle and increased tension within the fascia system. Presumably, these increases, if chronic, will contribute both to aberrant motor patterns that present as functional somatic symptoms and to symptoms of pain that accompany some of these patterns. For example, we can hypothesize that the recurrent abdominal and mediastinal pain (precordial catch syndrome) experienced by 15-year-old Evie (whom the reader met in Chapter 2) involved fascial tension patterns, much like the mechanisms that are hypothesized for chronic urogenital pain in women (Jantos, forthcoming 2020; Jantos and Stecco, forthcoming 2021).

In addition, because immune-inflammatory cells also reside within the fascia and because the fascia is rich is nerve receptors that carry interoceptive information (e.g., pain), activation of immune-inflammatory cells by stress (physical or psychological) is likely to contribute to chronic pain by secreting pro-inflammatory molecules that activate pain neurons from within the fascia (Jantos, forthcoming 2020) (see also Chapter 9).

For a simple-to-read article about fascia and references to science articles, see Online Supplement 7.1.

* * *

In this chapter we have examined the many different functional somatic symptoms that involve aberrant activation of the skeletomotor system. We have seen that the skeletomotor system works in close collaboration with the autonomic nervous system—increases in arousal are accompanied by activation of skeletal muscles—and that aberrant activation of the skeletomotor system/motor systems in the brain is maintained by activation of the brain stress systems. In the face of stress, whether physical or psychological, both systems activate together to manage threat. When these processes go awry—when the interplay between these systems becomes maladaptive—aberrant motor patterns that present as functional somatic symptoms may arise. In Chapter 8 we look at the role of the hypothalamic-pituitary-adrenal (HPA) axis in functional somatic symptoms.

References

Arnsten, A. F. (2015). Stress Weakens Prefrontal Networks: Molecular Insults to Higher Cognition. *Nature Neuroscience, 18,* 1376–1385.

Baker, J. (2017). *Psychosocial Perspectives on the Management of Voice Disorders.* Oxford: Compton.

Canning, B. J., Chang, A. B., Bolser, D. C., Smith, J. A., Mazzone, S. B., Mcgarvey, L., et al. (2014). Anatomy and Neurophysiology of Cough: Chest Guideline and Expert Panel Report. *Chest, 146,* 1633–1648.

Chen, Y. C., Xia, W., Chen, H., Feng, Y., Xu, J. J., Gu, J. P., et al. (2017). Tinnitus Distress Is Linked to Enhanced Resting-State Functional Connectivity from the Limbic System to the Auditory Cortex. *Human Brain Mapping, 38,* 2384–2397.

Chudleigh, C., Savage, B., Cruz, C., Lim, M., McClure, G., Palmer, D. M., et al. (2019). Use of Respiratory Rates and Heart Rate Variability in the Assessment and Treatment of Children and Adolescents with Functional Somatic Symptoms. *Clinical Child Psychology and Psychiatry, 24,* 29–39.

Demmink-Geertman, L., & Dejonckere, P. H. (2002). Nonorganic Habitual Dysphonia and Autonomic Dysfunction. *Journal of Voice, 16,* 549–559.

Dietrich, M., Andreatta, R. D., Jiang, Y., Joshi, A., & Stemple, J. C. (2012). Preliminary Findings on the Relation Between the Personality Trait of Stress Reaction and the Central Neural Control of Human Vocalization. *International Journal of Speech-Language Pathology, 14,* 377–389.

Dum, R. P., Levinthal, D. J., & Strick, P. L. (2016). Motor, Cognitive, and Affective Areas of the Cerebral Cortex Influence the Adrenal Medulla. *Proceedings of the National Academy of Sciences of the United States of America, 113,* 9922–9927.

Fleming, S., Thompson, M., Stevens, R., Heneghan, C., Plüddemann, A., Maconochie, I., et al. (2011). Normal Ranges of Heart Rate and Respiratory Rate in Children from Birth to 18 Years of Age: A Systematic Review of Observational Studies. *Lancet, 19,* 1011–1018.

Helou, L. B., Rosen, C. A., Wang, W., & Verdolini Abbott, K. (2018). Intrinsic Laryngeal Muscle Response to a Public Speech Preparation Stressor. *Journal of Speech, Language, and Hearing Research, 61,* 1525–1543.

Helou, L. B., Wang, W., Ashmore, R. C., Rosen, C. A., & Abbott, K. V. (2013). Intrinsic Laryngeal Muscle Activity in Response to Autonomic Nervous System Activation. *Laryngoscope, 123,* 2756–2765.

Jafari, H., Courtois, I., Van Den Bergh, O., Vlaeyen, J. W. S., & Van Diest, I. (2017). Pain and Respiration: A Systematic Review. *Pain, 158,* 995–1006.

Jantos, M. (forthcoming 2020). A Myofascial Perspective on Chronic Urogenital Pain in Women. In G. A. Santoro, A. P. Wieczorek, & A. H. Sultan (Eds.). *Pelvic Floor Disorders: A Multidisciplinary Textbook* (2nd ed.). Springer.

Jantos, M. & Stecco, C. (forthcoming 2021). Fascia of the Pelvic Floor. In R. Schleip, M. Driscoll, C. Stecco, & P. Huijing (Eds.), *Fascia: The Tensional Network of the Human Body* (2nd ed.). London: Elsevier.

Kain, K. L., & Terrell, S. J. (2018). *Nurturing Resilience: Helping Clients Move Forward from Developmental Trauma: An Integrative Somatic Approach.* Berkeley, CA: North Atlantic Books.

Koizumi, K., & Brooks, C. M. (1972). The Integration of Autonomic System Reactions: A Discussion of Autonomic Reflexes, Their Control and Their Association with Somatic Reactions. *Ergebnisse der Physiologie (Reviews of Physiology), 67,* 1–68.

Kozlowska, K. (2013). Stress, Distress, and Bodytalk: Co-constructing Formulations with Patients Who Present with Somatic Symptoms. *Harvard Review of Psychiatry, 21,* 314–333.

Kozlowska, K., Chudleigh, C., Cruz, C., Lim, M., McClure, G., Savage, B., et al. (2018a). Psychogenic Non-epileptic Seizures in Children and Adolescents: Part I—Diagnostic Formulations. *Clinical Child Psychology and Psychiatry, 23,* 140–159.

Kozlowska, K., Chudleigh, C., Cruz, C., Lim, M., McClure, G., Savage, B., et al. (2018b). Psychogenic Non-epileptic Seizures in Children and Adolescents: Part II—Explanations to Families, Treatment, and Group Outcomes. *Clinical Child Psychology and Psychiatry, 23,* 160–176.

Kozlowska, K., Rampersad, R., Cruz, C., Shah, U., Chudleigh, C., Soe, S., et al. (2017). The Respiratory Control of Carbon Dioxide in Children and Adolescents Referred for Treatment of Psychogenic Non-epileptic Seizures. *European Child and Adolescent Psychiatry, 26,* 1207–1217.

Kozlowska, K., Walker, P., McLean, L., & Carrive, P. (2015). Fear and the Defense Cascade: Clinical Implications and Management. *Harvard Review of Psychiatry, 23,* 263–287. https://www.ncbi.nlm.nih.gov/pmc/articles/PMC4495877/.

Leaver, A. M., Renier, L., Chevillet, M. A., Morgan, S., Kim, H. J., & Rauschecker, J. P. (2011). Dysregulation of Limbic and Auditory Networks in Tinnitus. *Neuron, 69,* 33–43.

Levine, P. (1997). *Waking the Tiger: Healing Trauma.* Berkeley, CA: North Atlantic Books.

Ogden, P., & Fisher, J. (2015). *Sensorimotor Psychotherapy: Interventions for Trauma and Attachment.* New York: Norton.

Payne, P., Levine, P. A., & Crane-Godreau, M. A. (2015). Somatic Experiencing: Using Interoception and Proprioception as Core Elements of Trauma Therapy. *Frontiers in Psychology, 6,* 93.

Roy, N., Dietrich, M., Blomgren, M., Heller, A., Houtz, D. R., & Lee, J. (2019). Exploring the Neural Bases of Primary Muscle Tension Dysphonia: A Case Study Using Functional Magnetic Resonance Imaging. *Journal of Voice, 33*, 183–194.

Schleip, R. (2003). Fascial Plasticity—A New Neurobiological Explanation: Part 1. *Journal of Bodywork and Movement Therapies, 7*, 11–19.

Schleip, R., & Klingler, W. (2019). Active Contractile Properties of Fascia. *Clinical Anatomy, 32*, 891–895.

Simons, D. G., Travell, J., & Simons, L. S. (1999). *Myofascial Pain and Dysfunction: The Trigger Point Manual*. Baltimore, MD: Williams & Wilkins.

Stecco, A., Stern, R., Fantoni, I., De Caro, R., & Stecco, C. (2016). Fascial Disorders: Implications for Treatment. *Physical Medicine and Rehabilitation, 8*, 161–168.

Stecco, C. (2015). *Functional Atlas of the Human Fascial System*. Edinburgh: Elsevier.

Tornblom, H., & Drossman, D. A. (2018). Psychotropics, Antidepressants, and Visceral Analgesics in Functional Gastrointestinal Disorders. *Current Gastroenterology Reports, 20*, 58.

Westgaard, R. H., Mork, P. J., Loras, H. W., Riva, R., & Lundberg, U. (2013). Trapezius Activity of Fibromyalgia Patients Is Enhanced in Stressful Situations, but Is Similar to Healthy Controls in a Quiet Naturalistic Setting: A Case-Control Study. *BMC Musculoskeletal Disorders, 14*, 97.

8

The HPA Axis and Functional Somatic Symptoms

Abstract In this chapter we continue our exploration of the neurobiology of functional somatic symptoms by considering the role of the hypothalamic-pituitary-adrenal (HPA) axis. It is a complicated system that helps to regulate energy, and that affects cell function and gene expression, throughout the body. In addition to playing a fundamental role in body regulation day to day, the HPA axis activates in response to stress and, when dysregulated (via either chronic hyper- or hypo-activation), plays a central role in all stress-related disorders. The vignettes in the chapter are designed to bring the neurobiology and dysregulation of the HPA axis, which are often difficult to detect, more into clinical focus.

As with all life processes, the body's efforts to regulate and maintain its internal environment—its *milieu intérieur* (see Online Supplement 1.2)—require energy. More broadly, *all* of the body's efforts to adapt to

Electronic supplementary material The online version of this chapter (https://doi.org/10.1007/978-3-030-46184-3_8) contains supplementary material, which is available to authorized users.

the everyday challenges, stress, and dangers of daily life require energy, and it is the *hypothalamic-pituitary-adrenal* (HPA) *axis* that makes the moment-by-moment adjustments required for that purpose.

The HPA axis is part of the body's energy-regulation system—a coordinated system that spans multiple system levels, from brain systems that continually anticipate the body's energy needs (Kleckner et al. 2017) to energy-regulation mechanisms in each individual cell (Picard et al. 2018). Any activation of the stress system in response to physical or psychological stress involves concomitant adjustments in energy regulation. The HPA axis relies on *hormones* for communication and signalling; these protein molecules serve 'as messengers between cells, telling them what's happening elsewhere and how they should respond' (Kushiro et al. 2003, p. 203) (see Fig. 8.1). This sort of chemical-communication system is thought to have originated

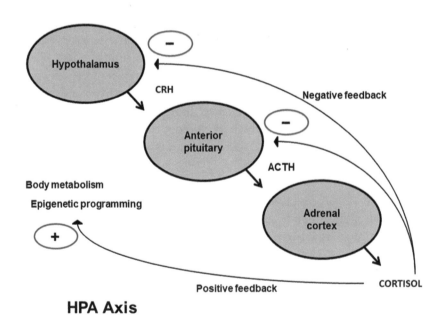

HPA Axis

Fig. 8.1   The HPA axis. Dysregulation of the HPA axis can occur on any level of the system. ACTH = adrenocorticotropic hormone. CRH = corticotropin-releasing hormone (© Kasia Kozlowska 2019)

primevally, before the plant and animal kingdoms separated from each other in evolutionary history (Kushiro et al. 2003). Within the body, hormones typically work relatively slowly—in a matter of minutes to hours.

Shifting Gear to Systems Thinking: A Few Tips to the Reader

The HPA system is immensely complex, and many imminent scientists have dedicated their lives to studying it (see Online Supplement 1.2). By the same token, clinicians from non-medical backgrounds may find this chapter challenging. While we do not expect the reader to master the science of the HPA axis (and we do not make any attempt to present it in any detail here), it is helpful to understand the fundamental processes and how they can go wrong.

In this context, it may be helpful for the reader to shift gear from linear to systems thinking, and to conceptualize the HPA system as having wide-ranging effects throughout the body, all the way down to the level of the individual cell. To capture this complexity, scientists use numerous expressions (e.g., *signalling cascades*) to communicate that HPA-axis activity cascades across, and affects, numerous body systems.

A key message that we want to communicate in this chapter is that stress—physical or psychological—contributes to the activation or dysregulation of the HPA axis. For most children (including adolescents), the effects of HPA-axis activation in the context of stress are immediate but temporary, with an appropriate short-term increase in available energy in the body. But for children with a history of stress that is chronic, uncontrollable, unpredictable, cumulative, recurrent, or overwhelming, the stress may dysregulate the HPA axis, with the consequence that healthy function is lost. For these children, the HPA axis may activate too much (pattern of overactivation) or too little (pattern of underactivation), or it may reprogram how the brain and other body systems (including the HPA axis itself) respond to stress encountered later in life. These various forms of HPA dysfunction contribute more broadly to the dysregulation of the stress system and the dysregulation of the body as a whole—conditions that set the stage for the emergence of functional somatic symptoms.

Cortisol/Glucocorticoids in Energy Regulation

The end product of activating the HPA axis is cortisol, a water-insoluble hormone that is the most important human glucocorticoid (when discussing the HPA axis in humans, the terms *cortisol* and *glucocorticoid* are often used interchangeably). Cortisol produced by the HPA axis—in the adrenal cortex (see Fig. 8.1)—is released in pulses, acting as a messenger that communicates through protein receptors (glucocorticoid receptors) that are present in every cell of the body, including in DNA (deoxyribonucleic acid) and mitochondria. DNA is the cell's genetic material, found in chromosomes within the cell nucleus and in the mitochondria. Genes are defined segments of DNA. Inside each cell, the mitochondria function as energy-producing machines; they regulate and produce energy for the cell and are, as such, a vital part of the body's energy-regulation system.

Patterns of HPA Dysregulation and the Role of Attachment Figures as Psychobiological Regulators

Dysregulation of the HPA axis can occur on one or more levels of the system (see Fig. 8.1). It may include a pattern characterized by hyper-activity and hyper-responsiveness (higher cortisol levels; enhanced cortisol awakening response; increased adrenocorticotropic hormone [ACTH]; insensitive negative glucocorticoid feedback of the HPA-axis loop; and increased cortisol responses to psychosocial stress or endocrine challenges). Alternately, it may include a pattern characterized by hypo-activity (lower cortisol levels; attenuated diurnal variation of cortisol; enhanced negative feedback within the HPA-axis loop; changed glucocorticoid-receptor sensitivity to cortisol;

and blunted HPA-axis responsiveness). Mounting evidence suggests that the age of exposure to stress may determine the pattern of HPA dysregulation (Agorastos et al. 2019) (see below). Studies from the maltreatment literature also suggest that the pattern of dysregulation can change from hyper-active to hypo-active during development (see Online Supplement 8.1).

The HPA axis is very sensitive to stress in early childhood. Children who experience significant stress early in development are likely to show a pattern of hyper-activation. Subsequently, as the child ages, the HPA axis may stay hyper-active or may transition to a hypo-active pattern (see Online Supplement 8.1). Importantly, because attachment figures function as biopsychosocial regulators, they are able to buffer HPA-axis activation through sensitive caregiving behaviours (Hostinar et al. 2014; Bernard et al. 2015). In this way, even though stressful events may take place in the life of the child and family, attachment figures can help prevent the child's HPA axis from becoming too activated, thereby buffering the child from the long-term effects of early-life stress. For the neurobiology of nurturing caregiver behaviours, see Online Supplement 8.2, which describes how licking behaviour by mother rats helps buffer HPA-axis activation in rat pups (and which also provides, in effect, a useful model for what happens in humans).

The HPA axis continues to be very sensitive to stress in adolescence. During adolescence the HPA-axis response to stress is more variable, however, and both hyper- and hypo-active patterns are common. Unfortunately, it seems that during adolescence, attachment figures are less able to buffer the HPA-axis response than they are in early childhood (Hostinar et al. 2015).

Cortisol/Glucocorticoids in Epigenetics (Gene Expression) and Plasticity Changes

In addition to mobilizing energy resources throughout the body, cortisol coordinates plasticity changes—via changes in gene expression—to help the brain and body adapt to stress during the individual's lifetime and across generations. For a brief summary of Michael Meaney's groundbreaking research pertaining to glucocorticoids, including changes in gene expression for the glucocorticoid receptor gene in baby rat pups, see Online Supplement 8.2.

Plasticity changes via cortisol's genomic mechanism can be adaptive or maladaptive. For example, regular exercise—a moderate form of pleasurable stress that temporarily increases blood cortisol levels—leads neurons in the hippocampus (a brain region involved in memory and learning) to grow more dendrites and to create more synapses, thereby increasing the size of the hippocampus and improving memory and learning (Erickson et al. 2011; Saraulli et al. 2017). In this way the inclusion of sport in school curricula is helpful for learning.

Another example is stress in utero or early childhood. In this scenario, changes in gene expression—coordinated by cortisol—function to reprogram the manner in which the brain and other tissues in the body (including the HPA axis itself) will respond to stress in the future. The HPA axis thus plays an important role in somatic memory (van der Kolk 1994): significant or cumulative stress in early childhood or adolescence can reprogram the way that the child's brain and body respond to future stress across the child's lifetime (Agorastos et al. 2019). The implication for children with functional somatic symptoms is that HPA-axis activation by past stress may change and intensify the way that each child's stress system responds to current and future stress, unrelated to circulating levels of cortisol at the time of that subsequent stress. This reprogramming can sometime be adaptive, as in cases where the more intensive response helps the child survive in the context of ongoing threat and danger. But it can be maladaptive in safe contexts, where even minor stress would potentially activate an overly robust, inappropriate stress response. In the group vignette below, we see reprogramming of the HPA axis in the context of severe trauma.

During the World Trade Center collapse on September 11, some women directly exposed to the terrorist attack were pregnant. Some of these women went on to develop post-traumatic stress disorder (PTSD), and some did not. When the babies reached one year of age, Rachel Yehuda and colleagues (2005) collected salivary cortisol samples in the babies and the mothers at waking up in the morning and at bedtime. Babies and mothers from the mother-with-PTSD group showed lower cortisol levels (a hypo-activity pattern). The lowest cortisol levels were found in babies who were in their third trimester at the time of the collapse. Reduced cortisol levels are linked to an increased vulnerability to PTSD in the face of future stress, and PTSD is associated with functional somatic symptoms. In this way, in the context of future stress, the babies with low cortisol have an increased risk of developing functional somatic symptoms (potentially those associated with a hypo-activity pattern [see below]), PTSD, or other stress-related disorders. For further reading see Yehuda and colleagues (2005) and Gupta (2013).

In the next group vignette, drawn from multiple studies, we see how the HPA axis can be reprogrammed to a hyper-activity pattern by stress.

Girls who are sexually abused show a hyper-activity pattern—overactivation of the HPA axis and too much cortisol—in the aftermath of the trauma. Across the lifespan, they also have higher rates of functional somatic symptoms, including pain, headache, stomachache, nausea, vomiting, eye problems, skin problems, dizziness, fatigue, and non-epileptic seizures. At some point in adulthood, the HPA axis normalizes and then shifts to a hypo-activity pattern—underactivation of the HPA axis and too little cortisol (Trickett et al. 2010). In adulthood the girls have higher rates of functional somatic symptoms—nonspecific chronic pain, functional gastrointestinal disorders, and chronic pelvic pain. Alongside HPA-axis dysregulation, sexually abused girls also show progressive activation, through adulthood, of both the autonomic nervous system and the immune-inflammatory system (for further discussion and additional references concerning this vignette, see Online Supplement 8.1).

In the next group vignette—also from a research study—we describe how psychological stress from adverse life events can reprogram the HPA axis, with the consequence that the individual is less able to fight off infection (in this case the common cold). Most readers will recognize themselves in this vignette because of the common knowledge that our susceptibility to viral infections increases in the context of life stress.

Activation of the HPA axis when the body is fighting infection helps to contain the immune-inflammatory response and keeps it from becoming too intense or prolonged. A study by Sheldon Cohen and colleagues (2012) looked at how healthy adults who had experienced recent major life stress (in the last year) responded to inoculation with the common cold virus, versus those who had not experienced such stress. The former group had a greater immune-inflammatory response—and symptoms and signs of illness (of the common cold). The explanation was the HPA axis, hypo-active in the wake of the recent stress, had been unable to appropriately dampen the immune-inflammatory response, with the consequence that the immune-inflammatory response was excessive: it rose to a level needed to combat a much more severe infection. Psychological stress had reprogrammed the HPA axis into a pattern of hypo-activity. For further reading see Cohen and colleagues (2012).

Farther along the maladaptive continuum, extreme, chronic, uncontrollable stress early in life can result in persistently high levels of cortisol and continually excessive energy use—called oxidative stress—causing, for example, dendrites in the vulnerable brain regions to shrink and to thereby impair function (McEwen et al. 2015). Stress-related decreases in brain volume in the hippocampus and brain regions that are part of the brain stress systems have been found in adults with PTSD and children with a history of physical or sexual abuse (for references see Online Supplement 1.3).

In these ways, even though the HPA axis may look like a simple system acting through hormone signals (see Fig. 8.1), it is actually a complicated system that, via glucocorticoid (cortisol) receptors, affects cell function and gene expression across the body.

HPA Dysregulation and Studies of Children with Functional Somatic Symptoms

Research pertaining to HPA-axis dysregulation in children with functional somatic symptoms is still in the early stages (for references and a summary of studies, see Online Supplement 8.1). We know, however, that in children, recurrent abdominal pain, non-neurological functional somatic symptoms (overtiredness, dizziness, headache, stomach pain, vomiting, nausea, and musculoskeletal pain [in the back, neck, shoulders, arms, or legs]), and chronic fatigue syndrome, as well as comorbid conditions such as PTSD and atypical depression, are associated with decreased cortisol levels and HPA-axis *hypo*-activation. From the adult literature we also know that non-epileptic seizures—as well as common comorbid conditions such as panic disorder and depression—are associated with increased cortisol levels and HPA-axis *hyper*-activation. Both patterns of HPA dysregulation are often accompanied by activation or dysregulation in other components of the stress system—in particular, the autonomic nervous system (see Chapter 6) and immune-inflammatory system (Agorastos et al. 2019) (see Chapter 9).

The Take-Home Messages About the HPA Axis for the Mental Health Clinician

Three key messages pertaining to the HPA axis are important to remember from a clinical perspective.

First, the HPA-axis profile, whether it is hyper- or hypo-active, may affect the child's symptom profile at presentation. For example, because HPA-axis activation suppresses sleep, a hyper-active HPA axis will contribute to sleep arousals and poor sleep (Chrousos et al. 2016) (see also Chapter 5). Alternatively, because cortisol is needed for release of energy resources, hypo-activation of the HPA axis may contribute to symptoms of tiredness and fatigue (Janssens et al. 2012).

Second, loss of synchrony within the HPA axis, between the HPA axis and other components of the stress system, or between the HPA axis and the circadian clock will also affect the child's subjective sense of vitality and well-being because body systems have lost the normal rhythms associated with wellness and energy regulation during the circadian cycle (see also Chapters 4 and 5).

Third, stress-related dysregulation of the HPA axis (as may be present in a child's hyper- or, over time, hypo-activation to stress) is likely to be associated with non-normative responses to future stress and with experience-dependent changes in the brain and body tissues. These experience-dependent changes may make the child vulnerable to aberrant responses that manifest as functional somatic symptoms in the context of future stress. In the following vignette of Bellynda, the reader can see how these processes may come into play—in clinical practice—in the case of an individual child.

Bellynda was an 11-year-old girl who presented with multiple somatic symptoms—tinnitus and hearing problems, dizziness, blurred vision, nausea, pain in the neck and back, abnormal gait and lack of coordination in the legs, and tremor and flapping of the hands—following three severe episodes of allergic rhinitis (allergic reaction in the nose) and a sudden growth spurt. Bellynda lived with her mother and had no contact with her father. From the family assessment interview, it was clear that Bellynda's symptoms had been triggered by activation of the immune-inflammatory system (via the allergic rhinitis) and dysregulation of the autonomic system (the autonomic system sometimes takes time to adjust following a growth spurt). Bellynda's standing test showed a stable blood pressure and a heart rate increase of 64 (from 80 to 144) beats per minute on standing, confirming the autonomic dysregulation (orthostatic intolerance; see Chapter 6). Her hyperventilation challenge showed chronic hyperventilation (activation of the respiratory motor system alongside the sympathetic system) (see Chapter 7). What was unusual was that apart from this physical stress, Bellynda's recent history was unremarkable: she did not report any other emotional or physical stress. She had, however, experienced significant early-life events in the perinatal period. First, Bellynda's mother had suffered from thyroid cancer and had been operated on during the third trimester of the pregnancy. After the operation Bellynda's mother had been given high doses of thyroxine hormone. Bellynda's mother remembered that she had been unable to sleep with the hormone and that she had felt baby Bellynda kicking and moving inside her in an unsettled way. Because thyroxine hormone is known to up-regulate the stress system, the therapist hypothesized that Bellynda's stress system may have been programmed—in utero—to respond to future stress in an excessively robust way, putting her at risk of developing functional somatic symptoms in response to minor stress. In addition to the exposure to high-dose thyroxine, Bellynda was separated from her mother at four weeks of age, when her mother received radioactive treatment for the thyroid cancer. The protective factor was that Bellynda was looked after by her grandmother, who, as an attachment figure, would have buffered the impact of the separation. Finally, the home environment was characterized by high levels of stress during Bellynda's first year of life; her parents separated when she was 11 months old. It is reasonable to hypothesize that the stress associated with these family events also affected the programming, sensitivity, and reactivity of Bellynda's stress system.

* * *

As we have seen in this chapter, stress—physical or psychological—contributes to activation or dysregulation of the HPA axis. For most children the effects of HPA-axis activation in the context of stress are immediate, with an appropriate increase in available energy in the body. That is exactly what is supposed to happen. But for children with a history of stress that is severe along any of various continuums, the pattern of activation of the entire stress system can be affected, with earlier stress leading to changes in how the body responds to stress encountered later. The exact pattern of HPA-axis activation or dysregulation varies across development and from individual to individual: it depends on both the quality of the stress and its timing. The advent of new technologies—including studies on a group level of analysis—has allowed researchers to begin to identify some of the neurobiological processes that underpin the contribution of HPA-axis activation and dysregulation to functional somatic symptoms. But much is still to be learnt. In Chapter 9, we look at another component of the stress system—the immune-inflammatory system—that is closely interconnected with the autonomic nervous system and HPA axis, and that is also involved in the production of functional somatic symptoms.

References

Agorastos, A., Pervanidou, P., Chrousos, G. P., & Baker, D. G. (2019). Developmental Trajectories of Early Life Stress and Trauma: A Narrative Review on Neurobiological Aspects Beyond Stress System Dysregulation. *Frontiers in Psychiatry, 10,* 118.

Bernard, K., Hostinar, C. E., & Dozier, M. (2015). Intervention Effects on Diurnal Cortisol Rhythms of Child Protective Services–Referred Infants in Early Childhood: Preschool Follow-Up Results of a Randomized Clinical Trial. *JAMA Pediatrics, 169,* 112–119.

Chrousos, G., Vgontzas, A. N., & Kritikou, I. (2016). HPA Axis and Sleep. In K. R. Feingold, B. Anawalt, A. Boyce, G. Chrousos, K. Dungan, A. Grossman, J. M. Hershman, G. Kaltsas, C. Koch, P. Kopp, M. Korbonits, R. McLachlan, J. E. Morley, M. New, L. Perreault, J. Purnell, R. Rebar, F. Singer, D. L. Trence, A.Vinik, & D. P. Wilson (Eds.), *Endotext: Comprehensive Free Online Endocrinology Book.* South Dartmouth, MA: MDText.com. https://www.ncbi.nlm.nih.gov/books/NBK279071/.

Cohen, S., Janicki-Deverts, D., Doyle, W. J., Miller, G. E., Frank, E., Rabin, B. S., et al. (2012). Chronic Stress, Glucocorticoid Receptor Resistance, Inflammation, and Disease Risk. *Proceedings of the National Academy of Sciences of the United States of America, 109,* 5995–5999.

Erickson, K. I., Voss, M. W., Prakash, R. S., Basak, C., Szabo, A., Chaddock, L., et al. (2011). Exercise Training Increases Size of Hippocampus and Improves Memory. *Proceedings of the National Academy of Sciences of the United States of America, 108,* 3017–3022.

Gupta, M. A. (2013). Review of Somatic Symptoms in Post-traumatic Stress Disorder. *International Review of Psychiatry, 25,* 86–99.

Hostinar, C. E., Johnson, A. E., & Gunnar, M. R. (2015). Parent Support Is Less Effective in Buffering Cortisol Stress Reactivity for Adolescents Compared to Children. *Developmental Science, 18,* 281–297.

Hostinar, C. E., Sullivan, R. M., & Gunnar, M. R. (2014). Psychobiological Mechanisms Underlying the Social Buffering of the Hypothalamic-Pituitary-Adrenocortical Axis: A Review of Animal Models and Human Studies Across Development. *Psychological Bulletin, 140,* 256–282.

Janssens, K. A., Oldehinkel, A. J., Verhulst, F. C., Hunfeld, J. A., Ormel, J., & Rosmalen, J. G. (2012). Symptom-Specific Associations Between Low Cortisol Responses and Functional Somatic Symptoms: The Trails Study. *Psychoneuroendocrinology, 37,* 332–340.

Kleckner, I. R., Zhang, J., Touroutoglou, A., Chanes, L., Xia, C., Simmons, W. K., et al. (2017). Evidence for a Large-Scale Brain System Supporting Allostasis and Interoception in Humans. *Nature Human Behaviour, 1,* 0069.

Kushiro, T., Nambara, E., & McCourt, P. (2003). Hormone Evolution: The Key to Signalling. *Nature, 422,* 122.

McEwen, B. S., Gray, J. D., & Nasca, C. (2015). 60 Years of Neuroendocrinology: Redefining Neuroendocrinology: Stress, Sex and Cognitive and Emotional Regulation. *Journal of Endocrinology, 226,* T67–T83.

Picard, M., McEwen, B. S., Epel, E. S., & Sandi, C. (2018). An Energetic View of Stress: Focus on Mitochondria. *Frontiers in Neuroendocrinology, 49,* 72–85.

Saraulli, D., Costanzi, M., Mastrorilli, V., & Farioli-Vecchioli, S. (2017). The Long Run: Neuroprotective Effects of Physical Exercise on Adult Neurogenesis from Youth to Old Age. *Current Neuropharmacology, 15,* 519–533.

Trickett, P. K., Noll, J. G., Susman, E. J., Shenk, C. E., & Putnam, F. W. (2010). Attenuation of Cortisol Across Development for Victims of Sexual Abuse. *Development and Psychopathology, 22,* 165–175.

Van Der Kolk, B. A. (1994). The Body Keeps the Score: Memory and the Evolving Psychobiology of Posttraumatic Stress. *Harvard Review of Psychiatry, 1,* 253–265.

Yehuda, R., Engel, S. M., Brand, S. R., Seckl, J., Marcus, S. M., & Berkowitz, G. S. (2005). Transgenerational Effects of Posttraumatic Stress Disorder in Babies of Mothers Exposed to the World Trade Center Attacks During Pregnancy. *Journal of Clinical Endocrinology and Metabolism, 90,* 4115–4118.

9

The Immune-Inflammatory System and Functional Somatic Symptoms

Abstract In this chapter we continue our exploration of the neuro-biology of functional somatic symptoms by considering the role of the immune-inflammatory system. This system functions like a watchdog that is gifted with prescience. It holds memory for past threats to the physical or psychological well-being of the child. It activates—into defensive mode—in response to both physical and psychological threats. If the child's life story has been marked by chronic, uncontrollable, unpredictable, cumulative, recurrent, or overwhelming stress, it maintains a state of readiness, a state of ongoing vigilance, alertness, or watchfulness, termed *low-grade inflammation*. Because it communicates with all other components of the stress system, the immune-inflammatory system can raise the first alarm to activate other stress-system components or the stress system as a whole, setting up the conditions that favour the generation of functional somatic symptoms. In clinical presentations that involve chronic/

Electronic supplementary material The online version of this chapter (https://doi.org/10.1007/978-3-030-46184-3_9) contains supplementary material, which is available to authorized users.

© The Author(s) 2020   **175**
K. Kozlowska et al., *Functional Somatic Symptoms in Children and Adolescents*, Palgrave Texts in Counselling and Psychotherapy,
https://doi.org/10.1007/978-3-030-46184-3_9

complex pain, the immune-inflammatory system keeps the pain system activated and signalling pain. In clinical presentations that involve persisting fatigue, the neurobiology is still in the process of being worked out, but clinicians can nevertheless avail themselves of three different metaphors or approaches that emerge from contemporary research.

All components of the stress system talk together and work—as an ensemble—to regulate body state and to coordinate the body's response to stress and threat. The *immune-inflammatory system* is part of this crosstalk. It is made up of cells that are scattered throughout the body or that reside in special tissues (e.g., immune cells in lymph glands or glial cells in the brain and spinal cord). The immune-inflammatory system uses cell-surface signalling molecules (immune signals), including a group of small proteins known as *cytokines*, to communicate cell to cell within the system. The evolutionary origins of the immune-inflammatory system are ancient (Flajnik and Kasahara 2010), with primitive systems present even in one-cell organisms (Janeway 2001).

The role of the immune-inflammatory system in infection, injury, and wound healing is well known. Immune-inflammatory responses promote the destruction and clearance of pathogens and enhance wound healing. Pro-inflammatory (defensive) cytokines function as messenger molecules to attract immune cells to sites of infection or injury, activating them to respond to the insult. Immune-inflammatory cells throughout the body retain memories of previous pathogens and facilitate rapid defensive responses if any particular pathogen is encountered again. In these ways, local inflammation enables the individual to fight infection and facilitates tissue healing.

But immune-inflammatory cells and their signalling messenger molecules are also involved in body regulation and protection more generally. They engage in intracellular communication day in and day out as the body works to regulate itself and to respond to the stress and challenges of daily life. Immune-inflammatory cells residing in the brain—glial cells (Fields 2009)—retain the memory of past stress, both physical and psychological (Brenhouse and Schwarz 2016; Frank et al. 2016). In this role the immune-inflammatory system is the body's watchdog: always vigilant for threat, and ready to rouse from sleep to attack an intruder in the blink of an eye. In this same role as watchdog, and in response to any new threat, the immune-inflammatory system further activates and also typically interacts with, activates, and modulates other components of the stress system. In most children (including adolescents), the stress system—including the immune-inflammatory system itself—will return to baseline once the threat has passed. Importantly for us, in some children, one or more components of the stress system may remain activated or dysregulated, thereby setting the stage for the emergence of functional somatic symptoms.

In this chapter we focus primarily on the way that stress can activate the immune-inflammatory system and on how the immune-inflammatory system's response to stress can, in turn, activate or dysregulate the stress system as a whole. Because the immune-inflammatory system is so complicated, we can only touch the surface of what is known, and share with the reader some of the key points that we raise in our discussions with children. A short, simple summary of the immune-inflammatory system is provided in a recent article by Heather Brenhouse and colleagues (2019). Further details (including reference articles) about the immune-inflammatory system—and the methodological difficulties of studying it—are provided in Online Supplement 9.1. An account of the discovery that glial cells—cells that were previously conceptualized as providing physical support to neurons—are also the brain's immune-inflammatory cells is provided by the neuroscientist Douglas Fields in his book *The Other Brain* (Fields 2009). Later in this book (see Chapter 11), we look at processes on the mind system level—for example, catastrophizing (Edwards et al. 2008; Lazaridou et al. 2018)—that also maintain the immune-inflammatory system in an activated state. Additional references are listed in Online Supplement 1.3.

Shifting Gear to Systems Thinking: A Few Tips to the Reader

Like the hypothalamic-pituitary-adrenal (HPA) axis, the immune-inflammatory system is immensely complex, and clinicians from non-medical backgrounds may find this chapter challenging. The interconnections between the immune-inflammatory system and the HPA axis, autonomic nervous system, and brain stress systems are indirect and non-linear. It may be helpful for the reader to shift gear from linear to systems thinking, and to conceptualize these interconnections not as involving specific pathways but rather as involving patterns of change and shifts in patterns of communication.

An easy way to keep these interactions in mind is to visualize the overlap between circles in the stress-system model (see Fig. 4.2) and to remember in a general way that, because of the cross-talk between the immune-inflammatory system and other components of the stress system, activation or dysregulation in one part of the system will have flow-on effects in other parts.

Alternatively, the reader can think of the immune-inflammatory system as a large fishing net. Just as a fish, caught in one part of a net, causes changes in tension in other parts of the net, so do changes in immune-inflammatory signalling lead to ripples of change across the broader immune-inflammatory system and also across the stress system as a whole. Likewise, changes in particular other components of the stress system will lead to ripples of changes throughout the rest of the stress system.

Attachment Figures and the Immune-Inflammatory System

Attachment figures, in their role as biopsychosocial regulators, help to regulate the immune-inflammatory system. The mother's exposure to stress in the prenatal period also has consequences for the development of the child's immune-inflammatory system (Brenhouse et al. 2019) (see epigenetic mechanisms in Chapter 8 and Online Supplement 8.2).

In animal studies, early separations from the attachment figure result in stress, activate and sensitize the immune-inflammatory system, and lead to increased vulnerability for maladaptive responses to future stress. In humans, warm, sensitive attachment relationships in childhood are associated with healthier levels of immune-inflammatory markers later in life, whereas at-risk childhood relationships (maltreatment), childhood sexual abuse, and adverse childhood experiences (ACEs) more generally are associated with chronic, low-grade inflammation. For references see Online Supplement 1.3. For a discussion of findings pertaining to the stress system in sexual abuse, see Online Supplement 8.1. For more on low-grade inflammation, see below.

Adolescence also appears to be a period of vulnerability in the development of the immune-inflammatory system and in the programming of the immune-inflammatory system for future health and well-being or ill health and dis-ease (Brenhouse and Schwarz 2016; Brenhouse et al. 2019). Adverse life events during adolescence appear to modulate persisting immune dysregulation, with far-reaching effects on the stress system as a whole—and with a lifelong impact on health and well-being. Whether the presence or availability of attachment figures during adolescence can buffer those stress-related effects is not known.

Immune-Inflammatory Cells Hold Immunological Memory for Past Stress

An exciting recent discovery is that *glial cells*—the immune-inflammatory cells of the brain—hold immunological memory for past stress and can both activate and proliferate in response to stress (Brenhouse and Schwarz 2016). In this way, stress that occurs early in development can sensitize the immune-inflammatory system, a process called *neuroinflammatory priming* (Frank et al. 2016). Each time the child experiences significant stress, the immune-inflammatory system is activated transiently—it undergoes a short-lived neuroinflammatory response—that functions to sensitize how the brain's immune-inflammatory cells will respond to subsequent stress (physical or psychological) in the future. With repeated activation, the child's immune-inflammatory system may be sensitized into a *state of increased readiness*—with increased and ongoing vigilance, alertness, and watchfulness. This state, called *low-grade inflammation*, involves a small but continuing degree of excessive activation over long periods of time. Using our watchdog metaphor, the immune-inflammatory system has become hyper-vigilant, hyper-reactive, and ultimately maladaptive. As an ongoing physiological burden, this state has long-term, adverse consequences for the child's health and well-being, and it also contributes to the generation and maintenance of functional somatic symptoms.

For example, in our studies of children presenting with functional neurological disorder (FND), 50 percent of children report a physical trigger to the illness, and 50 percent report a psychological trigger, with the majority also reporting cumulative past adverse life events (see Chapter 4). In chronic fatigue syndrome (CFS), a viral infection is the most common trigger, but psychological stress and other physical stress can also function as triggers; a history of early-childhood stress and past adverse life events are important risk factors that contribute to illness severity. For references see Online Supplement 1.3.

What is particularly important for us here is that very often, after the immune-inflammatory system has returned to baseline—or alternatively, has returned to a baseline state of ongoing readiness (low-grade inflammation)—other components of the stress system may remain activated in aberrant ways and may continue to maintain symptoms of pain, fatigue, autonomic system dysregulation, aberrant motor or sensory function, or difficulties with cognitive function. For example, in children who develop persistent fatigue following a viral infection, the autonomic nervous system remains in an activated state, and psychological factors, such as negative emotions, presence of anxiety, or depression, appear to contribute to the maintenance of stress-system activation (Pedersen et al. 2019; Kristiansen et al. 2019). Theoretically, implicit processes—for example, aberrant predictive coding (see Chapter 11)—could also contribute to stress-system activation. What this means is that, while either a physical or psychological stress can trigger the illness process via activation of the immune-inflammatory system, other factors can subsequently maintain stress-system activation or dysregulation, and also contribute to the emergence and maintenance of functional somatic symptoms. The implication for clinical practice is that treatment may require mind-body interventions that switch off the stress system, rather than interventions that target the original trigger event—for example, the viral event—which may no longer be relevant.

Inflammatory Markers Are Elevated in Patients with Functional Somatic Symptoms

Since immune-inflammatory cells hold immunological memory for past stress, and since all functional symptoms and syndromes show an association with ACEs, it is not surprising to find that inflammatory markers are elevated in patients with functional somatic symptoms. A mounting body of evidence documents that adult patients with chronic pain, fatigue, irritable bowel, musculoskeletal complaints, and other somatization syndromes have a sensitized immune-inflammatory system—an immune-inflammatory system in a state of readiness, or low-grade inflammation (increased levels of inflammatory markers compared to healthy controls). Studies with children are just beginning to emerge (for details see Online Supplement 9.1). For additional references see Online Supplement 1.3.

The term *low-grade inflammation* distinguishes this state of *readiness*, which is a characteristic feature across functional presentations, from high-level activation, as seen in response to infections or in rheumatology diseases. Low-grade inflammation is also seen when the stress to the body results from obesity, a poor diet, or disrupted sleep (see Online Supplement 9.1). As noted above, what this means in clinical practice is that, while an infection or minor injury may trigger stress-system activation in some patients (via the immune-inflammatory system component), this high-level activation of the immune-inflammatory system that is a marker of significant infection or rheumatological diseases is *not* present in patients with functional neurological symptoms. Standard laboratory tests, which are designed to detect inflammation infections and rheumatological diseases, will be normal. In other words, once a good medical assessment has been done—including the blood workup—and has shown nothing, the child and family have nothing to gain in going from doctor to doctor in search of 'better' test results.

Nonetheless, low-grade inflammation marks a shift from restorative mode to defensive mode. It reflects a subtle shift of the immune-inflammatory system: low-grade inflammation signifies that the prescient watchdog stands on guard in a state of hyper-vigilant readiness.

The Immune-Inflammatory System's Involvement in Chronic/Complex Pain

Chronic/complex pain, as we have seen in the vignettes throughout this book, is a common comorbid symptom across functional presentations. The pain is called chronic or complex because it exists in the absence of tissue injury or because, when tissue injury does initially trigger the pain, it persists long after the injury has healed or the infection has passed.

Pain has been an intense area of research over the last 60 years. One of the most exciting recent discoveries is that the immune-inflammatory system has a central role in maintaining chronic/complex pain: activated immune-inflammatory processes appear to potentiate pain in many different ways. In particular, chronic/complex pain is generated and maintained by immune-inflammatory mechanisms that sensitize neurons involved in sensing pain (in the tissues), carrying pain (through the spinal cord), and representing pain (in the brain, as *pain maps*). This sensitization process makes the pain neurons more excitable, with the consequence that they signal pain at the least provocation. Other names for this sensitization process in chronic pain include the following: in the *tissue*, neurogenic inflammation, peripheral sensitization, and visceral sensitization, and in the *spinal cord* and *brain*, central sensitization or neuroinflammation. For clinicians who commonly see children with complex/chronic pain, we explain these processes in more detail in the paragraphs below (for references on chronic/complex pain, see Online Supplement 1.3). For most readers, the simple explanation provided above (in this paragraph) may suffice; if so, skip right down to the section 'Activation and Sensitization of the Pain System at the Brain System Level', along with its vignette of Martin.

Activation and Sensitization of the Pain System at the Tissue Level

At the tissue level in chronic/complex pain, the endings of afferent nerves, which carry sensory and interoceptive information from the body to the spinal cord, secrete pro-inflammatory substances that cause a local inflammatory response (*neurogenic inflammation*). These pro-inflammatory substances attract other immune-inflammatory cells, which also secrete pro-inflammatory substances. Together, these pro-inflammatory substances irritate the pain-sensing receptors on pain neurons (*peripheral sensitization* or *visceral sensitization*), thereby activating the pain system from the periphery. See discussion of macrophages in 'How Exercise Works to Decrease Chronic/Complex Pain', below.

Clinically, this sensitization at the tissue level means that the child will experience pain in response to non-noxious stimuli such as a light touch to the skin (called *allodynia*) or the expansion of the gut lumen during normal digestion or defecation (*visceral sensitivity*). The child may also experience painful stimuli as more painful than they should be (*hyper-algesia*).

Activation and Sensitization of the Pain System at the Spinal Cord Level

At the spinal cord level in chronic/complex pain, there is also an increase in pain signalling (through a variety of processes). Pain neurons in the spinal cord release pro-inflammatory substances that function to amplify pain signals. Glial cells—the immune-inflammatory cells found throughout the central nervous system—contribute to the immune-inflammatory process of amplifying pain by also releasing pro-inflammatory molecules. Glial signalling via signalling molecules released into spinal fluid allows pain messages to be carried to distant sites, enabling the spread of pain sensitization at the spinal cord level. In addition, pain neurons sprout new axons (*feet*), a process that amplifies communication about pain between pain neurons (a plasticity phenomenon). It is hypothesized that the combination of these processes sensitizes and activates the pain neurons in the spinal cord segment— and possibly even segments below and above—that receives information from the affected tissue. It is also hypothesized that these processes may sensitize and activate other neurons lying in the same segment(s) that carry information about, or relate to, other parts of the body.

In this way, pain that was triggered by a local inflammatory response within some portion of the viscera—for example, the pelvic cavity— could also be associated with sensitization and activation of spinal segments representing and signalling pain or other sensory information from the skin (innervated via the same spinal segment) or with increased tone in skeletomotor muscles of the pelvic floor (again, innervated via that same spinal segment).

Activation and Sensitization of the Pain System at the Brain System Level

At the brain level in chronic/complex pain, activation of pain maps that underpin the subjective experience of pain is maintained and amplified by various processes: bottom-up signals from the tissues and spinal cord; activation of glial cells (immune-inflammatory cells in the brain); and activation of the brain stress systems (of which glial cells are also a part) (see also Chapter 11). By activating the brain stress systems—and then, in turn, the brain's pain maps—negative emotions, catastrophizing, anticipatory anxiety, and such processes can activate and maintain pain maps, resulting in or contributing to chronic/complex pain.

The following vignette of Martin highlights how a viral illness—which activates the immune-inflammatory system—can activate/dysregulate other components of the stress system. In Martin's case, the pain system and the autonomic nervous system were activated (see Chapter 6 for the role of the autonomic system in regulating the gut). It also highlights how the body may be unable to switch off the pain system and to re-regulate the autonomic nervous system over time, well after the infection has passed, and well after the immune-inflammatory system has settled back to baseline. In Martin's case, stress-system dysregulation was reflected in ongoing abdominal pain (activation of pain system) and recurring constipation (activation of autonomic nervous system [sympathetic activation causes constipation]). It also highlights how asking about the pain—bringing attention to it—can activate the pain via top-down mechanisms. Martin's presentation was complicated by the use of antibiotics that disrupt the microbiota—which may have contributed to stress-system dysregulation (see Chapter 10).

Martin, a 10-year-old boy who lived with his parents and younger sister, was an all-rounder: he enjoyed school work and sporting activities, and was in line for becoming house captain in his school. Martin's health had always been good, but his bowel had always been sluggish: he emptied his bowels three to four times a week. Just after the start of year 6, Martin came down with a viral illness characterized by high temperatures, fatigue, lethargy, sleepiness, nausea, and pain in his head and abdomen. In the months that followed, the abdominal pain came and went. Martin's family doctor gave him antibiotics in case he had parasites. His blood panel screening for ongoing infection or inflammation was normal. The abdominal pain still came and went. Martin then became constipated, and the constipation made the pain worse. He was admitted to hospital for disimpaction. A diagnosis of functional abdominal pain was made. Martin was referred to a therapist, who taught him hypnosis and other strategies to help him manage the pain. His capacity to manage the intermittent pain improved. Toward the end of year 6, Martin became very constipated, and his pain crescendoed. Again, he was admitted to hospital for disimpaction. From this point on, at repeated intervals throughout the day, Martin would scream suddenly and clutch his abdomen in pain. The pain would pass as suddenly as it had come, and Martin would continue on with whatever he was doing. Martin now experienced pain every time he passed a bowel motion or passed wind, and he would scream so loudly that it sounded as if he was being tortured or murdered. Sometimes the pain would wake him up at night—when he passed wind. He would scream and then go back to sleep. Martin was now worried about going to the toilet and spent a large part of the day anticipating his pain and worrying about what would happen if he needed to go or when he needed to pass wind. At school, the school counsellor, who was trying to be supportive, discovered that when she asked Martin about his pain, the question would trigger a pain episode for Martin.

Treatment involved, among other things, careful bowel management by Martin's paediatrician to make sure that Martin did not become constipated—which would further sensitize his existing visceral hypersensitivity. He took probiotics and ate yogurt to look after his microbiota. Slow-breathing training, which down-regulates autonomic system function, was timetabled into Martin's day. He also continued to practice the various mind-body strategies that he had learnt with his therapist. Martin was treated with an anti-anxiety mediation (20 mg fluoxetine in the morning) to help with his anxiety (which was activating the brain stress systems top-down). For a few months, Martin also used a small dose of quetiapine—a mood stabilizer with excellent anti-anxiety properties—to help him switch off the brain stress systems (6.25 mg three times a day, and 25 mg for pain that Martin could not manage). The quetiapine was particularly useful at school at those times that Martin was unable to regulate himself, had lost the capacity to control his pain and anxiety, and had lapsed into a prolonged state of screaming. The quetiapine also helped Martin sufficiently so that he could implement his mind-body strategies, even when the pain was very bad. Because a good explanation about the pain had been provided to Martin and his family, they understood how each intervention was helping to treat Martin's abdominal pain.

How Exercise Works to Decrease Chronic/Complex Pain

The story about how exercise works to decrease chronic/complex pain is a useful piece of research that we often share with children and their families (Sluka 2017). It provides a clear rationale (see below) as to why exercise is important and how exercise works to help chronic pain.

Macrophages are immune-inflammatory cells that eat up debris and that exist in all parts of the body. Exercise helps shift macrophages from defensive to restorative mode. When children exercise regularly, they keep their macrophages in restorative mode, in which they secrete anti-inflammatory molecules that promote analgesia (see Fig. 9.1). When children do *not* exercise regularly—for example, because of chronic/complex pain or symptoms of persisting fatigue—they keep their macrophages in defensive mode, in which they secrete pro-inflammatory molecules that promote pain and fatigue. When children understand how exercise will help them in the long run, even though it triggers more pain and fatigue in the short run, it helps children to push through the initial discomfort—and exacerbation of pain—and to implement exercise as part of their treatment regimes.

How Opioids Contribute to Chronic/Complex Pain

Children and their families also find it helpful to understand that opiate medications are contraindicated in chronic (vs. acute) pain because opiates irritate macrophage cells (and glial cells in the brain),

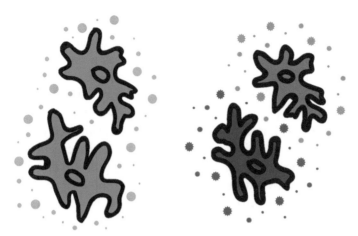

Fig. 9.1 Macrophages in restorative mode and defensive mode. Macrophages in restorative mode (blue, on left) promote analgesia by secreting anti-inflammatory molecules. Macrophages in defensive mode (red and purple, on right) maintain chronic pain by secreting pro-inflammatory molecules that activate pain neurons (© Kasia Kozlowska 2017)

putting them into defensive mode and thereby causing them to secrete pro-inflammatory molecules and to maintain chronic pain (for references see Online Supplement 1.3). For example, Jai—the boy with dystonia of the neck—and his family found this piece of information helpful during the painful process of trying to wean Jai off opiate medications (see Chapter 5 or, for a much more detailed account, Khachane et al. [2019]).

Sex Hormones and Chronic/Complex Pain

An emerging body of research has found that sex hormones—including oestrogen, progesterone, and testosterone—are involved in pain processing. Oestrogen, for example, acts on the oestrogen receptors on the nerve and immune-inflammatory cells that are part of body's pain system. Via activation of these receptors, oestrogen appears to play an important role in up-regulating and down-regulating pain. Of special importance for us, oestrogen can up-regulate the immune-inflammatory component of the pain system (and stress system more generally) to sustain chronic/complex pain (Chrousos 2010), and it generally has a pro-nociceptive role in visceral pain, intensifying the subjective experience of pain (Sun et al. 2019; Traub and Ji 2013). These findings are not surprising, given that chronic/complex pain is more common in girls/women than boys/men (Traub and Ji 2013), and as many women know from their own personal experience, the susceptibility to pain and the subjective experience of pain fluctuate with the menstrual cycle. By contrast, progesterone and testosterone appear to have anti-nociceptive effects. In this context, the research community is actively investigating the potential use of sex hormones or sex hormone analogues in treating chronic/complex pain. For additional references see Online Supplement 1.3.

The Immune-Inflammatory System and Fatigue

Efforts to understand the connection between activation of the immune-inflammatory system and the symptom of fatigue have become intertwined with an intriguing bit of recent medical history. Understanding short-lived fatigue in the context of acute infection is relatively simple and well established. Every reader can bring to mind a normally healthy child who suddenly becomes lethargic and sleepy when she comes down with an infection that activates her immune-inflammatory system when fighting off an infection (see also vignette of Martin, above). This lethargy and sleepiness are caused by high levels of signalling molecules that are produced by immune-inflammatory cells. Once the immune-inflammatory system has brought the infection under control, the immune-inflammatory system deactivates, and the child bounces back to normal.

But the story is less clear in relation to *persisting* fatigue, and the relative lack of clarity reflects two main factors. First, research efforts to understand fatigue are still in their early stages—reaching back 30 years compared to the 60 years of research on pain. Second, because the fundamental processes underlying fatigue are still being worked out, and because so many issues therefore have yet to be resolved, there is much more room for divergent interpretations of what is known and for divergent arguments concerning the appropriate direction for future research. What has happened, in particular, is that research efforts involving persisting fatigue have become entangled in what is perhaps best understood as an ideological struggle, with some insisting that fatigue needs to be understood exclusively in physical terms, and others highlighting that fatigue involves a significant psychological component (Maxmen 2018; Komaroff 2019). A clear conceptualization with which everyone agrees has yet to emerge.

Against this background, what we attempt to do here is to build upon what *is* known about fatigue while sidestepping the continuing controversies. In our central case (see below), the primary presenting problem is persisting fatigue—which typifies the children we see—and we share ideas and emerging findings from the current literature that we find useful in our own clinical practice. In line with all the material in this book, our perspective is systemic—or biopsychosocial—and we presume that to understand fatigue one needs to take into account factors across the full range of system levels: from the molecular, to the mind, to the level of interpersonal interactions with others.

Rudi was a 15-year-old Norwegian boy with a two-year history of disabling fatigue that had developed in the wake of a long-lasting respiratory infection. At the time that he contracted the infection, he was already a promising young hurdler who trained four days a week and competed almost every weekend. Even after becoming sick, Rudi pushed himself and continued training. At the end of one tough race, he collapsed at the finish line. In the aftermath, he was completely exhausted and stayed home from school for three weeks. In the following months he attended school and resumed his training, but felt constantly drained and began to experience problems such as headache, dizziness, and problems with concentration and memory. Any physical activity left him exhausted and needing days to recover. At one point, he could not even move from his bed. Fatigue dominated his life. Every effort—physical, cognitive, or emotional—made him feel worse. As a consequence, Rudi, with the support and assistance of his parents, tried to avoid anything that sapped his energy. He was caught in a downward spiral.

Despite seeing what turned out to be many doctors, Rudi and his family were always told the same thing: the medical assessments, from various specialists, disclosed no medical problem. But his parents were unable to accept these assessments; they were convinced that Rudi had some rare immune disease.

Eventually, Rudi's paediatrician referred Rudi and his family to the local mental health service, where they were seen by the psychiatrist and team. The family assessment interview identified a more complicated story of cumulative stress. When Rudi was born his mother had experienced a postpartum depression of one-year duration, and during that same year Rudi developed infection-triggered childhood asthma, with worsening episodes, sometimes accompanied by respiratory infections, every winter since. When he was 12, his parents underwent a difficult divorce following their conflict-filled marriage. During this same period, Rudi's grandmother, who lived next door and to whom he was very close, died unexpectedly. But because of the turmoil in the family, Rudi kept his grief to himself. And throughout this period, he continued his gruelling schedule for hurdling. It was in the aftermath of these events that Rudi developed the respiratory infection that triggered his symptoms of persisting fatigue.

Against this background, the psychiatrist and her team, in a joint consultation with Rudi's paediatrician, offered an alternative explanation of Rudi's fatigue. They suggested that Rudi's immune system appeared to be very sensitive to stress. They said that Rudi's pattern of presentation fit with what was known about the interconnections between the immune-inflammatory system, the HPA axis, emotional stress, and increased susceptibility to infection. Emotional stress and distress could temporarily disrupt immune-inflammatory function, making the individual more vulnerable to inflammatory illnesses such as asthma and respiratory infections. This pattern of response was common and has been well described in the literature (see Online Supplement 9.1 and the vignette pertaining to cold-virus inoculation in Chapter 8). The psychiatrist said that from the history given by the family, Rudi had followed this pattern across development.

- His initial bout of asthma developed during his mother's postpartum depression.
- His subsequent bouts of asthma and accompanying respiratory infections regularly emerged during the long Norwegian winter, when the family had to spend more time indoors and when Rudi was thus more exposed to his parents' chronic conflict.

- Given the above, Rudi's stress system was chronically activated/dysregulated by the parental conflict.
- At the age of 13, his infection and then disabling fatigue emerged in context of his parents' divorce and his grandmother's death, all while continuing to train for hurdling.

In the most recent illness, however—at the age of 15—the stress had been more pronounced, and other components of the stress system, as well as the pain system, had been activated. Autonomic nervous system activation was reflected in symptoms of orthostatic intolerance (dizziness and abnormal standing test completed by the psychiatrist). Activation of the brain stress systems was reflected in problems with memory and concentration (see Chapter 11). And activation of the pain system was reflected in his chronic headache.

In this context, the treatment offered to Rudi and his family was one that focused on rebuilding Rudi's physical strength, on switching off the stress and pain systems, and on improving his capacity to manage emotional stress. The intervention also helped the family address some of the family stress that had contributed to Rudi's illness.

After 14 months of treatment, Rudi had returned almost to 'normal'. The following interventions had been useful. Rudi had engaged in physiotherapy and occupational therapy to help him mobilize gradually and participate in activities of daily living. He had learnt breathing exercises to reduce and control his arousal (autonomic nervous system activation). He had learnt self-hypnosis, and he was able to visualize himself full of energy when recovered and to rediscover how an energetic body feels. He had been able to articulate, to his parents, his emotional distress in being constantly exposed to their fighting. He had been able to work through his grief about his grandmother's death. An individualized academic program and return-to-school plan were arranged. Finally, Rudi's parents had decided to join a program for parent counselling as an effort to reduce the devastating conflict that continued between them, even after the divorce.

Two years after the illness had started, Rudi felt fully recovered. He was back working at his hurdling but had left behind his dream of becoming a professional athlete.

Rudi's case highlights that, though infection may trigger activation or dysregulation of the immune-inflammatory system and set the illness process in motion, and though the immune-inflammatory system generally settles back to baseline (or nearly so, which may involve an ongoing state of readiness [low-grade inflammation]), persisting fatigue can be maintained by other factors (Russell et al. 2018). These other factors may include the following:

• Sensitization of the pain system (increased sensory sensitivity and pain severity) (Pedersen et al. 2019).
• Activation or dysregulation of the autonomic nervous system (Wyller 2019).
• Dysregulation of the HPA axis (hypo-activation) (Rimes et al. 2014) and other components of the body's energy-regulation systems.
• Changes in gene expression in tissues or the brain (e.g., dysregulated immune-gene networks [Nguyen et al. 2019]).
• Activation of the brain stress systems (suggested by decreased verbal memory) (Pedersen et al. 2019) (see Chapter 11).
• Activation of the brain stress systems (in particular, a shift from reflective to reflexive [defensive] modes of behaviour control [Arnsten 2015]). In defensive mode, implicit computation of salience within the brain stress systems—an evaluation of the child's behavioural repertoire in terms of costs and benefits—may result in a shutdown of behaviour because of the unacceptably high costs to energy resources (Boksem and Tops 2008; Kleckner et al. 2017).
• Aberrant predictive representations—namely, that the body needs much more energy than is being made available (Pedersen 2019).
• Psychological factors that activate the stress system, that shape expectancies, and that change subjective feelings of fatigue. These factors include attention to symptoms, catastrophizing, anxiety, perfectionism, depression, negative illness beliefs, maladaptive coping strategies, and negative emotions (Loades et al. 2019; Pedersen et al. 2019; Katz and Jason 2013) (see Chapter 12). Lessons learnt from athletics are relevant in this context; as a regular part of the training regime, athletic coaches encourage the use of mind strategies to help athletes overcome feelings of fatigue (Noakes 2012) (see Chapter 15).

The vignettes of Martin and Rudi (in this chapter) and Bellynda (Chapter 8) have highlighted how activation of the immune-inflammatory system by infection, allergy, or injury can trigger different patterns of functional symptoms: chronic abdominal pain and functional constipation (Martin); chronic/complex pain, autonomic dysregulation, and persisting and debilitating fatigue (Rudi); chronic/complex pain, autonomic dysregulation, and functional neurological symptoms (Bellynda). In this way, as described earlier in this chapter, while activation of the immune-inflammatory system may serve as the initial trigger, the persisting symptoms of pain, fatigue, autonomic dysregulation, or motor or sensory dysfunction are maintained by other processes. Of particular note in this context is the activation of multiple components of the stress system, coupled with the body's inability to *switch off* or *re-regulate* these systems back to *physiological coherence*.

Against this background, it is worth highlighting that when the functional presentation is triggered via activation of the immune-inflammatory system—whether or not any particular child meets the consensus diagnostic criteria for a particular functional disorder—each child and family should receive a comprehensive assessment that identifies all the relevant physical and psychological contributors to the persisting functional somatic symptoms. Regardless of the symptom pattern—which will vary from child to child—the treatment intervention needs to include targeted interventions that address all relevant areas of dysfunction, and on multiple system levels.

Different Metaphors That Clinicians Can Use When Working with Children with Persisting Fatigue

In recent years the research literature has produced several clinically useful metaphors for conceptualizing persisting fatigue.

Metaphor 1: Persisting Fatigue as a Biologically Ancient Response to Injury or as an Innate Defence Response

A number of clinicians and researchers have suggested that in cases in which the persisting fatigue is completely debilitating or nearly so, it is possible that the presentations reflect biologically ancient responses to stress or injury. Rudi's presentation could potentially be viewed in the light of this metaphor.

In 2015, the first author (KK) and colleagues suggested that that extreme cases of chronic fatigue can be understood in terms of *quiescent immobility*—or rather quiescent immobility in maladaptive form—one of the neurophysiological states that are part of the human (and animal) defence cascade. 'Quiescent immobility [in animals] is a reaction to "deep or inescapable" pain, chronic injury, injury by a predator, or defeat by a conspecific, and to states of exhaustion (where recuperation is needed) after a period of acute stress, once the animal has returned to a safe environment' (Kozlowska et al. 2015, p. 275). In this way the functional symptoms experienced by patients with debilitating chronic fatigue would sit on a continuum with other presentations related to activation of the defence cascade—freezing, flight or fight, tonic and collapsed immobility, and quiescent immobility. Each of these states has a signature neural pattern accompanied by a signature state of arousal and energy use.

In 2016, Robert Naviaux, Professor of Medicine, Pediatrics, and Pathology at the University of California, San Diego, suggested that some cases of persisting fatigue may be similar to entering *dauer*, 'a hypo-metabolic state capable of living efficiently by altering a number of basic mitochondrial functions, fuel preferences, behaviour, and physical features' in response to adverse environmental conditions (Naviaux et al. 2016, p. E5477). In this hypo-metabolic state, cells of the body enter a *cell danger response*, a state in which mitochondria—the organelles in the cell that regulate and produce energy on a cellular level—shift into a defensive mode in which they decrease mitochondrial metabolism to enable the organisms to survive a hostile environment. The changes described by Naviaux on the cellular level may also be part of the quiescent immobility state described above.

In 2019, Anthony Komaroff, Professor of Medicine and Senior Physician, Brigham and Women's Hospital, Harvard Medical School, suggested that persisting fatigue may reflect 'the activation of biologically ancient, evolutionarily conserved responses to injury or potential injury, a pathological inability to turn these responses off, or both' (Komaroff 2019, p. 500).

Referring back to our clinical vignette of Rudi, the reader can see that Rudi was exposed to multiple sources of stress that threatened his physical and psychological integrity, and that the combination of these threats could have activated the body's innate responses to threat, injury, and the sustained overuse of energy resources.

Metaphor 2: Persisting Fatigue as a Vitally Protective System Gone Wrong

From this perspective, persisting fatigue, like pain, is conceptualized as a subjective feeling with protective value, gone wrong (Pedersen 2019). Fatigue—like pain—functions as a *homeostatic emotion* (Craig 2003) or *biological alarm system* (Brodal 2017) that 'alert[s] the organism', whether accurately or erroneously, 'to urgent homeostatic imbalance' (Hilty et al. 2011, p. 2151; St Clair Gibson et al. 2003; Noakes 2012). In the case of persisting fatigue, the homeostatic alarm would be errone-ous. Fatigue, like pain, has protective survival value in acute situations, but it becomes maladaptive and debilitating when it becomes chronic. Using the watchdog metaphor, when the hyper-vigilant watchdog raises the alarm in response to events that have no threat value (or that no longer have any threat value), then the watchdog needs to be retired.

Metaphor 3: Persisting Fatigue as a Vitally Protective System Signalling Loss of Physiological Coherence

Yet another metaphor emerges from the perspective of this book—and the stress-system model—regarding the symptom of fatigue: fatigue as a vitally protective system working *just right*, signalling the loss of phys-iological coherence. In the stress-system model, we also conceptualize fatigue as a homeostatic emotion, a homeostatic alarm signal (see previous subsection). But we see the alarm as working *just right*. The fatigue alarm is signalling ongoing activation of the stress system, the body's shift into defensive mode (and failure to return to switch off and return to restora-tive mode), the concurrent increase in energy use, and the concurrent loss of physiological coherence. In the stress-system scenario, the metaphor of the homeostatic alarm is right on target—it is accurate. It signals a dysregulated stress system: one that has lost harmony and physiological coherence within and between its various components, along with its capacity for *efficient use of energy*. Because the easy flow of life processes that is associated with health and well-being is compromised (McCraty and Childre 2010), it is not surprising that the homeostatic alarms of fatigue and pain are activated in such a large number of children with functional somatic symptoms. This idea of fatigue as a *homeostatic alarm* signalling disturbed homeostasis has also been put forth by Vegard Wyller (2019, p. 6), a well-known Norwegian researcher in the field of chronic fatigue syndrome.

The Full Picture Pertaining to Fatigue Is Still Emerging

Whatever the final answers, the emerging picture suggests that patients with persisting fatigue—whether the illness is triggered by an infection or by other physical or psychological stress—show dysregulation in multiple components of the stress system (autonomic nervous system, HPA axis, immune-inflammatory system, brain stress systems) and in the energy-regulation system on the cellular level, as well as changes in the gene networks (epigenetic changes in gene expression) that regulate these systems (see Online Supplements 1.3 and 9.1). The overall result is that these patients are characterized by a loss of physiological coherence. The easy flow of their life processes, including the efficient use of energy, has been disrupted—and their health and well-being, severely compromised.

The Take-Home Messages About the Immune-Inflammatory System for the Mental Health Clinician

The immune-inflammatory system functions like a watchdog that is gifted with prescience. It holds immune-inflammatory memory for past stress and activates in response to physical and psychological stress. Of special importance to us, a sensitized or unrestrained immune-inflammatory system—in a state of low-grade inflammation—can respond to commonplace physical and psychological stress in an overly robust way. In so doing, it can activate other stress-system components or the stress system as a whole, thereby contributing to the generation of functional somatic symptoms, including persisting pain or fatigue. In extreme cases, persisting debilitating fatigue may represent an innate biologically ancient response to stress or injury.

Because of technological advances and interest in systems biology, we can look forward to many new findings about the immune-inflammatory system in the coming years. Some of those findings will help us better understand and treat children with functional somatic symptoms.

***

In Chapter 10, we look at the gut system, which is closely connected and overlaps with the stress system in many ways.

References

Arnsten, A. F. (2015). Stress Weakens Prefrontal Networks: Molecular Insults to Higher Cognition. *Nature Neuroscience, 18,* 1376–1385.

Boksem, M. A., & Tops, M. (2008). Mental Fatigue: Costs and Benefits. *Brain Research Reviews, 59,* 125–139.

Brenhouse, H. C., Danese, A., & Grassi-Oliveira, R. (2019). Neuroimmune Impacts of Early-Life Stress on Development and Psychopathology. *Current Topics in Behavioral Neurosciences, 43,* 423–447.

Brenhouse, H. C., & Schwarz, J. M. (2016). Immunoadolescence: Neuroimmune Development and Adolescent Behavior. *Neuroscience and Biobehavioral Reviews, 70,* 288–299.

Brodal, P. (2017). A Neurobiologist's Attempt to Understand Persistent Pain. *Scandinavian Journal of Pain, 15,* 140–147.

Chrousos, G. P. (2010). Stress and Sex Versus Immunity and Inflammation. *Science Signaling, 3,* pe36.

Craig, A. D. (2003). A New View of Pain as a Homeostatic Emotion. *Trends in Neurosciences, 26,* 303–307.

Edwards, R. R., Kronfli, T., Haythornthwaite, J. A., Smith, M. T., Mcguire, L., & Page, G. G. (2008). Association of Catastrophizing with Interleukin-6 Responses to Acute Pain. *Pain, 140,* 135–144.

Fields, R. D. (2009). *The Other Brain: The Scientific and Medical Breakthroughs That Will Heal Our Brains and Revolutionize Our Health.* New York: Simon & Schuster.

Flajnik, M. F., & Kasahara, M. (2010). Origin and Evolution of the Adaptive Immune System: Genetic Events and Selective Pressures. *Nature Reviews Genetics, 11,* 47–59.

Frank, M. G., Weber, M. D., Watkins, L. R., & Maier, S. F. (2016). Stress-Induced Neuroinflammatory Priming: A Liability Factor in the Etiology of Psychiatric Disorders. *Neurobiology of Stress, 4,* 62–70.

Hilty, L., Jancke, L., Luechinger, R., Boutellier, U., & Lutz, K. (2011). Limitation of Physical Performance in a Muscle Fatiguing Handgrip Exercise Is Mediated by Thalamo-Insular Activity. *Human Brain Mapping, 32,* 2151–2160.

Janeway, C. A. J. (2001). Afterword: Evolution of the Immune System: Past, Present, and Future. In C. A. J. Janeway, P. Travers, M. Walport, & M. J. Shlomchik (Eds.), *Immunobiology: The Immune System in Health and Disease* (5th ed.). New York: Garland Science.

Katz, B. Z., & Jason, L. A. (2013). Chronic Fatigue Syndrome Following Infections in Adolescents. *Current Opinion in Pediatrics, 25,* 95–102.

Khachane, Y., Kozlowska, K., Savage, B., McClure, G., Butler, G., Gray, N., et al. (2019). Twisted in Pain: The Multidisciplinary Treatment Approach to Functional Dystonia. *Harvard Review of Psychiatry, 27,* 359–381. https://pubmed.ncbi.nlm.nih.gov/31714467/.

Kleckner, I. R., Zhang, J., Touroutoglou, A., Chanes, L., Xia, C., Simmons, W. K., et al. (2017). Evidence for a Large-Scale Brain System Supporting Allostasis and Interoception in Humans. *Nature Human Behaviour, 1,* 0069.

Komaroff, A. L. (2019, July 5). Advances in Understanding the Pathophysiology of Chronic Fatigue Syndrome. *JAMA* (Epub ahead of print).

Kozlowska, K., Walker, P., Mclean, L., & Carrive, P. (2015). Fear and the Defense Cascade: Clinical Implications and Management. *Harvard Review of Psychiatry, 23,* 263–287. https://www.ncbi.nlm.nih.gov/pmc/articles/PMC4495877/.

Kristiansen, M. S., Stabursvik, J., O'Leary, E. C., Pedersen, M., Asprusten, T. T., Leegaard, T., et al. (2019). Clinical Symptoms and Markers of Disease Mechanisms in Adolescent Chronic Fatigue Following Epstein-Barr Virus Infection: An Exploratory Cross-sectional Study. *Brain, Behavior, and Immunity, 80,* 551–563.

Lazaridou, A., Martel, M. O., Cahalan, C. M., Cornelius, M. C., Franceschelli, O., Campbell, C. M., et al. (2018). The Impact of Anxiety and Catastrophizing on Interleukin-6 Responses to Acute Painful Stress. *Journal of Pain Research, 11,* 637–647.

Loades, M. E., Rimes, K., Lievesley, K., Ali, S., & Chalder, T. (2019). Cognitive and Behavioural Responses to Symptoms in Adolescents with Chronic Fatigue Syndrome: A Case-Control Study Nested Within a Cohort. *Clinical Child Psychology and Psychiatry, 24,* 564–579.

Maxmen, A. (2018). A Reboot for Chronic Fatigue Syndrome Research. *Nature, 553,* 14–17.

McCraty, R., & Childre, D. (2010). Coherence: Bridging Personal, Social, and Global Health. *Alternative Therapies in Health and Medicine, 16,* 10–24.

Naviaux, R. K., Naviaux, J. C., Li, K., Bright, A. T., Alaynick, W. A., Wang, L., et al. (2016). Metabolic Features of Chronic Fatigue Syndrome. *Proceedings of the National Academy of Sciences of the United States of America, 113,* E5472–E5480.

Nguyen, C. B., Kumar, S., Zucknick, M., Kristensen, V. N., Gjerstad, J., Nilsen, H., & Wyller, V. B. (2019). Associations Between Clinical Symptoms, Plasma Norepinephrine and Deregulated Immune Gene Networks in Subgroups of Adolescent with Chronic Fatigue Syndrome. *Brain, Behavior, and Immunity, 76,* 82–96.

Noakes, T. D. (2012). Fatigue Is a Brain-Derived Emotion That Regulates the Exercise Behavior to Ensure the Protection of Whole Body Homeostasis. *Frontiers in Physiology, 3,* 82.

Pedersen, M. (2019, June 29). Chronic Fatigue Syndrome and Chronic Pain Conditions—Vitally Protective Systems Gone Wrong. *Scandinavian Journal of Pain* (Epub ahead of print).

Pedersen, M., Asprusten, T. T., Godang, K., Leegaard, T. M., Osnes, L. T., Skovlund, E., et al. (2019). Predictors of Chronic Fatigue in Adolescents Six Months After Acute Epstein-Barr Virus Infection: A Prospective Cohort Study. *Brain, Behavior, and Immunity, 75,* 94–100.

Rimes, K. A., Papadopoulos, A. S., Cleare, A. J., & Chalder, T. (2014). Cortisol Output in Adolescents with Chronic Fatigue Syndrome: Pilot Study on the Comparison with Healthy Adolescents and Change After Cognitive Behavioural Guided Self-Help Treatment. *Journal of Psychosomatic Research, 77,* 409–414.

Russell, A., Hepgul, N., Nikkheslat, N., Borsini, A., Zajkowska, Z., Moll, N., et al. (2018). Persistent Fatigue Induced by Interferon-Alpha: A Novel, Inflammation-Based, Proxy Model of Chronic Fatigue Syndrome. *Psychoneuroendocrinology, 100,* 276–285.

Sluka, K. A. (2017). *Macrophages Are Key Players in Pain and Analgesia.* https:// bodyinmind.org/Macrophages-Pain-Analgesia/.

St Clair Gibson, A., Baden, D. A., Lambert, M. I., Lambert, E. V., Harley, Y. X., Hampson, D., et al. (2003). The Conscious Perception of the Sensation of Fatigue. *Sports Medicine, 33,* 167–176.

Sun, L. H., Zhang, W. X., Xu, Q., Wu, H., Jiao, C. C., & Chen, X. Z. (2019). Estrogen Modulation of Visceral Pain. *Journal of Zhejiang University Science, 20,* 628–636.

Traub, R. J., & Ji, Y. (2013). Sex Differences and Hormonal Modulation of Deep Tissue Pain. *Frontiers in Neuroendocrinology, 34,* 350–366.

Wyller, V. B. B. (2019). Pain Is Common in Chronic Fatigue Syndrome— Current Knowledge and Future Perspectives. *Scandinavian Journal of Pain, 19,* 5–8.

10

The Role of the Gut in the Neurobiology of Functional Somatic Symptoms

Abstract Functional somatic symptoms involving the gut are common in children and adolescents. The human gut has a close symbiotic relationship with the microorganisms that live inside it. When this relationship is going well, the microbiota—the community of organisms that live inside the gut—and the gut work together to break down food to provide both the microbiota and the body with energy, and to protect the integrity of the gut barrier (intestinal wall). Working together, the microbiota and gut also modulate set-points within the stress system and contribute to brain function and subjective experience. Because of these wide-ranging functions and because the gut talks to the brain and the brain talks to the gut, functional gut disorders are conceptualized as disorders arising from dysregulation of the *microbiota-gut-brain axis*. This axis overlaps, interconnects, and interacts with multiple components of the stress system. Activation or dysregulation of the stress system affects gut function and dysregulates the microbiota-gut-brain axis, which then affects stress-system function. In this chapter we examine the interactions between the stress system and microbiota-gut-brain axis. We also discuss the functional somatic symptoms that may arise when that axis is dysregulated.

© The Author(s) 2020   **203**
K. Kozlowska et al., *Functional Somatic Symptoms in Children and Adolescents*, Palgrave Texts in Counselling and Psychotherapy,
https://doi.org/10.1007/978-3-030-46184-3_10

Functional somatic symptoms involving the gut—abdominal pain, nausea, vomiting, irregular bowel function, and rumination—are common in children (including adolescents) and are a leading cause of functional impairment and school absenteeism (Varni et al. 2006). Functional gut symptoms sit on a continuum with other functional somatic symptoms and, like other functional somatic symptoms, show an association with adverse childhood experiences (ACEs) and with stress more generally (Bradford et al. 2012; Park et al. 2016; Michels et al. 2019) (for more references see Online Supplement 1.3). These gut symptoms can present as the primary presenting symptom, or they can present alongside other functional somatic symptoms (see, e.g., case of Paula in Chapter 2 or case of Jai in Chapter 5).

Consensus guidelines (the Rome IV Criteria) used by gastroenterologists cluster functional gut symptoms into 10 diagnostic entities in childhood and 33 diagnostic entities in adulthood (Hyams et al. 2016; Drossman and Hasler 2016) (see Text Box 10.1).

Text Box 10.1: Functional gut diagnoses

When the child with functional gut symptoms goes to see the paediatrician, she may receive a diagnosis that fits under one of three clusters (see Hyams et al. [2016]):

Cluster 1: Functional nausea and vomiting disorders
- Cyclic vomiting syndrome
- Functional nausea and functional vomiting
- Rumination syndrome (belch-like motor pattern)
- Aerophagia

Cluster 2: Functional abdominal pain disorders
- Functional dyspepsia
- Irritable bowel syndrome
- Abdominal migraine
- Functional abdominal pain not otherwise specified

Cluster 3: Functional defecation disorders
- Functional constipation
- Nonretentive faecal incontinence

Shifting Gear to Systems Thinking: A Few Tips to the Reader

As recently as two decades ago, the gut was considered an independent organ, and functional gut disorders were conceptualized as problems that related to the gut. Over the last decade, however, it has become clear that the gut is part of a complex system—what is known as the *microbiota-gut-brain axis*. This system includes the microbiota (the organisms living in the gut), the gut itself, the communication pathways between the gut and the brain, and relevant regions in the brain (including the brain stress systems). In turn, functional gut disorders have come to be conceptualized as complex disorders arising from dysregulation of the microbiota-gut-brain axis. This conceptualization reflects the introduction of systems thinking into gastroenterology. Gut doctors are now well aware that the gut does not function as an independent organ but that it must be understood as part of a complex system.

The idea of the microbiota-gut-brain axis brings together many processes on multiple system levels, from the gut lumen (i.e., the inside of the intestine) to the brain (Drossman 2016), including the following:

- The composition and health of the gut microbiota, the colony of organisms that live in the gut lumen.
- The health of the gut itself, including the following: the integrity of the mucosal barrier and immune function; gut motility; digestive processes; and gut signalling.
- The communication from the gut (and the microbiota) to the brain. Key communication pathways include the following: the autonomic nervous system (the vagal nerve carries information from the gut to the brain; see Chapter 6); immune-inflammatory signalling molecules, which are part of the immune-inflammatory system (see Chapter 9); and metabolites and neurotransmitters that are synthesized and processed by the gut (and microbiota). In this way the gut modulates brain function—and function of the HPA axis—bottom-up.
- The communication from the brain to the gut and top-down modulation of gut function (the autonomic nervous system modulates gut function top-down, see Chapter 6).

- Activation of the pain system on the gut, spinal cord, and brain system levels (see below and Chapter 9).

To add to the complexity, the microbiota-gut-brain axis overlaps, interconnects, and interacts with the stress system—the autonomic nervous system, HPA axis, immune-inflammatory system, and brain stress systems—in many ways. Activation of the stress system affects function within the microbiota-gut-brain axis, and dysregulation of this axis affects function within the stress system. For example, gut microbiota play a role in the programming and activity of the HPA axis—including gene expression—and influence neuronal activation and the brain stress systems (Butler et al. 2019; Bastiaanssen et al. 2020).

As we see from the above, the microbiota-gut-brain axis is immensely complex; clinicians from non-medical backgrounds may find this chapter challenging. In order to avoid being overwhelmed by the detail, it may be helpful for the reader to shift gear to systems thinking. In this way, the reader can hold in mind, in a general way, that dysregulation of any one of these processes can compromise both healthy gut function and healthy brain function, and can contribute to the generation of functional somatic symptoms. Or, in a nutshell, the reader can think of functional gut disorders as emerging from a 'combination of irritable bowel, [activated communication pathways,] and irritable brain' (Qin et al. 2014, p. 14126; Mayer et al. 2019).

See Online Supplement 1.3 for references to non-technical articles about the microbiota-gut-brain axis published either in the health sections of major newspapers or by other science writers.

What We Know About the Gut: The Gut as a Complex System

In the late 1990s, the neuroscientist Michael Gershon nicknamed the gut's nervous system *the second brain* (Gershon 1998). Gershon, who had spent his entire research career studying the gut, worked during an era in which the brain was seen as 'the central organ of stress and

adaptation' (McEwen 2009, p. 911)—a time when research on the gut
was somewhat disparaged. Through his play on words, Gershon wanted
to highlight the complexity of the gut system and its important role in
human health and disease. The intriguing comparison was also a way of
drawing attention, as well as the interest of young scientists, to his field.

The gut has its own nervous system, the *enteric nervous system*, which
includes both sensory and motor components. It is a network of nerve
fibres that respond to chemical and mechanical stimuli and that activate
smooth muscle in the gastrointestinal tract, pancreas, gall bladder, and
blood vessels to coordinate motility, endocrine secretions, and blood
flow—together, the gut's digestive and defensive programs. Historically,
the enteric nervous system was considered part of the autonomic nervous system, which innervates the viscera: all the organs and tissues
inside the body (see Online Supplement 1.2). The gut's motor system
is part of the visceromotor system, the efferent component of the autonomic nervous system (see Chapter 6). With the exception of the brain,
the gut contains the largest number of neurons in the body.

The gut also functions, in effect, as a barrier between the body and the
outside world. In this context, the 'outside world' comprises the *microbiota*, the colony of organisms that live inside the gut. A large proportion
of the body's immune-inflammatory cells reside in the gut lumen, where
they help maintain the integrity of the gut barrier. Any loss of gut-barrier
integrity can lead to the passage of organisms across the gut wall into the
inside of the body (organism translocation due to increased gut permea-
bility), which in turn activates the immune-inflammatory system (resulting in increased inflammation) and also disrupts nutrition, digestion, and
absorption (Osadchiy et al. 2019).

Each person's gut microbiota is the community of microorganisms—
including bacteria, fungi, and viruses—that live in that individual's gut
at any particular time. The genetic material carried by the microbiota—'the full collection of genes in all the microbes in a microbiota community' (Learn.Genetics, Genetic Science Learning Center 2020)—is
called the *microbiome*. The health and relative stability of the microbiota
are important to the health and well-being of the individual because the
microbiota lives in symbiosis with humans and works together with the

human body to maintain life processes. These symbiotic functions are so intertwined that some scientists have suggested that humans (and presumably, therefore, many other animals or at least primates) should be viewed as multi-species organisms and that the microbiome should be considered a second form of genetic inheritance, one that is acquired via the mother's birth canal, through subsequent close body contact during infancy (but also later), from the physical environment in early childhood, from the food that we eat, and from the microorganisms that we encounter in our daily lives, lifelong (Gilbert et al. 2012).

Among other things, a healthy and diverse microbiota helps in the digestion of food, contributes to the gut-barrier integrity by protecting the individual from pathogenic organisms, modulates the immune-inflammatory system and the HPA axis, and supports normal brain development and function (Osadchiy et al. 2019; Dominguez-Bello et al. 2019; Bastiaanssen et al. 2020). For example, lactobacilli—the bacteria found in yogurt and fermented milk—help in maintaining a healthy microbiota via their antimicrobial functions (production of antimicrobial molecules), anti-inflammatory functions, and gut-barrier functions (for references see Online Supplement 1.3). Disruption of lactobacillus populations via physical (bad diet or antibiotics) or psychological stress may, in turn, compromise the health and integrity of the gut, and increase its vulnerability to functional somatic symptoms.

Healthy eating contributes to the health and relative stability of the microbiota. In this context, the eating patterns in Western-style societies, with so much processed food and the decreased intake of fruits and vegetables, appears to be decreasing the biodiversity of the human gut microbiota. Some scientists propose that the dwindling health of the microbiota in modern, Western-style societies may, in part, explain their soaring rates of anxiety and depression, as well as the apparent increase in functional gut disorders, other functional somatic symptoms, and other forms of dis-ease (Zinocker and Lindseth 2018). Moderate pleasurable exercise also affects the health of the microbiota and is one of the mechanisms that increase the child's stress tolerance (Bastiaanssen et al. 2020).

Communication Between the Gut and the Brain

The microbiota-gut-brain axis, discussed at the outset and also known as the *gut-brain axis* or *brain-gut axis*, comprises the many different mechanisms through which the gut and brain communicate with each other. *Gut-to-brain* communication includes the following: the vagal nerve (the afferent part of the autonomic system) and other interoceptive afferents; messenger molecules secreted by the immune-inflammatory cells (part of the immune-inflammatory system); hormone messengers produced by gut endocrine cells (part of the endocrine system); and other messenger molecules (e.g., neurotransmitters and metabolites) produced by the microbiota or the gut (Foster et al. 2017). *Brain-to-gut* communication includes the following: the autonomic system (sympathetic, restorative parasympathetic, and defensive parasympathetic) and the HPA axis (see Chapter 6). Via these connections, disruptions of the axis on the gut level will affect brain function, and disruptions of the axis on the brain level will affect gut function.

The Gut and Pain

Pain is a common symptom in functional gut disorders. The mechanisms that underpin chronic/complex pain in the gut are the same as those that underpin chronic/complex pain elsewhere (see Chapter 9). In chronic or recurring gut pain, the pain system is activated on many levels.

- At the *tissue level*, pain-sensing nerve endings are kept in an activated state (known as *visceral sensitivity, visceral hypersensitivity,* or *neurogenic inflammation*).
- At the *spinal cord level*, nerve cells that receive and carry information about pain are activated (called *central sensitization* or *neuroinflammation*).
- At the *brain level, pain maps*—central representations of pain—are activated (also called *central sensitization* or *neuroinflammation*).

On all these levels, activation of neurons involved in sensing, carrying, or representing pain is maintained by aberrant activation of the immune-inflammatory system. Hence the idea that an irritable bowel exists alongside an irritable brain (Qin et al. 2014). For further details about chronic/complex pain, see Chapter 9.

Stress-System Activation Affects Healthy Gut Function

From reading the previous sections, the reader will already have noticed that the stress system and the microbiota-gut-brain axis share many components; they are overlapping systems.

- The autonomic nervous system—made up of the sympathetic system and the restorative parasympathetic and defensive parasympathetic systems—is part of both the stress system and the microbiota-gut-brain axis. Autonomic nerves provide communication from the gut to the brain and from the brain to the gut.
- The immune-inflammatory system is part of both the stress system and the microbiota-gut-brain axis, and a large number of immune cells reside in the gut and communicate to the brain via immune-inflammatory signalling molecules.
- The HPA axis communicates with the gut via hormone messengers. In addition, the gut microbiome affects both the development and the regulation of the HPA axis (Sudo 2014; Bastiaanssen et al. 2020).

Because of this close relationship between the stress system and the microbiota-gut-brain axis, activation or dysregulation of the former will affect the latter—including gut health and function, along with the well-being of the gut microbiota—and will potentially trigger, or contribute to the emergence of, functional gut symptoms (Foster et al. 2017; Osadchiy et al. 2019).

Of particular importance, changes in the activation of the autonomic system significantly affect gut health and well-being. As we saw in Chapter 6, activation of the sympathetic component of the autonomic system switches off normal digestive programs in both the upper and lower digestive tract, and activation of the defensive parasympathetic component of the autonomic system activates the defensive programs of nausea, vomiting, and diarrhoea. In addition, activation of the autonomic system during periods of stress may mediate changes that decrease gut-barrier integrity and lead to the loss of healthy microbiota species (Michels et al. 2019). Some of the factors that contribute to the decrease in gut-barrier integrity include the following: reduced secretion of gastric acid, reduced gastric emptying, slower transit in the small intestine, and reduced levels of anti-inflammatory antibodies that specialize in mucosal protection (Campos-Rodriguez et al. 2013). Taken together, the reduction of gut-barrier integrity and its consequences for the microbiota will decrease the health and well-being of the gut, and potentially lead to the emergence of functional gut symptoms. Dysregulation in one component of the microbiota-gut-brain axis can thus have potentially major flow-on effects in other components.

The Microbiota, Health, and Well-Being

The connection between the health of the microbiota and stress-induced symptoms was identified more than a century ago (for references see Online Supplement 1.3). In 1907, Ilya Metchnikoff, a Ukrainian-Russian biologist and the 1908 Nobel Prize winner in Physiology or Medicine, wrote about the health benefits of yogurt eating—and ingestion of lactobacilli—in rural Bulgaria. And in 1910, the physician George Porter Phillips reported that preparations rich in live lactic acid bacteria—for example, curdled milk or liquid solutions from malted grains—were helping to improve symptoms in his patients with melancholia (severe depression). Lactobacilli, as we saw previously, have multiple antimicrobial, anti-inflammatory, and gut-barrier functions that help in maintaining a healthy microbiota-gut-brain axis. More recently, a small number of randomized, controlled trials suggest that diet—in and of itself—can improve symptoms of depression (Parletta et al. 2019; Opie et al. 2018; Bastiaanssen et al. 2020). Probiotics—made up of live microbes that have a beneficial effect on the individual—also appear to have beneficial effects on mood, as reported by Phillips in 1910 (Bastiaanssen et al. 2020). In this context, and to help foster long-term health and well-being, a healthy diet—one that includes a regular top-up of lactobacilli—needs to be a key component in all clinical interventions for functional somatic symptoms.

The Foundation for the Microbiota Is Established Early in Life

Recent studies show that the health of the gut microbiota is established during the first days, weeks, and months of life. The baby is colonized by the correct type of microbes during the vaginal birth process (including from faeces), and also via microbes picked up from the environment and via breast feeding. The health of the baby's microbiota can be disrupted by maternal use of antibiotics, caesarean delivery, and antibiotic use during early development. The role of microbiota disruptions for subsequent health and disease across the lifespan is a topic of current research. For references see Online Supplement 1.3.

The Microbiota Modulates Set-Points Within the Gut System

The microbiota plays a centrally important role in the gut by modulating set-points for gut motility, visceral sensitivity, and thickness of the gut's mucosal barrier (Galley et al. 2014). Some of these functions are controlled via serotonin, a neurotransmitter synthesized in the gut and also in the microbiota. Too much serotonin in the gut lumen—because of too much production or inadequate reuptake—can cause abdominal pain and cramping, bloating, and, in some individuals, alternating diarrhoea and constipation (key symptoms of irritable bowel syndrome). Likewise, disruptions in the health of the microbiota presumably affect serotonin production and may contribute to functional presentations. It is notable in this context that many, though not all, studies of individuals with irritable bowel syndrome show unhealthy changes in microbiota composition (Osadchiy et al. 2019; Bastiaanssen et al. 2020).

In parallel, because serotonin is also a key neurotransmitter in the brain, changes in serotonin metabolism in the gut may affect anxiety, depression, and mood-related behaviours (Faure et al. 2010; O'Mahony et al. 2017). Indeed, some studies of probiotics in patients with high levels of stress, irritable bowel syndrome, and chronic fatigue syndrome have shown, respectively, decreases in stress-related gut symptoms and stress/anxiety measures, better mood scores and decreased responses to fear stimuli, and decreased anxiety symptoms.

For references see Online Supplement 1.3.

The Microbiota Modulates Set-Points Within the Stress System

The microbiota also modulates set-points within the stress system—for example, the reactivity of the HPA axis (Sudo 2014; Foster et al. 2017; Bastiaanssen et al. 2020). Children with a healthy microbiota may be less susceptible to HPA-axis hyper- or hypo-activation in the face of adversity (see Chapter 8). By keeping stress-system activation within a healthy range, these children may be less susceptive to a broad range of stress-related symptoms and disorders, including anxiety, depression, and functional somatic symptoms of all kinds. For references see Online Supplement 1.3.

Stress and Functional Gut Symptoms

As we have seen in previous sections, the health and well-being of the gut system relies on the health and well-being of all components that make up the microbiota-gut-brain axis and on communication and synchronization both within and between the microbiota-gut-brain axis and the stress system. In the vignettes below we provide some clinical examples so that the reader can see how these issues present in clinical practice.

In clinical practice, functional gut symptoms—like other functional symptoms—are often triggered by psychological stress. The vignette of

Tommie illustrates how psychological stress activated Tommie's stress system, which then activated his gut and led to his presentation with pain (headache) and gut symptoms.

> Tommie was an eight-year-old boy in primary school. He was a good student who liked to please his teachers. Tommie told the following story. In year 2 of primary school, he had had a 'nice' teacher and a good year at school (resulting in a stress rating of 1/10 for Tommie). In year 3 his teacher changed, and Tommie and the class did not like her (stress rating of 9/10 for Tommie). Tommie said that she disapproved of how the class dressed, and frequently made the children stay back at lunch. Among the many things she disliked were the bags that the children used to carry their things, the way that they placed their bags in the classroom, and the types of pens that they used. Tommie found himself unable to please his teacher. He began to worry about going to school, and he also began to suffer from headaches and nausea. He had butterflies and cramps in his stomach every day, and sometimes he also vomited. One day, the teacher lost her temper, and she expressed her disapproval of Tommie publicly in front of the class. That evening Tommie's mother brought him to the emergency department clutching his head in pain. When Tommie told the story, his body manifest its distress. Tommie first showed increases in both respiratory and heart rates. Then the headache increased in intensity, and Tommie clutched his head in distress. Then Tommie's abdomen made fluttering motions that were visible to the interviewer (presumably reflecting movement of smooth muscle that makes up the gut). A little later, Tommy retched into a vomit bag. Finally, Tommie's arms and legs went weak. His mother gathered him into her arms, and Tommie sobbed into her body.

In clinical practice, functional gut symptoms and the dysregulation of the microbiota-gut-brain axis can also be triggered by physical stress such as an illness or infection, as we saw in the vignette of Martin in Chapter 9. In this way, even though the infection or illness resolves, ongoing symptoms may be maintained by ongoing dysregulation of the microbiota-gut-brain axis or ongoing activation or dysregulation of the stress system (or components of the stress system). Ongoing dysregulation of the microbiota-gut-brain axis makes the child more susceptive to subsequent episodes of infection and to symptoms of anxiety and depression.

As we see in the following vignette of Emma, some patients walk a difficult path and demonstrate remarkable tenacity and resilience in the face of a series of physical insults involving the gut that have eventually triggered functional somatic symptoms. While the medical details of the presentation may be challenging to the reader, it is important to include them here because Emma's pattern of presentation is one that gastroenterologists encounter on a regular basis.

Emma was an 18-year-old woman with a five-year history of chronic abdominal pain and recurring episodes of nausea, bringing up food (sometimes via vomiting and sometimes via rumination [see Chapter 7]), and irregular bowel function. Emma's initial period of illness followed in the wake of various medical events: an episode of spontaneous peritonitis (inflammation of the inner lining of the bowel) diagnosed via laparoscopy (keyhole surgery using a camera), which was followed by multiple treatments with various antibiotics. The symptoms of severe vomiting and explosive diarrhoea—and the inability to keep food down—had worsened after a gastric-emptying study (study looking at mobility of the stomach) that used a radioactive preparation to which Emma had a serious adverse response. Investigations suggested that gut dysmotility (loss of normal speed and rhythm of bowel movements) and visceral hypersensitivity (activation of the pain system on the gut system level) contributed to the clinical picture. Emma also suffered from severe postural orthostatic tachycardia syndrome (POTS), a form of autonomic dysregulation that made it more difficult for her to mobilize from her bed (see Chapter 6). In the early stages of the illness, her respiratory motor system had been chronically activated (chronic hyperventilation with a slightly low pCO_2 [see Chapter 7]). Comorbid anxiety contributed to her difficulties with both falling asleep and remaining asleep at night. New episodes of illness were triggered by infections such as colds and bouts of gastritis. But Emma was keen to be well, and she had engaged actively in treatment, availing herself of all the suggested interventions for treating her symptoms: pharmacological (e.g., medications for gut function, POTS, and anxiety), physical (e.g., physiotherapy and nasogastric tube to top up her hydration status), and psychological (e.g., mind-body pain-regulation strategies). After each new bout of illness, Emma had to work extra hard to regain her previous level of function and to maintain periods of well-being. In the future, new options, such as faecal transplants and a targeted use of probiotics, may be added to treatment plans to help patients like Emma.

Throughout the book we have emphasized the interrelated nature of functional somatic symptoms and how different symptoms can exist one alongside the other. An additional feature of functional somatic symptoms is their propensity to change over time. In the following vignette of Morgan, we see how the somatic symptoms—including symptoms involving the microbiota-gut-brain axis—changed over time with exposure to new stress. The vignette highlights that failure to treat functional somatic symptoms—and to address issues in the child's family and social context—may result in a complex clinical picture in which symptoms layer over symptoms, leaving the child progressively more disabled. The vignette also highlights in a tangible way the connection between ACEs and increased risk for functional somatic symptoms in both children and adults (for a discussion of ACEs, see Chapter 4).

> Morgan, a 15-year-old girl living with her parents, had an eight-year history of functional gut symptoms: recurrent abdominal pain, nausea, and vomiting; ongoing difficulties with eating; and irregular bowel function. During the family assessment, Morgan and her family gave a history of chronic stress at home because her parents were always fighting. At the age of 12, Morgan experienced a sporting injury—a fall that involved a severe knock to the head—and her symptom pattern became more complicated. She developed chronic headache and fatigue, and began to suffer from intermittent non-epileptic seizures. Since she found the treatment interventions offered by her local hospital (involving a pain team and mental health team) unhelpful, she stopped attending appointments. At the age of 15, after a period of nasty bullying at school, she presented to hospital with functional hemiparesis and sensory loss of the left side of her face and body.

* * *

In this chapter we have seen that the human body is not all our own. We share this body with microscopic organisms that live on every crevice and contour of our body: on our skin, on all our mucous membranes, and, most especially, inside our gut. We have seen how gut doctors have had to shift their thinking from the gut as a single organ to the gut as part of a complex system, the microbiota-gut-brain axis. We have also seen that functional gut disorders—expressed in symptoms of nausea, vomiting, abdominal pain, cramping, bloating, irregular bowel function, alternating diarrhoea and constipation, and so on— are now conceptualized as disorders arising from dysregulation of the microbiota-gut-brain axis. Both physical and psychological stress can function as triggers that dysregulate the microbiota-gut-brain axis away from *physiological coherence* and health to a state of imbalance and disharmony that may be expressed in functional gut symptoms.

References

Bastiaanssen, T. F. S., Cussotto, S., Claesson, M. J., Clarke, G., Dinan, T. G., & Cryan, J. F. (2020). Gutted! Unraveling the Role of the Microbiome in Major Depressive Disorder. *Harvard Review of Psychiatry, 28,* 26–39.

Bradford, K., Shih, W., Videlock, E. J., Presson, A. P., Naliboff, B. D., Mayer, E. A., & Chang, L. (2012). Association Between Early Adverse Life Events and Irritable Bowel Syndrome. *Clinical Gastroenterology and Hepatology, 10,* 385–390.e3.

Butler, M. I., Cryan, J. F., & Dinan, T. G. (2019). Man and the Microbiome: A New Theory of Everything? *Annual Review of Clinical Psychology, 15,* 371–398.

Campos-Rodriguez, R., Godinez-Victoria, M., Abarca-Rojano, E., Pacheco-Yepez, J., Reyna-Garfias, H., Barbosa-Cabrera, R. E., & Drago-Serrano, M. E. (2013). Stress Modulates Intestinal Secretory Immunoglobulin A. *Frontiers in Integrative Neuroscience, 7,* 86.

Dominguez-Bello, M. G., Godoy-Vitorino, F., Knight, R., & Blaser, M. J. (2019). Role of the Microbiome in Human Development. *Gut, 68,* 1108–1114.

Drossman, D. A. (2016). Functional Gastrointestinal Disorders: History, Pathophysiology, Clinical Features and Rome IV. *Gastroenterology, 150,* 1262–1279.e2.

Drossman, D. A., & Hasler, W. L. (2016). Rome IV–Functional GI Disorders: Disorders of Gut-Brain Interaction. *Gastroenterology, 150,* 1257–1261.

Faure, C., Patey, N., Gauthier, C., Brooks, E. M., & Mawe, G. M. (2010). Serotonin Signaling Is Altered in Irritable Bowel Syndrome with Diarrhea but Not in Functional Dyspepsia in Pediatric Age Patients. *Gastroenterology, 139,* 249–258.

Foster, J. A., Rinaman, L., & Cryan, J. F. (2017). Stress & the Gut-Brain Axis: Regulation by the Microbiome. *Neurobiology of Stress, 7,* 124–136.

Galley, J. D., Nelson, M. C., Yu, Z., Dowd, S. E., Walter, J., Kumar, P. S., et al. (2014). Exposure to a Social Stressor Disrupts the Community Structure of the Colonic Mucosa–Associated Microbiota. *BMC Microbiology, 14,* 189.

Gershon, M. (1998). *The Second Brain: The Scientific Basis of Gut Instinct and a Groundbreaking New Understanding of Nervous Disorders of the Stomach and Intestine.* New York: HarperCollins.

Gilbert, S. F., Sapp, J., & Tauber, A. I. (2012). A Symbiotic View of Life: We Have Never Been Individuals. *Quarterly Review of Biology, 87,* 325–341.

Hyams, J. S., Di Lorenzo, C., Saps, M., Shulman, R. J., Staiano, A., & Van Tilburg, M. (2016). Childhood Functional Gastrointestinal Disorders: Child/Adolescent. *Gastroenterology, 150,* 1456–1468.e2.

Learn.Genetics, Genetic Science Learning Center. (2020). *The Human Microbiome.* https://learn.genetics.utah.edu/Content/Microbiome/.

Mayer, E. A., Labus, J., Aziz, Q., Tracey, I., Kilpatrick, L., Elsenbruch, S., et al. (2019). Role of Brain Imaging in Disorders of Brain-Gut Interaction: A Rome Working Team Report. *Gut, 68,* 1701–1715.

McEwen, B. S. (2009). The Brain Is the Central Organ of Stress and Adaptation. *Neuroimage, 47,* 911–913.

Michels, N., Van De Wiele, T., Fouhy, F., O'Mahony, S., Clarke, G., & Keane, J. (2019). Gut Microbiome Patterns Depending on Children's Psychosocial Stress: Reports Versus Biomarkers. *Brain, Behavior, and Immunity, 80,* 751–762.

O'Mahony, S. M., Dinan, T. G., & Cryan, J. F. (2017). The Gut Microbiota as a Key Regulator of Visceral Pain. *Pain, 158*(Suppl 1), S19–S28.

Opie, R. S., O'Neil, A., Jacka, F. N., Pizzinga, J., & Itsiopoulos, C. (2018). A Modified Mediterranean Dietary Intervention for Adults with Major Depression: Dietary Protocol and Feasibility Data from the Smiles Trial. *Nutritional Neuroscience, 21,* 487–501.

Osadchiy, V., Martin, C. R., & Mayer, E. A. (2019). The Gut-Brain Axis and the Microbiome: Mechanisms and Clinical Implications. *Clinical Gastroenterology and Hepatology, 17,* 322–332.

Park, S. H., Videlock, E. J., Shih, W., Presson, A. P., Mayer, E. A., & Chang, L. (2016). Adverse Childhood Experiences Are Associated with Irritable Bowel Syndrome and Gastrointestinal Symptom Severity. *Neurogastroenterology and Motility, 28,* 1252–1260.

Parletta, N., Zarnowiecki, D., Cho, J., Wilson, A., Bogomolova, S., Villani, A., et al. (2019). A Mediterranean-Style Dietary Intervention Supplemented with Fish Oil Improves Diet Quality and Mental Health in People with Depression: A Randomized Controlled Trial (Helfimed). *Nutritional Neuroscience, 22,* 474–487.

Qin, H. Y., Cheng, C. W., Tang, X. D., & Bian, Z. X. (2014). Impact of Psychological Stress on Irritable Bowel Syndrome. *World Journal of Gastroenterology, 20,* 14126–14131.

Sudo, N. (2014). Microbiome, HPA Axis and Production of Endocrine Hormones in the Gut. *Advances in Experimental Medicine and Biology, 817,* 177–194.

Varni, J. W., Lane, M. M., Burwinkle, T. M., Fontaine, E. N., Youssef, N. N., Schwimmer, J. B., et al. (2006). Health-Related Quality of Life in Pediatric Patients with Irritable Bowel Syndrome: A Comparative Analysis. *Journal of Developmental and Behavioral Pediatrics, 27,* 451–458.

Zinocker, M. K., & Lindseth, I. A. (2018). The Western Diet–Microbiome–Host Interaction and Its Role in Metabolic Disease. *Nutrients, 10,* 365.

11

The Brain Stress Systems I: The Implicit Level of Brain Operations

Abstract In this chapter we continue our exploration of the neurobiology of functional somatic symptoms by considering the role of the brain. The brain plays a key role in regulation, in coordinating the stress response, and in helping the child adapt to the circumstances of living over time. Every component of the body stress system—the HPA axis, autonomic nervous system, and immune-inflammatory system—is regulated by the brain or connected to it, or communicating with it, in some way. When a child is exposed to stress that is chronic, uncontrollable, unpredictable, cumulative, recurrent, or overwhelming, it leads to activation of brain systems that are involved in managing stress and in stress-related adaptations. Because these regions interact with and modulate motor-, sensory-, pain-, and fatigue-processing regions, the sustained activation of the brain stress systems changes patterns of neural activation and connectivity across and between these systems, and sets up the necessary conditions for generating functional

Electronic supplementary material The online version of this chapter (https://doi.org/10.1007/9e78-3-030-46184-3_11) contains supplementary material, which is available to authorized users.

K. Kozlowska et al., *Functional Somatic Symptoms in Children and Adolescents*, Palgrave Texts in Counselling and Psychotherapy, https://doi.org/10.1007/978-3-030-46184-3_11

somatic symptoms. All the processes discussed in this chapter are non-conscious—the implicit level of brain operations—and involve processes that the brain engages in spontaneously, by itself, without conscious control or conscious awareness.

The neuroscientist Bruce McEwen has called the human brain 'the central organ of stress and adaptation' (McEwen 2009, p. 911), and the neuroscientist Christof Koch has described the brain as 'the most complicated object we know of in the universe' (Koch 1993, p. 13). All functional somatic symptoms depend upon implicit—that is, automatic and unconscious—processes that involve the brain and its response to threat or perceived threat. But somehow, in talking with children (including adolescents) about their functional somatic symptoms, we need to bring that complexity down to earth. How is the clinician to do that?

In the stress-system model, we use the metaphor of the stress system as depicted by overlapping circles. The brain stress systems—the implicit processes that involve and occur in the brain—are represented by the top circle (see Fig. 4.2). This circle represents all the brain regions that are involved in stress regulation and the stress response, including the brain regions that underpin salience detection (stimuli and body sensations that have particular importance for the individual), arousal, pain, and emotional states. The brain stress systems play a key role in initiating, amplifying, and maintaining functional somatic symptoms.

The top circle and even the term *brain stress systems* are simple metaphors that we can use to communicate with children and their families about the brain's role in functional somatic symptoms. For readers interested in the details of the neuroscience, including basic science articles and the many different expressions used in the neuroscience literature to denote the brain stress systems, see Online Supplement 11.1.

The Brain in Maintenance and Restorative Mode

As we have seen throughout this book, body regulation is a never-ending task, much of which is framed within repeating patterns across the circadian cycle. In the normal course of events, when things are safe and going well, the brain stress systems maintain body function within normative physiological limits (homeostasis) and ensure that the child's body has access to sufficient energy resources to face the challenges of daily life (allostasis) (see Online Supplement 1.2). But in the face of threat or perceived threat, the brain stress systems can shift from maintenance and restorative mode—*restorative mode*, for short—into defensive mode. Rapid mobilization into *defensive mode* and, in turn, timely termination, with a consequent return to restorative mode, are adaptive responses to the challenges of daily life, to stressful experiences, and to situations that threaten the child's safety or well-being (see also Chapter 4).

The Brain in Defensive Mode

When events pose a threat to the body's internal environment or to the well-being of the child, the brain stress systems activate into defensive mode: this means that the brain shifts gears (organization) into a mode that prioritizes automatic (unconscious) responses and switches off the capacity for reflective (conscious) processes (Arnsten 2015). The activation of the brain stress systems is an implicit process that occurs automatically and without any conscious control. Differences in the intensity and pattern of activation are thought to reflect individual genetic and epigenetic variations as well as the degree to which the child's stress system has been primed—activated by stressful events—in the child's own lifetime.

   In that initial, threshold step of tagging the event as *salient*, the brain, which is continuously anticipating the body's energy needs, begins activating the stress system to meet those needs (Kleckner et al. 2017; Picard et al. 2018). All these processes occur without conscious awareness. Activation of the brain into defensive mode occurs in tandem with activation of the stress system as a whole. The brain secretes neurotransmitters (the brain's messenger molecules), including noradrenalin in the locus coeruleus (in the brain stem) and corticotropin-releasing hormone (CRH) in the hypothalamus, to facilitate processing in the brain, to change the pattern of neural activation and connectivity, and to activate the broader stress system (Chrousos and Gold 1998; Pervanidou and Chrousos 2018; Arnsten 2015). At the same time, the HPA axis is switched on (via the hypothalamus) to mobilize energy resources throughout the body (see Chapter 8); the sympathetic system is switched on (via the brain's autonomic centres) to increase arousal in the body (see Chapter 6); and the immune-inflammatory system is switched on (via immune-inflammatory cells that reside in the brain) to work with neurons to support the brain's response to stress (see Chapter 9).

Along with the change into defensive mode is a change in how information is processed and also how risk is assessed (for different terminologies in the neuroscience literature, see Online Supplement 11.1). States of calm and safety facilitate certain patterns of processing, and states of threat facilitate (and necessitate) others. An example from the animal kingdom will illustrate the point here.

> In the Canadian Rockies, the second author (SS) was, from a very safe distance, observing a grizzly bear eating dandelions (a dietary staple), seemingly without a care in the world and without taking much into account except the location of the next dandelion. But then, the bear stumbled, likely because of some unpredicted unevenness in the ground. With a suddenness that was actually frightening, the bear's body tensed, and he seemed to grow in size. He jerked his head around, looked to the rear, scanned the environment for potential threats, and gave every appearance of being the dangerous, aggressive predator that one hears so much about (whether true or not). In that instant, everything about the bear's stress system and how the bear processed information had changed. While focused on dandelions, information from the environment—noises, smells, colours—was presumably scanned only for major or surprising changes. But after the bear stumbled, many of the previously disregarded details suddenly became salient. All the bear's energy was now focused on identifying and assessing potential threats.

What we see here is a dramatic (and frightening) change in the bear's brain-body state, moving from restorative mode (while eating dandelions) to defensive mode (prepared to defend itself from potential danger). And what we see in the bear is basically what we see when humans encounter threats. The relevant systems have a long evolutionary history. From the particular perspective of the stress system, we are no more than just another mammalian species.

Innate Defence Responses and Functional Somatic Symptoms

One potential manifestation of the brain in defensive mode is activation of innate defence responses. Evolution has endowed all humans with a continuum of innate, hard-wired, automatically activated defence behaviours triggered by extreme danger or threat to self (Kozlowska et al. 2015). These very primitive responses involve activation of evolutionarily old regions in the brain: the brain stem and amygdala. *Flight or fight* is an active defence response for dealing with threat; *freezing* is a flight-or-fight response put on hold; *tonic immobility* and *collapsed immobility* are responses of last resort to inescapable threat, when active defence responses have failed; and *quiescent immobility* is a state of quiescence that promotes rest and healing. Arousal is the first step in activating any of these automatic defence responses. Each response has a distinctive neural pattern mediated by a common neural pathway: activation or inhibition of particular functional components within the brain stress systems (the amygdala, hypothalamus, periaqueductal grey, and sympathetic and vagal nuclei [the brain component of the autonomic nervous system]).

Innate defence responses are usually time-limited; they are switched on in response to extreme threat and then switched off when the threat has passed. We mention them briefly here because a small percentage of children who present with functional somatic symptoms present with innate defence responses that are being activated frequently or that fail to resolve in a timely manner.

For example, children who frequently activate the tonic immobility defence response (long periods of immobility and non-responsiveness) or the collapsed immobility defence response (episodes of collapse or fainting) are often referred for neurological assessment. The neurologist will typically diagnose non-epileptic seizures (NES), a subtype of functional neurological disorder (FND). In our own clinical practice, most

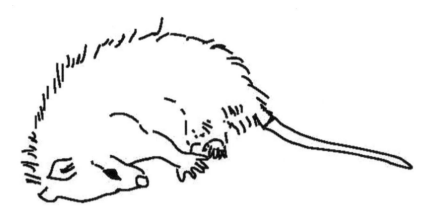

Fig. 11.1 Opossum in collapsed immobility. The opossum's trunk and limbs are limp and immobile. The animal has the appearance of being dead. The terms *death feint* and *playing dead* have been used to describe collapsed immobility in animals. In actual fact, the animals are not playing at anything. Collapsed immobility in animals and humans is totally automatic (unconscious) (*Source* This figure was first published in Kozlowska and colleagues [2015]. © Kasia Kozlowska 2015)

of the children who have presented in this way have a past history of maltreatment or brain pathology that compromises their capacity, in a neurological sense, to respond to stress. See, for example, the case of BJ, a 16-year-old adolescent who manifests a range of innate defence responses in the context of a history of childhood maltreatment, as discussed in Ratnamohan and colleagues (2018), or the vignette of Danae, a 14-year-old adolescent with left cerebral atrophy of unknown origin, as discussed in Kozlowska and colleagues (2015).

When explaining tonic immobility and collapsed immobility to children and their families, we often use videos of animals—for example, the American opossum, which uses the collapsed immobility defence response to protect itself from predators (Fig. 11.1).

We can see the same sort of collapsed immobility in the following vignette of a young boy.

Frank was an 11-year-old boy who lived with his mother. Frank had been exposed to significant domestic violence that had occurred between his mother and one of her previous partners, Don. Frank described one episode of domestic violence in the following words:

Then mum like hit him. Then Don pushed her, then they started hitting each other and slapping each other and hitting. And Don held her around here (pointing to neck) and smashed her into a shelf and walked off and all my stuff fell down on top of her. So then Don, they went to the lounge room and Don, and mum came back in and got the coffee table lid like since it opened up had all this stuff in pulled it back so it smashed down on top of Don's laptop. Then I could hear lots of smashing and lots of stuff being thrown around. Then my mum screamed out 'let go' 'cause she was getting literally pushed down like up against the couch, pushed down in a lock so she couldn't get away. And then um last when Don was about to leave, he had a bleeding lip and mum had bruises all up her arm and stuff. And um we [Frank and his siblings] were just standing there crying.

In the years following the domestic violence, when Frank got stressed, he experienced intrusive memories of the violence. At those times he suffered from disrupted sleep, headaches, vomiting attacks, and bouts of hyperventilation, and sometimes he would collapse to the ground and remain inert for a long period of time. His mother would find him lying collapsed in some part of the house or yard, sometimes in a pool of blood, from a cut on the head or face.

Finally, as noted in Chapter 9, it is possible that children, or at least some children, presenting with fatigue that is unrelenting and completely debilitating have activated the *quiescent immobility* defence response—a biologically ancient response to stress or injury—and have been unable to switch it off (see Chapter 9 for a discussion of chronic fatigue as a homeostatic alarm and for a clinical case scenario). In animals, 'quiescent immobility involves the cessation of all ongoing spontaneous activity, hypo-reactivity (absence of orientation, startle response, and vocalization), hypotension, and bradycardia' (Kozlowska et al. 2015, p. 275). Patients who meet criteria for chronic fatigue syndrome may likewise manifest cessation of spontaneous activity, enter a hypo-metabolic state (Komaroff 2019; Naviaux et al. 2016), and experience autonomic dysregulation that manifests as difficulties in appropriately adjusting blood pressure and heart rate when standing upright or when exercising (see Online Supplement 6.1).

For a detailed description of the way that the innate defence responses present in clinical practice, see 'Fear and the Defense Cascade' (Kozlowska et al. 2015).

The Brain Stuck in Defensive Mode and the Generation of Functional Somatic Symptoms

More commonly, functional somatic symptoms do not involve activation of innate defence responses. Instead, they are generated when the brain stress systems get stuck in defensive mode, setting in motion a range of processes, involving other brain regions, that are maladaptive and that enable functional somatic symptoms to occur. These brain processes are interrelated, interact in non-linear ways, and contribute to changes in brain function and, on a cellular and molecular level, also in brain structure. In this section we briefly discuss some of these interrelated processes. For additional information and references to basic science articles pertaining to each of these subsections, see Online Supplement 11.1.

Aberrant Changes in Neural Activation and Connectivity

A recurring theme from neuroscience studies of patients with functional somatic symptoms is that when the brain stress systems become overactive and over-dominant—that is, get stuck in defensive mode—they over-connect with and disrupt brain regions for motor, sensory, pain, and fatigue processing (Pick et al. 2019; Blakemore et al. 2016; Vachon-Presseau et al. 2016; Sun et al. 2020). Disrupted or aberrant processing within these regions is, in turn, expressed in the individual's *body* as aberrant motor patterns or in her *subjective experience* as aberrant sensory experiences or as feelings of persisting pain or fatigue. Because this aspect of the neuroscience research is easily depicted in visual metaphors, we use it as a foundation for our explanations to children and their families (see later section, 'Metaphors for Explaining Changes in Brain Function to Children with Functional Somatic Symptoms').

Dysregulated Immune-Inflammatory Mechanisms That Amplify and Perpetuate Pain

As we have seen in the clinical vignettes peppered throughout this book, children can present with pain either as the primary presenting symptom or as one among other functional somatic symptoms. When the brain stress systems are stuck in defensive mode, they can maintain activation of the brain's pain maps and the subjective experience of pain (Vachon-Presseau et al. 2016; Ji et al. 2018; Li et al. 2019). Because the brain's immune-inflammatory cells and immune-inflammatory signalling molecules work in tandem with neurons on all levels of the nervous system to activate the pain system, these processes are referred to as *central sensitization* or *neuroimmune dysregulation* on the brain and spinal cord levels, as *neurogenic inflammation* on the tissue level, or simply as *neuroinflammation* within the pain system as a whole (see Chapter 9). Activation of the immune-inflammatory processes at all these levels is implicated in the initiation, amplification, and maintenance of musculoskeletal pain and chronic/complex pain felt in the viscera (abdominal or pelvic cavity).

Plasticity Changes in the Brain and Epigenetics

In Chapter 8 (about the HPA axis), we discussed how cortisol, the end product of the HPA axis, was involved in coordinating plasticity changes—via changes in gene expression (epigenetic mechanisms)—to help the brain and body adapt to stress during the individual's lifetime and across generations. Here we remind the reader that when a child is exposed to stress that is cumulative, recurrent, or overwhelming, the brain itself begins to change in order to make sure that it is adapting to the child's actual life experience and that it is ready to respond to future stress in a robust way. This process, called *experience-dependent plasticity*, involves functional and structural changes of neurons, glial cells, and neuronal circuits that occur in response to experience. It is also part of the brain's adaptive response to chronic stress. Although plasticity changes are occurring in the brain all the time in everyone—which is how cell differentiation, development, and learning take place—plasticity changes acquired in the context of extreme stress can become maladaptive by continuing to affect brain function even when the level of threat has abated. When that happens, the brain stress systems are sensitized to stress and remain ready to respond robustly to each new threat that arises. Even seemingly minor stress, such as a minor injury, an illness, or an event associated with negative emotions, can trigger a stress response far in excess to what is required. In this manner, plasticity changes can contribute to and help maintain maladaptive activation of the brain stress systems, thereby setting the stage for the generation of functional somatic symptoms (Bègue et al. 2019; Ji et al. 2018).

Inefficient Use of Energy Resources

Energy underpins all life processes. *Defensive mode* involves increased utilization of energy resources and a decreased capacity for energy renewal, tissue regeneration, and repair (see also Chapter 4). The use of energy is even greater (and under the circumstances, excessive) when defensive mode persists beyond the presence of the immediate threat. The continuing activation of the brain stress systems requires excess energy, and the patterns of information processing characteristic of defensive mode (think about the grizzly, above) are also associated with increased energy use. Contemporary researchers propose that the brain is well equipped to perform non-conscious analyses pertaining to the energy-related costs and benefits of behaviour. These researchers suggest that the information that an action is not worth performing—that the energy costs involved outweigh benefits—is signalled as the feeling of fatigue (Boksem and Tops 2008, p. 130). In this context, fatigue functions as an adaptive signal—and as an *alarm* signal. When the brain is stuck in defensive mode, and when functional somatic symptoms are being generated, feelings of fatigue may serve as an adaptive signal—an alarm signal (Pedersen 2019) or homeostatic alarm (Wyller 2019) (see Chapter 9)—that activation of the stress system into defensive mode is depleting energy resources and is no longer adaptive.

Aberrant Predictive Representations

The processes of energy regulation and allostasis—the ongoing changes of stress-system activation in response to the challenges of daily living—require the brain to assess information about the external environment and the state of the body, and to predict what is likely to happen next. In the science literature, these initial predictions—which the brain generates automatically without any conscious awareness—are often referred to as *predictive representations*, and the process of generating these representations, as *predictive coding* (Kleckner et al. 2017). This process of predictive coding enables the brain to work efficiently and to conserve energy resources, and the predictive representations generated by this process are continually (and non-consciously) adjusted as the brain compares them to real-time sensory and interoceptive inputs from the world and the body, respectively. By identifying when something new or different or unexpected has occurred, these representations enable the brain to make appropriate adjustments.

Predictive representations contribute to the regulation of, and ongoing changes in, body state. They also contribute to the child's subjective experience of body state, including the homeostatic emotions of pain and fatigue. But like all biological processes, predictive coding can go awry. If the predictions of body state been made by the brain are erroneous—because, for example, they are tailored for a threat-related context that is no longer present—then these erroneous representations will hold priority over afferent inputs, the actual sensory and interoceptive information coming from the body. This priority will hold even when there is a significant mismatch between the erroneous predictive representations and actual body state. Threat-related information is always prioritized by the brain because the consequences of failing to respond to threat may be irreversible—and include the death of the organism.

Although the predictive-coding framework involves predictions that are made by the brain without conscious awareness, the mismatch of the brain's erroneous representations and actual body state sometimes comes into conscious awareness, as we see in the following vignette.

Jai, the 14-year-old boy whom we met in Chapter 5, presented with painful fixed dystonia in the neck, motor weakness and lack of coordination in the legs, and a pain-related curve of the body to the left. He consequently both sat and slept in a C-shape. He could not walk, sit up straight in the wheelchair, or toilet or shower himself. After the clinical team determined that Jai was highly hypnotizable—he could enter the trance state easily—hypnosis was integrated into his occupational therapy and physiotherapy sessions. While Jai was in a trance state, his psychotherapist made suggestions to Jai about his body state—that his body was deeply relaxed, that he could disconnect from the pain, that he could image that his body was bendable like a reed, or that his body could sway like a tree. These suggestions enabled the physiotherapist and occupational therapists to straighten and reposition Jai in the wheelchair. At the end of each session, when Jai was guided out of the trance state, he would suddenly find himself in the non-C-shaped position, and he would panic. He reported that he perceived his body—temporarily straight in the wheelchair—as being bent and wrong. By contrast, his internal perception of the C-shaped position was that his body was straight. Jai was initially unable to utilize any interventions to manage his panic—including suggestions during the trance state that he stay calm—but the length and intensity of the panic gradually settled as he habituated himself to the process of emerging from a trance.

As Jai got better, his subjective experience of his body shape—when straight or bent—progressively normalized. For additional reading material about predictive coding, see Online Supplements 1.3 and 11.1. For a full description of Jai's treatment, see Khachane and colleagues (2019).

Stress-Related Wear and Tear

Stress-related wear and tear is best documented in stress-related conditions such as post-traumatic stress disorder (PTSD) (Miller et al. 2018). Because functional somatic symptoms also involve activation of the brain stress systems into defensive mode over significant periods of time, and because chronic activation of the brain (and body) uses considerably more energy than the brain (and body) in restorative mode, the brain's opportunities for energy renewal, tissue regeneration, and repair are also likely to be restricted. The long-term cost of this activation is known as *wear and tear*, and scientifically as *allostatic load* (see Online Supplement 1.2). Major contributors to this wear and tear in the brain are the adrenal cortisol secreted by the HPA axis in response to prolonged stress (Miller et al. 2018) and the free radicals that are the natural byproduct of energy metabolism in the brain (Salim 2017). These free radicals are more difficult to neutralize when energy use remains high and restorative processes are compromised. Other interrelated processes will no doubt be identified. What is already known and clear, however, is that in the short term, stress-related plasticity changes increase the brain's implicit (non-conscious and automatic) processing capacity, enabling it respond to stress more effectively. If defensive mode is maintained over long periods of time, however, wear and tear may occur, compromising the brain's capacity to regulate body state and to respond to stress in the future.

Key Lessons from This Body of Work

A fundamental lesson from this body of work is that the brain—both brain function and brain structure on the micro level—can change in the context of both positive and adverse experiences. Positive experiences promote good regulation, health, and learning. Adverse experiences— excessive physical or psychological stress—activate changes that are adaptive in the short term but can become maladaptive in the long term, especially if the brain stress systems become stuck in defensive mode. What this means from a practical point of view is that clinicians need to support interventions that will help the child's stress system, including the brain stress systems, shift from defensive mode back to restorative mode. Such interventions may involve the body system level (promoting body states that mobilize restorative and repair processes; see Chapter 14), the mind system level (interventions that use the mind to mobilize restorative and repair processes; see Chapter 15), or the relational system level (interventions that use co-regulation between the child and her caregivers and siblings to mobilize restorative and repair processes; see Chapter 16).

Metaphors for Explaining Changes in Brain Function to Children with Functional Somatic Symptoms

In this section we present some of the visual metaphors that we use with children and their families to communicate key themes from the neuroscience literature concerning the changes in brain function that are associated with functional somatic symptoms. In this context, we discuss three types of functional neurological symptoms (motor symptoms, sensory symptoms, and NES), chronic/complex pain (including syndromes such as fibromyalgia and chronic tension headache), and symptoms of persisting fatigue that accompany other functional somatic symptoms. Our visual metaphors are simple: they try to capture key themes in a way that is, at least in general terms, clinically and scientifically accurate, that is useful for clinicians in their discussions with patients and families, but that avoids details that would likely muddy that communication with unneeded complexities. The goal is to keep one's eye on the ball, and in this context the challenge is to promote shared understandings that enable clinicians, patients, and families to work together and to promote healing. For further reading and basic science articles pertaining to each subsection, see Online Supplement 11.1.

Activation of Brain Stress Systems and Functional *Motor* Symptoms

Functional motor symptoms include limb paralysis, limb weakness, tremor, tic-like movements, functional cough, and dystonia. They fall under the umbrella of FND. When talking to children who have presented with functional motor symptoms, we use the visual metaphor in Fig. 11.2 to discuss research findings from neuroscience and to provide an explanation of what is happening in the brain. The key message for children and families is that functional motor symptoms emerge when the brain stress systems are overactive and over-dominant, and when they over-connect with and disrupt—hijack—motor-processing regions and motor function. Neuroscientist Valerie Voon and colleagues first used the term *hijack* in her wonderful study of motor preparation in patients with functional motor symptoms (Voon et al. 2011). Other references that underpin this visual metaphor are available in Online Supplement 11.1.

Our conversation—in effect, a step-by-step commentary on Fig. 11.2, with the details filled in as we draw—proceeds along the following lines:

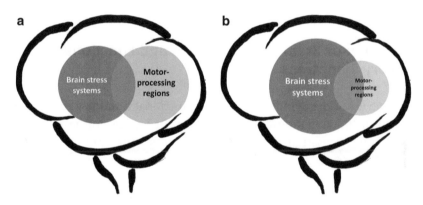

Fig. 11.2 Overactive brain stress systems and motor function. *Frame A*. The red ball represents the brain regions that underpin salience detection, arousal, pain, and emotional states—the *brain stress systems*, for short. The pink ball represents brain areas involved in motor processing—*motor-processing regions*, for short. When all is well, the brain stress systems get on with their job, as do the motor-processing regions, and they interact together in a balanced way (see Online Supplement 11.1 for the brain regions that lie at the intersection of the *brain stress systems* and motor processing). *Frame B*. In functional motor symptoms, the relationship between the brain stress systems and motor-processing regions changes and becomes unbalanced, disrupting or hijacking motor function and activating aberrant motor patterns (functional motor symptoms) (© Kasia Kozlowska 2017)

When everything is going well, the brain stress systems and motor-processing regions in the brain work together in a balanced equal way [draw Frame A]. Sometimes, however, illness, injury, emotional stress, or trauma can *switch on* the brain stress systems and make them bigger and stronger. When this happens, they take over and disrupt the motor-processing regions, and they disrupt motor function and cause all sorts of motor symptoms [draw Frame B]. In your case, the brain stress systems were switched on by [event or series of events from child's history]. They are still switched on now, and they are disrupting your [describe the motor function]. They should have *switched off* when the [trigger or other recent stress] had passed, but they didn't. They have stayed *switched on*. So, we need to do that ourselves, using different types of interventions: *mind-body* interventions help to *switch off* the brain stress systems; *physiotherapy* interventions help your [arms or legs] start working normally again; and *psychological, family*, and *school* interventions help to address the stress in your life.

Activation of Brain Stress Systems and Functional *Sensory* Symptoms

Functional sensory symptoms include functional blindness (or changes in vision), functional deafness (or tinnitus or changes in hearing), and loss of touch sensation in the limbs. Like functional motor symptoms, they fall under the umbrella of FND. The key message for children and families is that functional sensory symptoms emerge when the brain stress systems are overactive and over-dominant, and when they over-connect with and disrupt sensory-processing regions and sensory function (see Fig. 11.3). When using this metaphor, the reader can adapt the language that we set forth above in our example for functional motor symptoms.

Loss of Top-Down Executive Control in Non-epileptic Seizures

NES also fall under the umbrella of FND. Other names for NES are *psychogenic non-epileptic seizures*, *functional seizures*, and *dissociative*

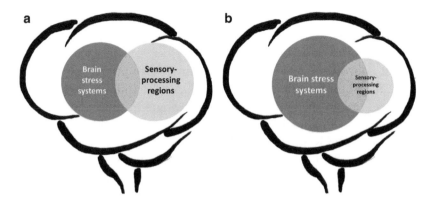

Fig. 11.3 Overactive brain stress systems and sensory function. *Frame A.* The red ball represents the brain stress systems. The yellow ball represents brain areas involved in sensory processing—*sensory-processing regions*, for short. When all is well, the brain stress systems get on with their job, as do the sensory-processing regions, and they interact together in a balanced way. *Frame B.* In functional sensory symptoms, the relationship between the brain stress systems and sensory-processing regions changes and becomes unbalanced, disrupting or hijacking sensory function and activating aberrant sensory patterns (functional sensory symptoms) (© Kasia Kozlowska 2019)

seizures (Asadi-Pooya et al. 2020). NES can occur alongside motor and sensory neurological symptoms, or they may be the sole presenting symptom. NES are paroxysmal: they occur suddenly, in time-limited episodes. Many children are able to identify the approaching onset of NES because they can feel somatic sensations that reflect sudden increases in arousal, what we call their *warning signs*. Common warning signs include increased heat in the chest, sweatiness, nausea, butterflies in the abdomen, feelings of tension or sudden pain in the muscles of the head (or elsewhere), buzzing in the head, muscle twitching or motor agitation (jiggling legs), breathing too fast, dizziness, blurry vision, visual blackout, wobbly legs, being unable to think clearly, an altered state of consciousness (e.g., feeling fuzzy, foggy, disconnected, or floaty, or 'spacing' or 'vagueing out'). Because children can learn to identify interoceptive sensations associated with mounting arousal/motor activation and can then implement arousal-decreasing interventions—before the specific mechanisms that generate their NES are activated—they are able to avert most potential episodes of NES.

In this context, the working hypothesis of the first author (KK) is that sudden increases in arousal disrupt normal brain processes in the prefrontal cortex and also the connectivity between the prefrontal cortex and subcortical regions, and that these disruptions result in the release of motor programs in the basal ganglia, midbrain, and brain stem, resulting in the body movements, changes in tone, and time-limited alterations in consciousness that present as NES (Kozlowska et al. 2018a). For details about the various mechanisms that are thought to contribute to disruption of brain function in NES, see Kozlowska and colleagues (2018a, b) and Szaflarski and LaFrance (2018).

When talking to children who have presented with NES, we use the visual metaphor in Fig. 11.4 to discuss the above-described, hypothetical explanation of what is happening in the brain. For a summary of different types of NES presentations, see Kozlowska and colleagues (2018a).

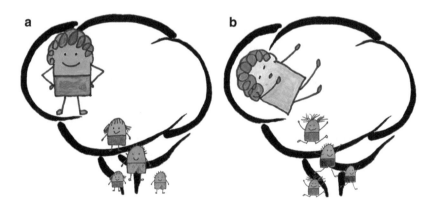

Fig. 11.4 Visual representation of the hypothesized mechanism underpinning non-epileptic seizures. *Frame A.* The mother figure represents the prefrontal cortex, the control area of the brain. The child figures represent motor programs in the basal ganglia, midbrain, and brain stem. When all is well, the mother (prefrontal cortex) maintains control over the children (the motor programs). *Frame B.* In NES, the mother (prefrontal cortex) goes offline in the context of stress-related changes, and the children (motor programs) activate and present as NES (© Kasia Kozlowska 2017)

Our conversation proceeds along the following lines:

In this cartoon the mother figure represents the prefrontal cortex—the control centre of the brain—and the child figures represent motor programs in the lower regions of the brain: the basal ganglia, midbrain, and brain stem. When things are going well, the mother keeps control of the children; that is, the prefrontal cortex maintains control over the motor programs in the basal ganglia, midbrain, and brain stem. But in NES, the mother figure—the prefrontal cortex—gets really stressed, gets overwhelmed, cannot function, and goes *offline*. When this happens, the mother loses control of the children; the motor programs in the basal ganglia, midbrain, and brain stem are out of control. They activate and produce NES. There are lots of things that stress out the prefrontal cortex. In your case, [Here insert the presentation that is relevant for the child. Possibilities include the following: breathing too fast in response to stress (hyperventilating); worrying or recalling bad memories or feelings; sudden pain; or closing vocal cords and shutting off the air passage in response to stress (causing hypoxia).] The team will help you work on catching the warning signs that an NES is coming and on making your brain and body calm, so that you can prevent the NES from happening.

Activation of Brain Stress Systems and Chronic/Complex Pain

The neurobiology of chronic/complex pain that occurs in the absence of tissue injury is complex. Pain is a homeostatic emotion (Craig 2003), an alarm (Wyller 2019) that signals, whether accurately or erroneously, that the body or the self needs protection from threats to its physical or psychological integrity (Moseley and Butler 2015; Brodal 2017). Pain signals are carried by afferent nerves from the body to the spinal cord and by special pain pathways within the spinal cord to the brain. In the brain, pain processing involves a widely distributed network of regions that, in our work with children, we refer to as *pain maps* (for other terminology see Online Supplement 11.1). Pain maps function as an alarm signal. They can be activated by pain signals from the body and by signals from the brain itself—from the brain stress systems. Because of their role as an alarm signal, they are often activated alongside other components of the stress system to signal that the body or the self needs protection from threat. For basic science references about pain-related processes on the brain system level, see Online Supplement 1.3.

Complex/chronic pain is maintained by a number of different inter-acting processes. As we saw, for example, in Chapter 9, chronic/complex pain is maintained when the immune-inflammatory system keeps the pain system activated, across multiple levels of the body system. This process is also known as *neuroimmune dysregulation* because the nervous system and the immune-inflammatory system activate together to maintain a vicious cycle of changes that maintain chronic/complex pain.

Chronic/complex pain is also maintained by (non-conscious) activa-tion of the brain stress systems: when these systems become overactive and over-dominant—that is, get stuck in defensive mode—they over-connect with and activate brain regions involved in pain process-ing. In this way, the subjective experience of pain is both maintained and amplified.

Finally, chronic/complex pain can also be maintained by factors on the mind level of operations—attention to pain, catastrophizing, and negative emotions—because these processes operate in a top-down manner to activate the brain stress systems, which, in turn, maintain activation of pain maps (see Chapter 12).

When talking to children who present with chronic/complex pain, we use the visual metaphor depicted in Fig. 11.5.

Our conversation proceeds along the following lines:

When everything is going well, the pain maps in the brain, the parts of the brain that allow us to feel pain, are switched off. When everything is going well, the brain stress systems, the parts of the brain that switch on with stress, are also switched off. When I say *stress*, I mean anything that is stressful for the body, including illness, injury, emotional stress, or trauma. But when we experience stress, we *switch on* the brain stress sys-tems. They become active, big and strong. And then after the stress has gone, the brain stress systems should switch off. But sometimes they fail to switch off, and because they have a close relationship with the pain maps, they can switch them on, too (or keep them switched on)—even when your body has healed or is not injured at all. And the pain maps make you feel pain. From the story you told me, it seems that in your

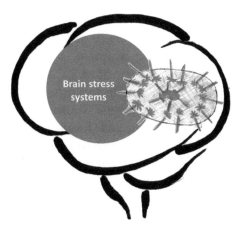

Fig. 11.5 Overactive brain stress systems and the subjective experience of pain. The red ball represents the brain stress systems. The spiky ball represents pain-processing regions—*pain maps*, for short. The overlap between the balls represents what the pain literature sometimes refers to as the emotional, affective, or aversive dimension of pain (see Online Supplement 11.1). In chronic/complex pain the brain stress systems become overactive and over-dominant, and they drive and amplify the pain experience (© Kasia Kozlowska 2019)

case the brain stress systems were switched on by [event or series of events from child's history]. They are still switched on now, and they are keeping your pain maps activated and signalling pain: like a pain-alarm system that cannot be switched off. So, treatment involves *mind-body* interventions that help to *switch off* the brain stress systems, because they are keeping the pain maps switched on; *physiotherapy* interventions that help you to keep up your level of fitness and to assist your body in fighting—switching off—the pain maps [see discussion of macrophages in Chapter 9]; *psychological* interventions that help switch off the pain maps and help to address the stress in your life; and family and school interventions that help support you in the best way possible.

Activation of Brain Stress Systems and Fatigue

Fatigue is a common comorbid symptom in children presenting with functional somatic symptoms. For example, in the clinical practice of the first author, fatigue is also reported by a quarter to half of the children presenting with FND and two-thirds of children presenting with chronic/complex pain. The term *chronic fatigue syndrome* is used when fatigue is the primary presenting symptom, and when the child meets the available symptom-based criteria (of which there are several versions) (Gluckman 2018; Knight et al. 2019). In this section we discuss fatigue in a general way and not chronic fatigue syndrome per se (see Chapter 9 for a discussion of persisting fatigue and chronic fatigue syndrome).

In the brain, fatigue processing involves a widely distributed network of regions (Boksem and Tops 2008; Noakes 2012), which, in our work with children, we refer to as the *fatigue alarm system* or the *fatigue alarm*. Fatigue, like pain, is a homeostatic alarm (Wyller 2019) that signals, whether accurately or erroneously, either an urgent homeostatic imbalance (Hilty et al. 2011, p. 2151) or an urgent need to protect the body's energy resources (Boksem and Tops 2008). In the context of stress, whether physical or psychological, and when the brain stress systems shift into and get *stuck* in defensive mode, the fatigue alarm is frequently activated. The fatigue alarm signals the loss of physiological coherence: the easy flow of life processes, harmony between body systems, and efficient utilization of energy are all lost when the stress system shifts from restorative mode and gets stuck in defensive mode. In this way, the fatigue alarm signals that the brain stress systems have been activated too much, for too long, or too frequently and that they need assistance to help them shift back into restorative mode and regain physiological coherence (as described above). For other metaphors for discussing persisting fatigue, see Chapter 9.

When talking to children who present with comorbid fatigue, we use the visual metaphor depicted in Fig. 11.6.

Our conversation proceeds along the following lines:

The biology of fatigue is very complicated, and scientists are still trying to work it out. The current thinking is that fatigue—like pain—is one of the body's alarm systems. The fatigue alarm allows us to feel fatigue. And the feeling of fatigue tells us many things. Sometimes the fatigue alarm tells us when the body has used up too much energy and it is time to stop. Sometimes the fatigue alarm tells us that it is time to go to sleep— to rest and to make energy for the next day. Sometimes the fatigue alarm tells us that our brain stress systems and our body stress systems have been

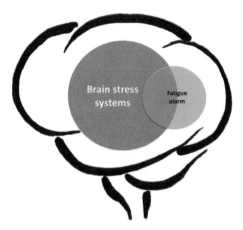

Fig. 11.6 Overactive brain stress systems and the fatigue alarm. The red ball represents the brain stress systems. The green ball represents the fatigue alarm. When the brain stress systems (and other components of the stress system) are activated by infection, illness, injury, or emotional stress, and when they get stuck in defensive mode, the fatigue alarm activates to signal the loss of physiological coherence—the loss of easy flow of life processes, harmony between body systems, and efficient utilization of energy—that occurs when the stress system shifts from restorative mode and gets stuck in defensive mode (© Kasia Kozlowska 2019)

activated too much and too long. As you already know, the brain stress systems and body stress systems include all the parts of the brain and body that activate with physical or emotional stress—illness, injury, emotional stress, or trauma. The stress system uses a lot of energy. That's why, when the stress system is switched on, the fatigue alarm is often switched on, too. The fatigue alarm signals that the stress system is hard at work (and maybe even a bit too hard at work) and that we need to take care of the stress and also to help the stress system switch off. This is why fatigue is so common in children who have [put in child's presentation, such as FND, chronic/complex pain, autonomic activation/dysregulation]. The treatment for your fatigue involves *mind-body* interventions that help to *switch off* the brain-body stress systems; *physiotherapy* interventions that help you keep up your level of fitness, that switch off pain, and that promote health and well-being; *psychological* interventions that help address the stress in your life; and family and school interventions that help support you in the best way possible. Once the brain-body stress systems have switched off, and your body has returned to a healthy way of being, your fatigue alarm will also switch off, and your feelings of fatigue will go away, too.

Combining Metaphors

In the previous subsections we have provided metaphors for different types of functional somatic symptoms. In real life, however, children present with multiple somatic symptoms. It may therefore be necessary to combine metaphors or even to use two different types of metaphor together—for example, the circles metaphor of the stress system, together with one of the metaphors specific to FND, pain, or fatigue. Figure 11.7 shows the combination of metaphors for a child presenting

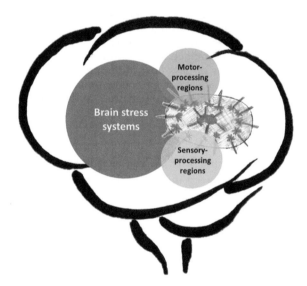

Fig. 11.7 Overactive brain stress systems, disrupted motor and sensory function, and the subjective experience of pain. The red ball represents the *brain stress systems*. The pink ball represents *motor-processing regions*; the yellow ball represents *sensory-processing regions*; and the spiky ball represents *pain maps*. When the *brain stress systems* are activated by infection, illness, injury, or emotional stress, they become overactive and over-dominant, disrupt motor and sensory processing, and amplify pain processing, causing functional motor and sensory symptoms and amplifying feelings of pain (© Kasia Kozlowska 2019)

with functional motor symptoms, functional sensory symptoms, and chronic/complex pain.

Problems with Memory and Concentration

Many patients with functional somatic symptoms report problems with memory and concentration, and families frequently ask about these symptoms. For example, in our study cohorts of children with FND, approximately one-fifth of children present with some sort of memory loss—failing to recognize their parents, siblings, or friends—or showing a sudden loss in some aspect of their academic function, as in speaking, reading, or writing. Likewise, memory and concentration difficulties are a key element in children whose main presenting symptom is persistent fatigue.

When talking to children whose presentations include difficulties with memory and concentration, we discuss the many different ways in which an activated stress system can interfere with cognitive function. We also tell families that this is an area of current research. Factors that are known to contribute to cognitive difficulties include the following:

- disturbed sleep (see Chapter 5)
- increased cortisol levels secondary to HPA-axis activation (high cortisol levels disturb functioning in the executive regions of the brain) (see Chapter 8)
- increased levels of stress hormones (noradrenalin, endogenous opioids, endogenous cannabinoids, and other anaesthetic neurochemicals) that are secreted as part of the brain's stress response during states of high arousal (these stress hormones likewise disturb functioning in the executive regions of the brain) (Lanius et al. 2014)
- chronic or episodic hyperventilation (see Chapter 7).

For additional reading materials pertaining to the impact of stress on cognitive function, see Online Supplement 11.1.

* * *

In this chapter we have highlighted that all functional somatic symptoms involve activation or dysregulation of the brain stress systems. The brain stress systems play a key role in initiating, amplifying, and maintaining functional somatic symptoms. We have also provided clinicians working with children and families with simple metaphors to discuss research findings from neuroscience and to provide an explanation of what is happening in the brain. All the processes discussed in this chapter have been non-conscious—the implicit level of brain operations—and have involved processes that the brain engages in spontaneously, by itself. Humans also have the capacity, however, to generate conscious representations that affect body state and that contribute to the generation of functional somatic symptoms. We look at this mind level of brain operations—psychological factors—in the next chapter.

References

Arnsten, A. F. (2015). Stress Weakens Prefrontal Networks: Molecular Insults to Higher Cognition. *Nature Neuroscience, 18,* 1376–1385.

Asadi-Pooya, A. A., Brigo, F., Mildon, B., & Nicholson, T. R. (2020). Terminology for Psychogenic Nonepileptic Seizures: Making the Case for "Functional Seizures". *Epilepsy & Behavior, 104,* 106895.

Bègue, I., Adams, C., Stone, J., & Perez, D. L. (2019). Structural Alterations in Functional Neurological Disorder and Related Conditions: A Software and Hardware Problem? *NeuroImage. Clinical, 22,* 101798.

Blakemore, R. L., Sinanaj, I., Galli, S., Aybek, S., & Vuilleumier, P. (2016). Aversive Stimuli Exacerbate Defensive Motor Behaviour in Motor Conversion Disorder. *Neuropsychologia, 93,* 229–241.

Boksem, M. A., & Tops, M. (2008). Mental Fatigue: Costs and Benefits. *Brain Research Reviews, 59,* 125–139.

Brodal, P. (2017). A Neurobiologist's Attempt to Understand Persistent Pain. *Scandinavian Journal of Pain, 15,* 140–147.

Chrousos, G. P., & Gold, P. W. (1998). A Healthy Body in a Healthy Mind—And Vice Versa—The Damaging Power of "Uncontrollable" Stress. *Journal of Clinical Endocrinology and Metabolism, 83,* 1842–1845.

Craig, A. D. (2003). A New View of Pain as a Homeostatic Emotion. *Trends in Neurosciences, 26,* 303–307.

Gluckman, S. J. (2018). *Clinical Features and Diagnosis of Myalgic Encephalomyelitis/Chronic Fatigue Syndrome.* https://www.uptodate.com/contents/clinical-features-and-diagnosis-of-myalgic-encephalomyelitis-chronic-fatigue-syndrome.

Hilty, L., Jancke, L., Luechinger, R., Boutellier, U., & Lutz, K. (2011). Limitation of Physical Performance in a Muscle Fatiguing Handgrip Exercise Is Mediated by Thalamo-Insular Activity. *Human Brain Mapping, 32,* 2151–2160.

Ji, R. R., Nackley, A., Huh, Y., Terrando, N., & Maixner, W. (2018). Neuroinflammation and Central Sensitization in Chronic and Widespread Pain. *Anesthesiology, 129,* 343–366.

Khachane, Y., Kozlowska, K., Savage, B., McClure, G., Butler, G., Gray, N., et al. (2019). Twisted in Pain: The Multidisciplinary Treatment Approach to Functional Dystonia. *Harvard Review of Psychiatry, 27,* 359–381. https://pubmed.ncbi.nlm.nih.gov/31714467/.

Kleckner, I. R., Zhang, J., Touroutoglou, A., Chanes, L., Xia, C., Simmons, W. K., et al. (2017). Evidence for a Large-Scale Brain System Supporting Allostasis and Interoception in Humans. *Nature Human Behaviour, 1,* 0069.

Knight, S., Elders, S., Rodda, J., Harvey, A., Lubitz, L., Rowe, K., et al. (2019). Epidemiology of Paediatric Chronic Fatigue Syndrome in Australia. *Archives of Disease in Childhood, 104,* 733–738.

Koch, C. (1993). When Looking Is Not Seeing: Towards a Neurobiological View of Awareness. *Engineering & Science,* Spring, 2–13.

Komaroff, A. L. (2019, July 5). Advances in Understanding the Pathophysiology of Chronic Fatigue Syndrome. *JAMA* (Epub ahead of print).

Kozlowska, K., Chudleigh, C., Cruz, C., Lim, M., McClure, G., Savage, B., et al. (2018a). Psychogenic Non-epileptic Seizures in Children and Adolescents: Part I—Diagnostic Formulations. *Clinical Child Psychology and Psychiatry, 23,* 140–159.

Kozlowska, K., Chudleigh, C., Cruz, C., Lim, M., McClure, G., Savage, B., et al. (2018b). Psychogenic Non-epileptic Seizures in Children and Adolescents: Part II—Explanations to Families, Treatment, and Group Outcomes. *Clinical Child Psychology and Psychiatry, 23,* 160–176.

Kozlowska, K., Walker, P., Mclean, L., & Carrive, P. (2015). Fear and the Defense Cascade: Clinical Implications and Management. *Harvard Review of Psychiatry, 23,* 263–287. https://www.ncbi.nlm.nih.gov/pmc/articles/PMC4495877/.

Lanius, U. F., Corrigan, F. M., & Paulsen, S. L. (2014). *Neurobiology and Treatment of Traumatic Dissociation: Toward an Embodied Self.* New York: Springer.

Li, T., Chen, X., Zhang, C., Zhang, Y., & Yao, W. (2019). An Update on Reactive Astrocytes in Chronic Pain. *Journal of Neuroinflammation, 16,* 140.

McEwen, B. S. (2009). The Brain Is the Central Organ of Stress and Adaptation. *Neuroimage, 47,* 911–913.

Miller, M. W., Lin, A. P., Wolf, E. J., & Miller, D. R. (2018). Oxidative Stress, Inflammation, and Neuroprogression in Chronic PTSD. *Harvard Review of Psychiatry, 26,* 57–69.

Moseley, G. L., & Butler, D. S. (2015). Fifteen Years of Explaining Pain: The Past, Present, and Future. *Journal of Pain, 16,* 807–813.

Naviaux, R. K., Naviaux, J. C., Li, K., Bright, A. T., Alaynick, W. A., Wang, L., et al. (2016). Metabolic Features of Chronic Fatigue Syndrome. *Proceedings of the National Academy of Sciences of the United States of America, 113,* E5472–E5480.

Noakes, T. D. (2012). Fatigue Is a Brain-Derived Emotion That Regulates the Exercise Behavior to Ensure the Protection of Whole Body Homeostasis. *Frontiers in Physiology, 3,* 82.

Pedersen, M. (2019, June 29). Chronic Fatigue Syndrome and Chronic Pain Conditions—Vitally Protective Systems Gone Wrong. *Scandinavian Journal of Pain* (Epub ahead of print).

Pervanidou, P., & Chrousos, G. P. (2018). Early-Life Stress: From Neuroendocrine Mechanisms to Stress-Related Disorders. *Hormone Research in Paediatrics, 89,* 372–379.

Picard, M., McEwen, B. S., Epel, E. S., & Sandi, C. (2018). An Energetic View of Stress: Focus on Mitochondria. *Frontiers in Neuroendocrinology, 49,* 72–85.

Pick, S., Goldstein, L. H., Perez, D. L., & Nicholson, T. R. (2019). Emotional Processing in Functional Neurological Disorder: A Review, Biopsychosocial Model and Research Agenda. *Journal of Neurology, Neurosurgery and Psychiatry, 90,* 704–711.

Ratnamohan, L., MacKinnon, L., Lim, M., Webster, R., Waters, K., Kozlowska, K., et al. (2018). Ambushed by Memories of Trauma: Memory-Processing Interventions in an Adolescent Boy with Nocturnal Dissociative Episodes. *Harvard Review of Psychiatry, 26,* 228–236.

Salim, S. (2017). Oxidative Stress and the Central Nervous System. *Journal of Pharmacology and Experimental Therapeutics, 360,* 201–205.

Sun, X., Pan, X., Ni, K., Ji, C., Wu, J., Yan, C., et al. (2020). Aberrant Thalamic-Centered Functional Connectivity in Patients with Persistent Somatoform Pain Disorder. *Neuropsychiatric Disease and Treatment, 16,* 273–281.

Szaflarski, J. P., and LaFrance, W. C., Jr. (2018). Psychogenic Nonepileptic Seizures (PNES) as a Network Disorder—Evidence from Neuroimaging of Functional (Psychogenic) Neurological Disorders. *Epilepsy Currents, 18*, 211–216.

Vachon-Presseau, E., Centeno, M. V., Ren, W., Berger, S. E., Tetreault, P., Ghantous, M., et al. (2016). The Emotional Brain as a Predictor and Amplifier of Chronic Pain. *Journal of Dental Research, 95*, 605–612.

Voon, V., Brezing, C., Gallea, C., & Hallett, M. (2011). Aberrant Supplementary Motor Complex and Limbic Activity During Motor Preparation in Motor Conversion Disorder. *Movement Disorders, 26*, 2396–2403.

Wyller, V. B. B. (2019). Pain Is Common in Chronic Fatigue Syndrome—Current Knowledge and Future Perspectives. *Scandinavian Journal of Pain, 19*, 5–8.

12

The Brain Stress Systems II: The Mind Level of Brain Operations

Abstract In this chapter we continue our exploration of the neuro-biology of functional somatic symptoms by considering the mind level of brain operations. Consciousness—the state of being aware, especially (for our purposes) of something within oneself—adds another dimension to the neurobiological systems that regulate body state. Among the objects of consciousness are feelings such as those pertaining to well-being and to dis-ease: pain, nausea, malaise, and fatigue. These feelings are mental representations of body state, a gestalt-like summary that integrates information from all levels of body regulation and that reflects the sum and substance of the individual as a whole. Feelings are consequently the end result of myriad interrelated processes: homeostatic information from the body itself (Chapters 6–10); spinal cord and implicit brain processes involved in both representing and regulating body state (Chapter 11); and—the subject of the present chapter—the

Electronic supplementary material The online version of this chapter (https://doi.org/10.1007/978-3-030-46184-3_12) contains supplementary material, which is available to authorized users.

© The Author(s) 2020   **251**
K. Kozlowska et al., *Functional Somatic Symptoms in Children
and Adolescents*, Palgrave Texts in Counselling and Psychotherapy,
https://doi.org/10.1007/978-3-030-46184-3_12

mind level of brain operations, including cognitive and attentional processes. These mind-level operations affect all of those other processes in a top-down manner and can alter feelings of body state in powerful ways that incline the child either toward health and well-being or toward ill health and dis-ease.

Perceiving the Body: The Role of Feelings

Consciousness refers to our state of being aware—especially (for our purposes) of something within oneself; it adds another dimension to the neurobiological systems that regulate body state. Among the objects of consciousness are *feelings*. Following Antonio Damasio's terminology, we conceptualize feelings as mental representations of body states: the idea, thought, or perception of the body being in a certain way (Damasio 2003). *Homeostatic feelings* are the particular focus of our attention here. They are mental representations regarding the safety and stability of the body's internal state, such as temperature, pain, nausea, fatigue, itch, visceral distension, muscle ache, hunger, thirst, and 'air hunger' (Craig 2002; Pace-Schott et al. 2019). 'They translate the ongoing life state in the language of the mind' (Damasio 2003, p. 85). These feelings, together with thoughts, mental and sensory images, and other conscious mental phenomena, make up what we recognize as the 'stream of mind' (Damasio 2003, p. 197). Throughout this chapter we use the terms *mental representations of body state, perceptions of body state*, and *feelings* interchangeably. For reading materials about consciousness, see Online Supplement 12.1.

In the normal course of events, the neurophysiological processes that support feelings are ones that function in the background, with no conscious awareness. These processes involve the following structures: nociceptors, thermoreceptors, osmoreceptors, and metaboreceptors; afferent nerve fibres that carry their signals; brain regions that map body state at different levels of processing; and brain regions that check and make adjustments for any discrepancies between the brain's predictions regarding the upcoming needs of the body and the actual incoming information about body state. When feelings emerge, they flag, in effect, that a given situation is important in one way or another.

> They signify physiological need (for example, hunger), tissue injury (for example, [acute] pain), optimal [well-regulated] function (for example, well-being), threats to the organism (for example, fear or anger) or specific social interactions (for example, compassion, gratitude or love). Feelings constitute a crucial component of the mechanisms of life regulation, from simple to complex. Their neural substrates can be found at all levels of the nervous system, from individual neurons to subcortical nuclei and cortical regions. (Damasio and Carvalho 2013, p. 143)

Damasio's systemic framework provides us with a way of thinking about feelings on different levels of complexity (see Damasio [2003]). On the simplest level, the feeling may be solely the perception of a certain body state (Damasio 2003, p. 89). Here, feelings function to 'amplify the impact of a given situation, enhance learning, and increase the probability that comparable situations can be anticipated' (Damasio 2001, p. 781). For example, when our child (including adolescent) patients experience symptoms related to hyperventilation, the feelings they experience and describe all reflect the conscious perception of the physiological changes in body state caused by hyperventilation. These homeostatic feelings may include one of more of the following: buzzing in the head; varying degrees of reduction in the level of consciousness, described as dizziness, lightheadedness, giddiness, or faintness; blurring of vision; dryness of the mouth; numbness and tingling of the hands, feet, and face; stiffness of the muscles; and tetany. As the children learn to attend to these changes in body state and, in turn, to recognize the changes as a product of hyperventilation, they can undertake measures—mind-body interventions learnt as part of their treatment process—to control their dysregulated breathing, to change their physiological state, and to rid themselves of the particular homeostatic feeling (see Chapter 14).

On the next level, 'a feeling is the perception of a certain state of the body along with the perception of a certain mode of thinking and of thoughts with certain themes' (Damasio 2003, p. 86). Here, mental representations of body state are modulated by other processes that occur on the mind level of operations—processes that occur as part of a person's stream of mind. Examples from athletics are helpful in this context. A person who runs daily might, at some point, feel (on the first level, as above) somewhat fatigued but might also recognize that she is running especially well on that particular day. This additional layer will likely enable her to keep running and to actually feel less fatigued than she would on a 'standard' day of running. Going one step further, it has been shown that athletes have greater endurance when they are timing their efforts against a clock that has been calibrated to run slowly, creating the false impression that they have not been exercising as long as they actually have. Even intentional, known distractions or deceptions have an impact. Athletes are able to modify their feelings of fatigue by distracting themselves with music or by using a mirror to observe the non-fatigued arm when working with the opposite arm (see Noakes [2012] for review). Evie—the 15-year-old girl presenting with precordial catch syndrome and non-epileptic seizures (NES) whom we met in Chapter 9—described how her feelings of extreme pain were always accompanied by thoughts with certain themes.

> When Evie experienced the bubble feeling of exploding pain in her chest, she would experience a negative mode of thinking and thoughts with negative themes: 'I can't stand this; I want to die; I hate myself; who invented this stupid thing; of all people I got this; I want to kill myself.' The pain and thoughts combined would trigger an NES. When the NES was over, the negative feelings remained. It would take some hours before the feelings of being overwhelmed and suicidal actually ebbed. [See Chapter 2 for history of Evie's presentation.]

On the final level, feelings can be generated by the brain itself—what Damasio calls the *as-if-loop mechanisms*. In this scenario, the brain can create mental representations of body state that do not correspond to the current reality of the body. This capacity enables us to feel empathy with others, to feel hope for the future, to shift our mind into 'wellness-thinking', and to use the felt experience of an anticipated future event to help optimize decision making (see vignette of Evie, below). Nevertheless, this same capacity to simulate feelings can contribute to feelings of pain when no injury exists, feelings of fatigue when exertion has been minimal, and feelings of nausea unconnected to current experience. The simulation of feelings can also shift one's mind into 'illness thinking' or generate felt fears or concerns about the future that impair or distort decision making.

In the following vignette, we see how a child used an as-if-loop mechanism to disrupt an emerging body state top-down.

> Together with her therapists (the first author [KK] and a psychologist), Evie sequenced the temporal order of sensations: hot inside/cold outside, followed by tingling in the left arm, blurred vision, and perceived shortness of breath, along with burning in the throat and lump in throat, culminating in the pain bubble 'exploding' in her chest (*precordial catch pain*). Evie then practiced the implementation of a visualization—which invoked pleasant feelings via the *as-if-loop mechanism*—and was able, with time, to avert the tension pattern that progressed within her mediastinum and that culminated in the bubble feeling of exploding pain in her chest.

Cognitive processes appear to have a profound impact on body state in and of themselves. Anticipation of pain activates the amygdalae (part of the brain stress systems) (Strigo et al. 2010). Negative appraisals of a situation can activate the autonomic system top-down (Gianaros and Wager 2015). Catastrophizing activates posterior regions of the brain stress systems (Lee et al. 2018). In patients with chronic/complex pain, catastrophizing and attention to pain increase activation in the insulae (also part of the brain stress systems) (Kim et al. 2015). And in the case of patients who persistently worry about body symptoms that resemble, and are misinterpreted as, known medical diseases, findings on functional MRI (fMRI) show that the brain stress systems are overactive and over-dominant, and over-connect with motor- and sensory-processing regions (Kim et al. 2019b).

What emerges from these examples and this three-tiered typology of feelings is a recognition that feelings, except at the lowest level involving direct perception of body state, are the product of dynamic interactions between physiological states, neural maps of physiological states, perceptions of physiological states, and wide-ranging cognitive processes. More concretely, the mind level of brain operations—how the child thinks about herself and her functional somatic symptoms, how she processes the stressful events in her life, how she is influenced by her own moods, and the role of previous experience and learning—has a potentially profound impact on the child's perceptions (feelings) of body state, on the body state itself, and even on her functional somatic symptoms. These interconnections among feeling, thinking, and functional somatic symptoms are the focus of the present chapter.

The Influence of Conscious Processes on Functional Somatic Symptoms

Within the field of developmental psychology, a child's ability to control her thoughts, feelings, and focus of attention using top-down cognitive processes falls under the umbrella term of *self-regulation* (Posner 2012). By now the reader is well aware that in this book we use the term *self-regulation* much more broadly to include both top-down and bottom-up processes. In Chapters 5–11, we have already seen that children with functional somatic symptoms show significant difficulties with self-regulation on the body level and on the implicit level of brain operations. In the following subsections we shall see that children with functional somatic symptoms also struggle with regulation on the mind level of brain operations and that these difficulties contribute to the children's perceptions (feelings) of body state. Although we discuss conscious processes using commonly used constructs, it is important to emphasize that many of the constructs are overlapping and interdependent, and that in clinical practice they are often impossible to separate and need to be managed in tandem.

Attention

'Everyone knows what attention is. It is the taking possession by the mind, in clear and vivid form, of one out of what seem several simultaneously possible objects or trains of thought' (James 1890, pp. 403–404). In this statement, William James was referring to what researchers now refer to as focal attention mediated by the executive attention network (Posner 2012), a network of brain regions that enable attention to be voluntarily directed and sustained on the mind level of brain operations, thereby bringing objects of consciousness into focus.

Attention plays a key role in determining how information about body state is processed. Focusing one's attention onto a body part increases blood flow in that part of the body (Darwin 1872). Bringing attention to body sensations biases the processing of selected stimuli, increases neural mapping at multiple levels, and is accompanied by changes the individual's perception (feelings) of body state (Bauer et al. 2014; Kim et al. 2019a). By filtering out competing sensory inputs, attention facilitates synchrony between groups of neurons; attentional processes can enhance sensory, motor, and cognitive processes by activating and strengthening synaptic linkages between neurons and by enhancing communication (connectivity) between brain regions. But attentional processes can also be maladaptive. In children with functional somatic symptoms, attention to symptoms can presumably enhance aberrant interoceptive, sensory, motor, and perceptual processes by activating and strengthening aberrant synaptic linkages between groups of neurons and by enhancing connectivity between brain regions involved in symptom production. These linkages will need to be weakened or deactivated if health and well-being are to be restored.

The important role of attention in worsening or maintaining functional somatic symptoms in children is well documented (Walker et al. 2006; Palermo et al. 2014). For example, functional neurological symptoms typically increase in severity with attention and decrease in severity or even disappear when the child is paying attention elsewhere (Faust and Soman 2012; Stone 2014). A similar pattern is typical in children who present with chronic pain or persisting fatigue. Very often the pain or fatigue is most evident when the child is attending to the symptom or when a parent or doctor is asking about it, and least evident when the child is engaged in, and attending to, an activity that she enjoys. In this context, once the diagnostic assessment has been completed, an explanation and diagnosis has been provided, and treatment has been initiated, ongoing attention to functional symptoms, rather than to the interventions that can make the symptoms better, is generally counter-productive. Such symptom-focused attention, whether by the child, parent, doctors, or self-help group, will have the effect of making the symptoms worse and potentially chronic.

Johnny was a 9-year-old boy with a three-year history of functional gut symptoms (abdominal pain, nausea, and diarrhoea), six-month history of whole-body jerking, and three-month history of episodes of chest pain during which Johnny felt he could not breathe, was dizzy and light-headed, and had intermittent loss of vision. More recently, Johnny's pain had begun to migrate over his whole body, and he began to experience periods of arm and leg paralysis that lasted up to six hours. Despite Johnny's many visits to the family doctor, emergency department, and paediatrician, the doctors said that Johnny's physical examination was normal, that all his tests were normal, and that they could find noth-ing wrong. Johnny's parents were unable to accept the medical verdict because they had to manage Johnny's symptoms on a daily basis and knew that the symptoms were real and functionally impairing. Despite repeated physical examinations and tests, Johnny's parents became more and more worried that some serious medical condition had being missed. They paid Johnny's symptoms more and more attention; they asked about the symptoms many times a day; and when new symptoms appeared, they filmed them. Johnny also was worried about his symptoms. He did not tell his parents, but secretly he thought he had some terrible disease and was going to die. In this highly charged context, in which Johnny's symptoms received constant attention, the symptoms progressively wors-ened, and with increasing frequency Johnny used a wheelchair to move around at school.

Raymond was a 12-year-old boy with a long history of anxiety, begin-ning with severe separation anxiety at ten months of age. Two years ago, prior to admission to the Mind-Body Program, he started to experience transient, recurring functional somatic symptoms—joint pains, bilat-eral leg weakness, and losses of vision—all in the context of significant family stress related to parental illness. Six months prior to admission, he began to experience stronger, more persistent pain in his right knee. Because weight bearing caused Raymond pain, he avoided using his right leg whenever possible, keeping it still and also elevating it if possible. With time, Raymond developed chronic regional pain syndrome (CRPS) with secondary complications related to his avoidance of weight bearing on his right leg (loss of bone density in the right femur and decreased range of movement in the ankle joint, documented under general anaesthetic). Raymond was admitted into the Mind-Body Program to treat his CRPS and transient losses of vision. Raymond now also reported severe pain in his right foot, and he refused to put any weight on it. His anticipatory anxiety was so great that he would begin to yell and scream—and to hide from the physiotherapist—as the time of his physiotherapy session approached. During some of these episodes, he also reported a loss of vision: 'I can't see, I can't see.'

Despite all the above, Raymond enjoyed therapy sessions with his psychologist, especially those in which his therapist used hypnosis. In one hypnosis session the role of attention in amplifying Raymond's pain was made especially clear. After inducing a trance state, the therapist suggested that Raymond relax his body and let the tension go. Raymond's body became progressively more relaxed. When the therapist focused Raymond's attention to the right foot—by making a direct suggestion pertaining to the foot—Raymond became agitated, his body made small jerky movements, and he began to pick at his arms, legs, and face. After coming out of the trance state, Raymond noted that as soon as the therapist had shifted his attention to his foot, the pain in the leg had spiked.

Hypervigilance to Threat, Negative Appraisal Processes, and Rumination

The appraisal and coping framework was put forward by Lazarus and his colleagues in a number of landmark publications (Lazarus 1966; Lazarus and Folkman 1984). *Appraisal processes* ascribe meaning, including threat-related meaning, to events in the external world, to body sensations, and to other images in the stream of mind—thoughts, memories, narratives, or other images—that arise at the mind level of brain operations. Primary appraisal processes include magnification and rumination, and secondary appraisal processes include helplessness. In this framework, these two types of processes work together to determine whether—and, if so, which—coping strategies will be employed.

Since the introduction of the appraisal and coping framework in the 1960s, rapid advances have been made in understanding the neurobiology of appraisal processes. We now know that the medial prefrontal cortex (part of the brain stress systems) is involved both in appraising information and in activating the efferent component of the autonomic system that fine-tunes body state on a second-by-second basis. What this means in practice is that when a child ascribes a threat-related meaning to an event, body sensation, or mental image, the prefrontal cortex will automatically *switch on* the autonomic nervous system component of the stress system and activate the body to prepare it for the upcoming threat (see Gianaros and Wager [2015] for review). These couplings between appraisals and body states establish brain-body pathways linking psychological stress—the threat-related meaning ascribed to events and mental images—and body state. In this way, the cognitive act of appraising events and mental images as threatening will activate the brain-body stress systems and, in particular children, will contribute to the generation and maintenance of functional somatic symptoms. By the same token, altering the cognitive appraisal of events and mental images—so that they are no longer seen as threatening—will help to decrease and even extinguish functional somatic symptoms. Accordingly, maladaptive appraisal processes are an important target of therapeutic intervention.

An ample literature suggests that maladaptive patterns of stress appraisal by children or their parents are associated with less healthy coping strategies, the development of functional somatic symptoms, and greater functional disability (Williams et al. 2011; Walker et al. 2007; Wallrath et al. 2019). Likewise, the importance of maladaptive appraisal processes and rumination has also been documented in adult patients with NES (see summary in Testa et al. [2012]), in patients with chronic fatigue (see summary in Meeus et al. [2010]), and chronic pain conditions more generally (see Jackson et al. [2014] and Kim et al. [2015]). In patients with chronic pain, threat appraisals have positive overall correlations with pain intensity, impairment, affective distress, and passive coping, and such appraisals are negatively related to active coping (Jackson et al. 2014).

In the vignettes below, we highlight how these processes emerge in daily clinical practice. For more about meaning making as part of family or individual narratives about the meaning of certain events (whether single events or longer series of interconnected events, as in a family history or one's life story), see Online Supplement 12.1.

Hypervigilance to threat. Zia was a 13-year-old girl who presented with headaches, dizziness, recurrent fainting and collapse events, and weakness in her legs. Zia lived with her father and her three brothers. During Zia's preschool years, all the children had been exposed to substantial abuse and neglect. Each morning, Zia and her siblings made the ten-minute walk from the family home to the bus station to catch a bus to school. Before leaving the house each morning, Zia's father would warn his children to stick together and keep an eye out for one another. Upon walking out the front door of their home, Zia was immediately on high alert for any unusual or sudden noises or dangerous-looking strangers. At the bus station and on the bus itself, she would scan the street and the bus for any person who appeared dangerous or threatening, for anyone who could hurt or threaten her brothers, and for anyone who looked like a potential child molester. If a stranger looked dangerous, Zia would move her brothers away. On the way home from school, Zia remained on high alert. Once home, Zia would collapse in a heap on the couch, with an intense headache and feeling exhausted from the day.

Negative appraisals. Anne-Marie was a 10-year-old girl with a 13-month history of pain and weakness in her legs; she was confined to a wheelchair. Through her various illness behaviours, Anne-Marie engaged her mother and siblings in fetching and carrying for her. She had previously experienced domestic violence, including her father's verbal abuse and his threats to kill the family. Her mother and siblings eventually fled the family home to obtain refuge (and safety) from the father. In the Mind-Body Program, because standing on her legs caused her pain, Anne-Marie appraised land-based physiotherapy as threatening and unacceptable. She therefore blankly refused to engage in physiotherapy or any activity that included weight bearing on land. If pushed to do so, she would become increasingly anxious and would go into shutdown as a defence mechanism, a state in which no one could reach her. By contrast, Anne-Marie appraised water-based physiotherapy as safe; in water-based sessions she swam around like a fish, with no pain in her legs.

Rumination. Owen was an 11-year-old boy with functional neurological disorder—shaking in the arms and legs, and weakness and loss of coordination in the legs—who presented in the context of severe bullying at school. When walking, Owen made his way slowly in a bizarre, laborious, wide-based, shaky gait. On admission to the Mind-Body Program, he was particularly worried about going to the hospital school. The night before his first attendance, he ruminated about the hospital school throughout the night—'I don't want to go', 'I don't know anyone', 'It's a new place', 'It will be awful'—and was unable to sleep. When he arrived at the hospital school, he kept thinking about how awful it was to be there, and he spent considerable time texting his ruminations to his parents. The never-ending stream of rumination meant that Owen never actually stopped to notice that hospital school was not as awful as he expected. Managing his ruminations became a key part of the psychological component of his treatment intervention. By the end of the admission, Owen loved the hospital school and was very sad to leave.

Rumination. Raymond—the boy with CRPS whom we met earlier in the chapter—was not the only anxious member in the family. Raymond's mother was also a worrier. In a discharge-planning meeting, when the discussion turned to Raymond's return to school, the mother voiced all the worries that had been running through her mind with regard to Raymond's return to school: 'He's not physically or mentally ready to go back to school'; 'If his foot gets knocked, he will not be able to manage his distress'; 'He might get teased'; 'He might be seen as different'; 'The teachers and other students might see him as a student with special needs'; 'He might feel uncomfortable in a role where he was dependent on others'; and so on. Raymond's father, who was well familiar with his wife's anxious thoughts, referred to this process as 'building bridges', a process by which his wife expended much mental energy rehearsing all possible future scenarios—all possible bridges that she might have to cross.

Catastrophizing

A related construct is that of catastrophizing. To *catastrophize* means 'to imagine the worst possible outcome of an action or event: to think about a situation or event as being a catastrophe or having a potentially catastrophic outcome' (Merriam-Webster's Online Dictionary). When catastrophizing, the individual engages in a process that involves active rumination and excessive magnification of negative cognitions and feelings—typically feelings of helplessness, often coupled with feelings of pain, fatigue, nausea, and so on—with regard to an approaching situation. In this way, the act of catastrophizing invokes the human ability to create mental images that symbolize potential future outcomes. Even though the mental images generated in catastrophizing are imaginary—they are generated by the brain—they engage the attentional and appraisal processes described earlier in this chapter. In addition, when articulated aloud, catastrophic thoughts help maintain the unhealthy dynamics by which parental attention and responsiveness to the child's symptoms are maintained (Williams et al. 2011) or by which a parent's own catastrophizing contributes to the maintenance of the child's symptoms (Palermo et al. 2014; Frerker et al. 2016). Catastrophizing is another example of an adaptive process—the capacity to anticipate and plan responses in order to facilitate survival—gone awry.

While catastrophizing about pain has received most attention in the literature—showing a clear impact of catastrophizing on the severity of symptoms and illness—catastrophizing is common across functional somatic presentations. Imaging studies of catastrophizing suggest that it contributes to symptom persistence and amplification because it activates the brain stress systems and increases connectivity between the brain stress systems and sensory-processing regions, which is a pattern that occurs across functional presentations (see Chapter 11). For references see Online Supplement 12.1.

> Morgan, the adolescent whom we met in Chapter 10, was a 15-year-old girl with a four-week history of hemiparesis and sensory loss on the left side of her face and body, a three-year history of chronic headache, fatigue, and intermittent NES, and a nine-year history of functional gut

symptoms (recurring abdominal pain accompanied by nausea, difficulties eating, and irregular bowel function). Morgan was a catastrophizer. With her therapist, Morgan tracked her thoughts about an upcoming test: 'If I don't study now, I will fail my English test; if I fail my English test, this will mean that I keep going badly in English until I get a bad mark in the HSC [Australian examination for university admission]; if I get a bad mark in the HSC, then I won't get into university; without skills, I will end up being a checkout chick; but because I am not good with numbers, they would sack me; and so I will end up homeless, depressed, on drugs, and living on the street.'

Feelings and Thoughts in Regulating Body State

Negative Feelings, Anxiety, and Depression

Negative feelings—fear, anger, and sadness—as well as anxiety and depression, also affect the perception (feelings) of body state and the manner in which children with functional somatic symptoms perceive and manage their symptoms (see second-level feelings described within Damasio's framework, above). Very often it is not possible to effectively treat the somatic symptoms unless the comorbid negative feelings, anxiety, or depression are addressed. Readers interested in this area of research may like to look up the references provided in Online Supplement 12.1. In the vignettes below, we provide some examples of how negative feelings crop up in clinical practice with children.

> *Hopelessness.* Morgan, the catastrophizing 15-year-old girl with functional neurological disorder whom we met above, felt hopeless about her situation and did not think that anything could change for her. Her stream of mind included a constant stream of rumination about her helplessness and the futility of the medical profession: 'The doctors can't help'; 'Nobody knows what's wrong with me'; 'You don't believe that there's anything wrong'; 'Yet another doctor has said they can't fix me'. Despite repeated conversations about Morgan's diagnosis and prognosis with her therapist, she kept returning to these thoughts. All attempts to use cognitive strategies to modify this stream of rumination made little difference.

It was only after Morgan had been on a therapeutic dose of an antidepressant (a selective serotonin reuptake inhibitor [SSRI]) for some time that these thoughts started to decrease in intensity. Whenever Morgan became stressed and her mood dipped, however—because of a setback in her progress or because of social or exam stress at school—her hopeless thoughts would return, and she had to work hard to manage the thoughts so that they did not overwhelm her.

Fear. Raymond, the 12-year-old boy with CRPS whom we met earlier in the chapter, had an intense fear of movement, weight bearing, and bumping his leg. In the initial stages of Raymond's admission, this fear blocked all treatment efforts. When Raymond woke up in the morning, he was conscious of his fear of the physiotherapy that was to happen that day. Lying in bed he would begin to ruminate and catastrophize: 'I don't want to go to physio'; 'They're going to set unrealistic goals for me'; 'I'll never be able to reach them'; 'Everyone is going to be disappointed in me'; 'I'll never walk again'; 'I won't be able to make it home by Christmas; I'll be in hospital forever'. By the time the physiotherapist arrived, Raymond was in a state of panic characterized by an elevated heart rate, elevated respiratory rate, and raw fear that led him to hide under the sink in the bathroom while shaking in fear. If the physiotherapist tried to lure Raymond out from under the sink, he would begin a long period of loud, distressed screaming.

Anger. Taylor was a 15-year-old girl with a three-year history of anxiety and recurring diarrhoea and abdominal pain, a two-year history of dizziness and fainting, and a two-week history of NES that had begun after Taylor had been prescribed an SSRI for her anxiety by her referring doctor. Increased too quickly—and at doses that were too large—the SSRI had agitated Taylor and increased her physiological arousal. During her hospital admission, Taylor experienced prolonged NES, during which she shook and from which she could not be roused. In her work with her psychotherapist, Taylor identified that a feeling of anger preceded all her NES. Taylor was especially angry with her mother, who had high expectations for Taylor's performance at school and who pushed her ruthlessly and relentlessly to do well. Taylor came to recognize that any interaction with her mother or hospital staff that triggered intense anger—for example, being told that she had to go to the hospital school—triggered an NES.

Putting Unwanted Material Out of Mind

Some children try to put unwanted negative thoughts, feelings, and memories out of mind. Different psychotherapy traditions have used different words for this phenomenon, including inhibition, suppression, and denial and avoidance of unwanted thoughts, feelings, and memories. A robust body of work now shows that putting unwanted negative thoughts, feelings, and memories out of mind is associated with increased physiological arousal and with increased activation of the brain stress systems. And when the unwanted material does come to mind, it can also be associated with very significant arousal. Further, a number of studies highlight that the cognitive process of putting unwanted negative material out of mind can contribute to functional somatic symptoms. For references see Online Supplement 12.1. Below we provide some vignettes of how putting *unwanted material out of mind* crops up in clinical practice with children.

Putting feelings into the box. Evie is the 15-year-old girl with precordial catch syndrome (sharp exploding pain in chest) and NES whom we met earlier in the chapter (see Chapter 2 for details of Evie's presentation). When asked about her mood during the family assessment interview, Evie said that she was 'fine'. Later it emerged that when Evie experienced the sharp exploding pain in her chest, she experienced suicidal ideation and wanted to kill herself. When asked why she had not mentioned this information, Evie said she had put the thoughts into her 'box'. When the feelings were in the box, she did not think about them, and they did not exist. In addition, Evie's relationship with her father—with whom she had been very close—had broken down 18 months before. But on the Early Life Stress Questionnaire (ELSQ), a checklist of 19 stress items, Evie had not ticked the section pertaining to family conflict. When asked why she had not included her conflicted relationship with her father on the questionnaire, Evie said that she no longer considered her father as part of her family and had therefore not ticked the questionnaire section. She had also put the conflict with her father in her 'box'.

Inhibition/suppression/denial/avoidance of unwanted thoughts, feelings, and memories. Victoria was a 17-year-old girl who presented with intense fatigue, amnesia (e.g., lack of recognition of her parents and siblings), clouded thinking, violent episodes of trembling, and pain and weakness in the legs after falling down some stairs near the school playground. Victoria also suffered from symptoms of post-traumatic stress disorder in relation to a sexual assault by a sports coach two years previously, which she had recently disclosed to her youth group leader. Even when Victoria's amnesia and clouded thinking began to clear, she refused to discuss the assault with anyone (including the police). She told her therapist that she did not want to think about the assault and that she would continue to manage the memories by blocking them out of mind. Despite all of Victoria's efforts, the unwanted material emerged at night—in the form of nightmares—and during the day in the form of fear: fear that people were looking at her, fear of men, and fear of being touched in any way. Victoria's body was also permanently activated in a state of high arousal, which was reflected in an elevated respiratory rate (20–30 breaths per minute with a pCO_2 of 23–29 mm Hg), a heart rate frequently in the range of 95–120 beats per minute, nights that were punctuated by night-mares, and frequent panic attacks during the day and night, during which her heart rate, respiratory rate, and trembling reached their maximum levels.

Expectations

Perceptions (feelings) of body state are significantly modulated by expectations—by what the child anticipates/expects to happen. Sometimes the anticipated body state—of pain or nausea or fatigue or motor difficulties—can be triggered in the absence of any sensory input. This is an example of feelings from the third tier of Damasio's typology of feelings, where the brain creates mental representations of body state that do not correspond to the current reality of the body. In this way, negative expectations play an important role in triggering and maintaining functional somatic symptoms—in maintaining dis-ease—whereas positive expectations contribute to the process of getting well (Benedetti et al. 2013).

Positive expectations are part of the placebo effect. Research studies demonstrate that placebos work best when they activate already existent neural pathways—that is, pathways that have been primed by past experience. For example, when treating pain, the positive expectations that are activated as part of the placebo response reduce activity in pain-processing regions and brain stress systems, and increase activity in prefrontal cortical networks (which support positive expectations and the brain's dopamine reward systems) and subcortical regions (which support experience-dependent learning) (Wager and Atlas 2015; Dodd et al. 2017). Negative expectations or the nocebo response—an increase of symptoms following an intervention in the context of negative expectations (expectations that promote pain, distress, and dis-ease)—have the opposite effect; they decrease signalling in prefrontal cortical networks and the brain's dopamine reward system (Dodd et al. 2017).

Expectations of pain. During the family assessment, the power of Raymond's expectations of pain—the boy with CRPS whom we met earlier in the chapter—were enacted in the session. At one point in the interview, Raymond's sister, who was perched on a chair near the head of Raymond's bed, leaned her body slightly toward Raymond. As his sister leaned in, Raymond yelled, 'Ow, your hurting me, move away.' Raymond felt his anticipated pain even though his sister had not touched him.

Expectations of nausea and pain. Zack was a 17-year-old boy with a three-year history of nausea, feeling unwell following eating, recurrent abdominal pain, and difficulties maintaining his weight and nutritional status. Zack tried to eat as little as possible to avoid precipitating his symptoms. On admission to hospital Zack had strong expectations that feeds given via a nasogastric tube would trigger his symptoms. Zack's treating team knew that in the normal course of a day, the stomach secretes approximately 1500 ml of fluid into the gastric lumen. In this context, the team examined the contribution of Zack's expectations by passing 1 ml of fluid into his gastric lumen via the nasogastric tube. When 1 ml of fluid was administered, Zack became white as a sheet; he began to sweat; and his heart rate and respiratory rate went up. He clutched his stomach, complained of excruciating pain, reached for his vomit bag, and begged for medication to relieve his pain. Following the 1 ml trial, Zack began to understand the power of his own mind. He realized that he could trigger his symptoms with just his mind. With the help of his psychologist, he worked on using his mind—via hypnosis, imagery, and other cognitive and body-regulation strategies—in more helpful ways, enabling him to manage his expectations and his symptoms.

∗∗∗

In this chapter we have examined how cognitive processes—the mind level of brain operations—can be used in maladaptive ways and can contribute to the shaping and maintenance of functional somatic symptoms. All of the cognitive processes that we have discussed in this chapter are available to conscious awareness, and they make up what we recognize as the 'stream of mind' (Damasio 2003, p. 197). Because conscious processes are amenable to conscious manipulation, they also provide a therapeutic window for change. In Chapter 13, we look at principles of treatment that are built upon our systemic model, and in the chapters after that (14–16), we examine therapeutic interventions on different system levels: the body level, the mind level of brain operations, and the family and behavioural system levels.

References

Bauer, C. C., Diaz, J. L., Concha, L., & Barrios, F. A. (2014). Sustained Attention to Spontaneous Thumb Sensations Activates Brain Somatosensory and Other Proprioceptive Areas. *Brain and Cognition, 87,* 86–96.

Benedetti, F., Thoen, W., Blanchard, C., Vighetti, S., & Arduino, C. (2013). Pain as a Reward: Changing the Meaning of Pain from Negative to Positive Co-activates Opioid and Cannabinoid Systems. *Pain, 154,* 361–367.

Craig, A. D. (2002). How Do You Feel? Interoception: The Sense of the Physiological Condition of the Body. *Nature Reviews Neuroscience, 3,* 655–666.

Damasio, A. (2001). Fundamental Feelings. *Nature, 413,* 781.

Damasio, A. (2003). *Looking for Spinoza: Joy, Sorrow, and the Feeling Brain.* Orlando, FL: Harcourt.

Damasio, A., & Carvalho, G. B. (2013). The Nature of Feelings: Evolutionary and Neurobiological Origins. *Nature Reviews Neuroscience, 14,* 143–152.

Darwin, C. (1872). *The Expression of the Emotions in Man and Animals.* London: John Murray.

Dodd, S., Dean, O. M., Vian, J., & Berk, M. (2017). A Review of the Theoretical and Biological Understanding of the Nocebo and Placebo Phenomena. *Clinical Therapeutics, 39,* 469–476.

Faust, J., & Soman, T. B. (2012). Psychogenic Movement Disorders in Children: Characteristics and Predictors of Outcome. *Journal of Child Neurology, 27,* 610–614.

Frerker, M., Hechler, T., Schmidt, P., & Zernikow, B. (2016). Pain-Related Parental Behavior: Maternal and Paternal Responses to Chronic Pain of Their Child and Modifications Following Inpatient Interdisciplinary Pain Treatment. *Schmerz, 30,* 241–247.

Gianaros, P. J., & Wager, T. D. (2015). Brain-Body Pathways Linking Psychological Stress and Physical Health. *Current Directions in Psychological Science, 24,* 313–321.

Jackson, T., Wang, Y., & Fan, H. (2014). Associations Between Pain Appraisals and Pain Outcomes: Meta-analyses of Laboratory Pain and Chronic Pain Literatures. *Journal of Pain, 15,* 586–601.

James, W. (1890). *The Principles of Psychology* (Vol. 1). New York: Henry Holt & Co.

Kim, J., Loggia, M. L., Cahalan, C. M., Harris, R. E., Beissner, F. D. P. N., Garcia, R. G., et al. (2015). The Somatosensory Link in Fibromyalgia: Functional Connectivity of the Primary Somatosensory Cortex Is Altered by Sustained Pain and Is Associated with Clinical/Autonomic Dysfunction. *Arthritis & Rheumatology (Hoboken, NJ), 67,* 1395–1405.

Kim, J., Mawla, I., Kong, J., Lee, J., Gerber, J., Ortiz, A., et al. (2019a). Somatotopically Specific Primary Somatosensory Connectivity to Salience and Default Mode Networks Encodes Clinical Pain. *Pain, 160,* 1594–1605.

Kim, S. M., Hong, J. S., Min, K. J., & Han, D. H. (2019b). Brain Functional Connectivity in Patients with Somatic Symptom Disorder. *Psychosomatic Medicine, 81,* 313–318.

Lazarus, R. S. (1966). *Psychological Stress and the Coping Process.* New York: McGraw-Hill.

Lazarus, R. S., & Folkman, S. (1984). *Stress, Appraisal, and Coping.* New York: Springer.

Lee, J., Protsenko, E., Lazaridou, A., Franceschelli, O., Ellingsen, D. M., Mawla, I., et al. (2018). Encoding of Self-Referential Pain Catastrophizing in the Posterior Cingulate Cortex in Fibromyalgia. *Arthritis & Rheumatology (Hoboken, NJ), 70,* 1308–1318.

Meeus, M., Nijs, J., Van Oosterwijck, J., Van Alsenoy, V., & Truijen, S. (2010). Pain Physiology Education Improves Pain Beliefs in Patients with

Chronic Fatigue Syndrome Compared with Pacing and Self-Management Education: A Double-Blind Randomized Controlled Trial. *Archives of Physical Medicine and Rehabilitation, 91,* 1153–1159.

Noakes, T. D. (2012). Fatigue Is a Brain-Derived Emotion That Regulates the Exercise Behavior to Ensure the Protection of Whole Body Homeostasis. *Frontiers in Physiology, 3,* 82.

Pace-Schott, E. F., Amole, M. C., Aue, T., Balconi, M., Bylsma, L. M., Critchley, H., et al. (2019). Physiological Feelings. *Neuroscience and Biobehavioral Reviews, 103,* 267–304.

Palermo, T. M., Valrie, C. R., & Karlson, C. W. (2014). Family and Parent Influences on Pediatric Chronic Pain: A Developmental Perspective. *American Psychologist, 69,* 142–152.

Posner, M. I. (2012). *Attention in a Social World.* New York: Oxford University Press.

Stone, J. (2014). Functional Neurological Disorders: The Neurological Assessment as Treatment. *Neurophysiologie Clinique, 44,* 363–373.

Strigo, I. A., Simmons, A. N., Matthews, S. C., & Craig, A. D. (2010). The Relationship Between Amygdala Activation and Passive Exposure Time to an Aversive Cue During a Continuous Performance Task. *PLoS ONE, 5,* e15093.

Testa, S. M., Krauss, G. L., Lesser, R. P., & Brandt, J. (2012). Stressful Life Event Appraisal and Coping in Patients with Psychogenic Seizures and Those with Epilepsy. *Seizure, 21,* 282–287.

Wager, T. D., & Atlas, L. Y. (2015). The Neuroscience of Placebo Effects: Connecting Context, Learning and Health. *Nature Reviews Neuroscience, 16,* 403–418.

Walker, L. S., Smith, C. A., Garber, J., & Claar, R. L. (2007). Appraisal and Coping with Daily Stressors by Pediatric Patients with Chronic Abdominal Pain. *Journal of Pediatric Psychology, 32,* 206–216.

Walker, L. S., Williams, S. E., Smith, C. A., Garber, J., Van Slyke, D. A., & Lipani, T. A. (2006). Parent Attention Versus Distraction: Impact on Symptom Complaints by Children With and Without Chronic Functional Abdominal Pain. *Pain, 122,* 43–52.

Wallrath, M. K., Rubel, J., Ohls, I., Demiralay, C., & Hechler, T. (2019, November 29). Bottom-up or Top-down? The Role of Child and Parent Chronic Pain and Anxiety in the Context of Parental Catastrophizing and Solicitousness. *European Journal of Pain (London, England)* (Epub ahead of print).

Williams, S. E., Blount, R. L., & Walker, L. S. (2011). Children's Pain Threat Appraisal and Catastrophizing Moderate the Impact of Parent

Verbal Behavior on Children's Symptom Complaints. *Journal of Pediatric Psychology, 36,* 55–63.

Part III
The Treatment of Functional Somatic Symptoms

Building on the initial formulation and the clinician's own understanding of the stress system and its relation to functional somatic symptoms, Chapters 13 to 16 focus on the treatment of functional somatic symptoms.

Chapter 13 summarizes the main treatment principles that guide our clinical practice day to day. The chapter is meant to function like a map that the clinician can consult when the treatment has stalled and it's not clear what to do next. We ourselves often consult the map when challenged by a particular clinical situation or to double-check whether we have overlooked some important principle that could help the treatment process get back on track.

An important theme that emerges from Chapter 13 is that the focus of the treatment intervention for functional somatic symptoms is the child's stress system and all the factors that activate and dysregulate the stress system—and not the symptoms per se. This theme runs contrary to much of contemporary clinical practice, in which the focus is on treating symptoms (in this case, the expression of stress-system dysregulation) or disorders (in this case, the expression of stress-system dysregulation that fits a commonly seen pattern). Because children with functional somatic symptoms often present with multiple somatic symptoms, and because their symptoms often shift and change over time, it is much more useful for the clinician to conceptualize the somatic narrative in terms of the underlying biological systems and the manner in which these systems embody the child's physical and emotional stress. Working from this perspective, the clinician will not be surprised or confused when child's symptoms shift and change. For example, when the child's symptoms include various combinations of abdominal pain, dizziness and nausea on standing (orthostatic intolerance), and panic and anxiety, the clinician will conceptualize all these symptoms as involving activation and dysregulation of the autonomic nervous system and will implement interventions that target this system. Based on a shared working formulation, the clinician, child, and family will implement interventions from multiple system levels to address the problem area. In most clinical situations, the interventions will involve multiple system levels—the body, mind, relationships in the family, and issues in the school—to address the broad range of factors that contribute to the activation and dysregulation of the child's stress system.

Chapters 14, 15, and 16 are organized by system levels. Chapter 14 outlines treatment interventions at the body system level. In our day-to-day clinical practice, given that the child is presenting with symptoms in the body, we always begin treatment at the body system level. Interventions at the body system level have an inherent acceptability for children and their families, and they allow the intervention to gain momentum, moving from interventions that are easy to implement (e.g., a sleep intervention) to those that are more challenging and confronting (e.g., addressing loss, trauma, or parental conflict). Chapter 15 moves onto the mind system level, the many different ways in which humans can use their minds to activate and dysregulate the stress system. Chapter 16 addresses social aspects of the intervention: the family system, behavioural interventions, and (in the online supplemental material) issues at school. In all three chapters we share with the reader the broad range of interventions that we and our clinical teams integrate, as needed, into an overall treatment program.

13

Principles of Assessment and Treatment

Abstract In this chapter we outline the key principles that are built into the structure of our Mind-Body Program and into the interventions we undertake with any particular child. The principles are especially useful in the following circumstances: in assessing a referral for treating functional somatic symptoms; in setting up the multidisciplinary team around a given patient; in explaining to the child and family the overall goals and structure of the treatment approach to be used; in determining the details of the therapeutic interventions to be used; in discussing and initiating those particular interventions with the child and family; in periodically assessing the success or failure of ongoing therapeutic interventions; and when confronting situations in which the therapy feels stuck and the treatment interventions that should be working are not working. In addition, the principles make key processes explicit and can be used as *touchstones* for teaching and for learning. As touchstones, the principles can be used to identify dynamics both within the family and between the clinician and the family, and to help to open space for reflection about

---

Electronic supplementary material The online version of this chapter (https://doi.org/10.1007/978-3-030-46184-3_13) contains supplementary material, which is available to authorized users.

© The Author(s) 2020   **275**
K. Kozlowska et al., *Functional Somatic Symptoms in Children and Adolescents*, Palgrave Texts in Counselling and Psychotherapy,
https://doi.org/10.1007/978-3-030-46184-3_13

different aspects of the therapeutic process. Specific interventions, organized by system levels, are discussed in Chapters 14–16.

The treatment of children (including adolescents) with functional somatic symptoms and their families ranges from straightforward to fraught with difficulty, and anywhere in between. To understand and manage this complexity, the mental health clinician—or more commonly, the multidisciplinary clinical team (from now on, simply the *clinician*)—needs to keep in mind some key principles. The principles help make key processes explicit—those that take place in the paediatric setting, the mental health setting, and between the clinician and family to support a path to health and well-being (versus illness and dis-ease). The principles also help us, the clinician, to effectively conceptualize and reflect about processes and patterns of communication between the family and medical system, within the family itself, and between the clinician and family. Keeping these principles in mind is helpful because their implementation increases the likelihood that the child will return to a state of health and well-being. We discuss these principles one by one, clustered under headings that approximate the temporal order of the therapeutic process. The reader will notice, however, that some of the principles are overlapping and interdependent, and that in clinical practice they are applied in tandem. Notwithstanding, we provide all the principles here as a sort of map that clinicians can use to guide the treatment process or that they can consult when they feel lost or when the therapeutic process is not going well.

Setting Things Up in the Broader Health Care System: Principles Concerning the Paediatrician and the Medical Assessment Process

Principle 1: Completion of a Thorough Medical Assessment

This principle pertains to processes in the health care system that take place before the mental health clinician accepts a referral. As we have noted throughout the book, best practice in the field of functional somatic symptoms requires that a thorough medical assessment—by a paediatrician or family doctor—be completed prior to referral to a clinician for treatment. As part of the medical assessment, the paediatrician needs to have ruled out an organic cause for the symptoms, identified any concomitant medical factors that are part of the child's presentation, and identified the pattern of symptoms and signs that enabled the paediatrician to provide the child and family with a positive diagnosis of a functional disorder (for positive diagnosis, see Chapter 2 and Online Supplement 2.1). In providing a positive diagnosis, the paediatrician needs to tell the child and family explicitly that the child's pattern of symptoms and signs has a name—for example, functional abdominal pain or functional neurological disorder—and that specific treatment is required. Via this medical process that precedes the referral to the mental health clinician, the paediatrician contributes to the creation of a *secure base* from which the child, family, and clinician can feel safe enough to explore the various factors that contributed to the child's presentation. Without this *secure base*, neither the family nor the mental health clinician can engage in the therapeutic process, because they will remain concerned that an organic condition may have been missed.

Principle 2: Early Referral for Mind-Body Treatment by the Paediatrician Leads to Good Outcomes and a Return to Health

The literature suggests that children with functional somatic symptoms have better outcomes than adult patients and that their functional symptoms are more likely to remit. Our own clinical experience is that when children are referred early to established programs—or treatment teams or settings—specifically developed for, or designed to include, children with functional somatic symptoms, they achieve much better clinical outcomes than children whose referrals for treatment have, for one reason or another, been significantly delayed. From the perspective of the stress-system model, it seems likely that early referral and treatment facilitate settling of the child's stress system to a more regulated state, preempt the decline into chronicity, and prevent the establishment of illness-reinforcing patterns within the family, school, and medical systems (see Chapter 2). Clinicians working in hospital settings and those who have ongoing relationships with paediatricians should advocate for, and take every opportunity to advocate for, early referral of functional disorders to appropriate mental health clinicians (Tot-Strate et al. 2016; Garralda 2016).

Setting Things Up in Psychological Medicine or the Mental Health System: Principles Concerning the Mental Health Clinician and Mental Health Setting

Principle 3: Maintaining a Systems Perspective

Thinking systemically about the problem of functional somatic symptoms involves 'thinking in terms of relationships, patterns, and contexts' (Capra and Luisi 2014, p. xii). The activation and dysregulation of the child's stress system, along with the emergence of functional somatic symptoms, occur in the context of interactions between the child (her body, brain, and mind) and the world outside (her experience of, and interactions within, the home, school, and broader sociocultural contexts)—interactions that Hans Selye referred to as *the stress of life* (Selye 1956) (see Online Supplement 1.2). In this context, the clinician needs to be able to hold in mind different system levels and the relationships between them. Rather than focusing on the symptoms(s) and treating the symptoms per se, with each new patient the clinician is challenged to identify and address the specific areas of dysfunction—on the body, individual, family, school, and social-system levels—that contribute to stress-system activation and dysregulation. In this way, the treatment may potentially involve interventions that engage and target all these system levels. While each intervention on its own will effect only a small change within the stress system, multiple targeted interventions across system levels will achieve considerable change. In addition, because components within the stress system are interrelated and interconnected, change in one component can lead to changes in other components—what are sometimes referred to as *ripple effects* (Guite et al. 2012).

See Online Supplement 13.1 for the many different terms have been used to describe this broader (systemic) way of working with children and their families and for published case studies using the systems approach to treatment.

Principle 4: The Goal of Treatment Is to Re-establish Regulation, Harmony, and Coherence Within the Child's Stress System

Principle 4 follows on directly from Principle 3. Clinicians who work with functional somatic symptoms using a systemic perspective see the overarching goal of the therapeutic intervention as helping the child to re-establish regulation, harmony, and coherence within her stress system, enabling the functional somatic symptoms to resolve (see Fig. 13.1). Put simply, the clinicians are treating a system—the child's stress system and all the factors that activate the stress system—and not the symptoms per

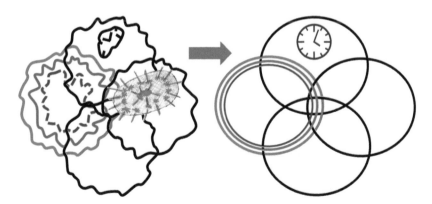

Fig. 13.1 Treatment and healing depicted using the circles metaphor of the stress system. With appropriate interventions, a dysregulated stress system that supports and generates functional somatic symptoms shifts to a regulated stress system that supports health and well-being (© Kasia Kozlowska 2017)

se. If all goes well, the child will develop an increased capacity for managing stress and distress; nurturing relationships will have been strengthened; the family will have made changes that support health and the child's well-being; and the stress in the family, school, and broader social environment will have been resolved. The overall result will be to build the child's resilience and to buffer her from future stress.

Principle 5: Establishing a Multidisciplinary Team to Work with the Child and Family

A multidisciplinary team is formed to enable the implementation of a therapeutic intervention on multiple system levels. Because the interventions at different system levels involve different skill sets, the treatment team for the child with functional somatic symptoms typically includes a diverse range of professionals who work together in a coordinated way. In the inpatient setting where the first author (KK) works, the multidisciplinary team always consists of a psychiatrist, a clinical psychologist, a physiotherapist, a paediatric resident on rotation, nursing staff from the ward, and school staff from the hospital school. When the need arises, an occupational therapist, neurologist, or paediatrician will also join the team.

Principle 6: Begin the Treatment Process with Interventions That Target the Body, and Move On to Interventions That Target the Mind and the Family System

Because the child presents with symptoms that pertain to the body, both the child and family usually find it easier to become engaged in the treatment—which will eventually reach multiple systems—when the clinician begins with an intervention targeting the body system. For example, in the first author's program, the interventions implemented first include stabilization of sleep, mind-body interventions designed to ameliorate the child's physical well-being, physiotherapy to address functional neurological symptoms or to build resilience, and attendance at the hospital school. Once the child's symptoms have been stabilized to some degree—and everyone can see that the child's physical well-being is on the mend—both the child and family find it easier to move on to interventions at the mind and family system levels (see, for example, the vignette of Paula in Chapter 3). Using family systems parlance, this is a strategic systemic approach in which the clinician begins with interventions on a system level that is more intuitive and acceptable for the child and family and then moves to system levels that are more challenging.

Principle 7: The Goal of Treatment Is a Return to Health/Well-Being and Normal Activities

For clinicians working with children, the goal of treatment should be a full return to health (for outcome data see Online Supplement 2.1). This principle is stated explicitly because the situation is different in adult practice, in which chronic functional presentations are more common and in which the probability that the symptoms will fully remit is lower. Clinicians working with adults often focus on helping the patient accept the illness; they support the patient in engaging in treatment to modify the symptoms to some degree; and they support the patient to accept that she or he may have to continue living with some degree of disability. By contrast, clinicians working with children should focus on getting the child *well*. In other words, in working with children, the clinician should voice the expectation that the treatment will enable the child to shift her stress system from defensive to restorative mode and that her functional somatic symptoms will resolve. During the treatment process, the child will begin the process of resuming her normal activities and should expect, with time, to return to a state of health and well-being. Of course, if there are comorbid chronic health concerns or unresolvable predicaments that cannot be modified, this expectation about returning to full health may itself need to be modified. In such scenarios the working goal may be a return to the child's previous level of function and activities, or alternatively, to her best possible level of function.

Principle 8: Understanding and Managing Attention Plays a Central Role in Achieving and Maintaining Progress Across System Levels and Across Treatment Interventions

Attention to functional somatic symptoms amplifies such symptoms, and attention away from the symptoms diminishes them (see Chapter 12). In this context, careful management of attention is a key element across all treatment components during the treatment intervention. In the first author's Mind-Body Program, the change in focus of attention is reflected in the very structure of the program (Kozlowska et al. 2012). Parents are asked to give the child space by absenting themselves from the hospital during the daytime hours that the child is engaged in the program. In this way, parents no longer attend to the child's symptoms day in and day out. Instead, the child is helped to attend to normal daily activities such as attendance at school and to activities that take place in physiotherapy and psychotherapy sessions. Likewise, the transition from assessment to treatment involves a shift in the focus of attention: the clinician shifts the focus of attention away from the symptoms to the mind-body strategies that the child is learning to use in managing the symptoms and also to the goals pertaining to functional gains (e.g., getting up in the morning, walking for longer distances, and going to school). For this attentional component of the intervention to work, parents must likewise learn (as part of the family-level intervention) to shift their attention away from the symptoms, to focus on supporting the child in implementing her new mind-body strategies, and to attend to the factors within the family system contributing to the child's symptoms. Likewise, the management of attention is a key component of physiotherapy (Gray et al. 2020) (see vignette of Jai in Chapter 15).

Principle 9: Clinicians Need to Remain Adaptable, Flexible, Creative, and Open to New Information

Openness and adaptability to new information are important for professionals working with functional somatic symptoms; the current knowledge base is limited and ever evolving, and all current models and theories reflect approximate truth (Capra and Luisi 2014).

Meeting the Family and the Engagement Process: Listening to the Story, Co-constructing a Formulation, Treatment Planning, Setting Expectations, and Agreeing to a Treatment Contract

Principle 10: Establishing a Therapeutic Relationship with the Multidisciplinary Team

Establishing a therapeutic relationship with the child and family is fundamental. A solid relationship enables the child's parents to give their unqualified approval (consent) to the treatment intervention (thereby giving the child explicit permission to be open and honest in her individual work); it bolsters the parents' effort to support the child throughout the treatment process (especially when the going gets tough); and it enables the clinician to address parental and family behaviours and factors that contribute to the child's illness. In building a therapeutic relationship, the clinician continues the process of solidifying the secure base—as initially set in motion by the paediatrician (see Chapter 2)—that is a prerequisite for a successful therapy intervention.

When parents and the child with functional somatic symptoms connect emotionally with the clinicians who make up the treatment team, anxiety within the family system settles to some degree. This settling of anxiety facilitates the parents' regulation of their own body states—the degree to which their stress systems are activated—and increases the probability that the parents will be able to support their child and efforts to settle the child's stress system.

A good therapeutic relationship also promotes positive and playful interactions between the child, family, and treatment team. Positive interactions work to counteract the defensive body state in which the child finds herself. In this way, positive interactions contribute to the neurophysiological conditions that Stephen Porges refers to as the *neural platform*—the range of body states underpinning better regulation and associated with health and well-being (Porges and Furman 2011).

Principle 11: Using a Working Formulation to Hold in Mind Information from Different System Levels

The *formulation*—the creative synthesis of a clinical case—draws on elements from all system levels, including the child's stress system, the child's mind, interactions between the parent and child, the contribution of the family, and experiences in the school context (Ross 2000; Winters et al. 2007). As we saw in Chapter 3, the formulation is co-constructed: it is worked out collaboratively in the conversation with the child and family during the assessment process. In this way, the formulation is a story that integrates, in chronological order, all the factors that contributed—and that currently contribute—to the child's functional illness and her clinical presentation. It is unique and specific to a child and her family. The formulation is always *a working formulation*; that is, it is modified during the treatment process as the clinician learns more about the child and family, and as trust is established and the family becomes more willing to reveal more about themselves and about their understanding of the factors that contributed to the child's presentation. In this way, as with all working hypotheses, the formulation is updated and changed—by the clinician and family members—as new information comes to light.

Principle 12: Use the Formulation to Guide the Choice of Treatment

In collaboration with the child and family, the clinician uses the formulation to guide the choice of treatment strategies, techniques, and interventions to promote change on the body, brain, mind, behavioural, family, and school and social-system levels. The *process of implementing* the multifaceted intervention involves the specific strategies, techniques, and interventions that are implemented—by the child, family, school, and clinical team—on each of those separate system levels. Each intervention is chosen because it targets a problem area identified in the co-constructed formulation (see the case of Paula in Chapter 3), because it represents a nodal point for intervention (see below), or because it is seen as essential to health and well-being, both now and in the long term. See Online Supplement 13.1 for published case examples as to how the formulation is used to guide the choice of treatment.

Principle 13: Identify Nodal Points for Intervention and Achieving Change

The notion of *nodal points* of change is helpful when the treatment involves interventions that engage and target multiple system levels. Nodal points are interventions that result in a greater degree of change than others or are so fundamental that without them, the desired progress will not be achieved. Understanding the nodal points for any particular patient not only facilitates the choice of treatment but helps the clinician (and family) decide the temporal order in which the interventions will be implemented. For example, interventions that stabilize sleep—the circadian clock—are powerful because the circadian clock regulates all the components of the stress system, and regulation of the circadian clock is likely to increase coherence of the stress system as a whole. Good sleep also increases the child's capacity to regulate more generally and to engage in positive interactions with others. Another example pertains to maltreatment. A child who continues to be exposed to ongoing maltreatment—for example, cyberbullying that involves texts telling her to kill herself or telling her that she is worthless and should die—will not be able to down-regulate her stress system. Establishing safety is fundamental; other interventions cannot be expected to work until safety had been established. Yet another example pertains to a good diet. Maintaining the health of the gut microbiota is essential to the health and well-being of the individual because the microbiota lives in symbiosis with humans and works together with the human body to maintain life processes (see Chapter 10).

Principle 14: Engage Hope and Positive Expectations at Assessment and Throughout the Treatment Process

The expectations and hopes that the clinician voices to the child and family—about the positive expectations for a successful outcome, about how the therapy achieves its results and how it will help the child to build her skills in managing her symptoms, and about the family's crucial role in supporting the child—are important because they function to activate the placebo effect in both the child and the family. Positive expectations and the placebo effect increase the likelihood that each component of the treatment program will have its maximal benefit (Benedetti 2011a, b, 2013). Because engagement of positive expectations is both a principle and an intervention, it is further discussed in Chapter 14.

Principle 15: Agree to a Treatment Contract Before Treatment Begins

The contract outlines expectations, roles, and responsibilities for the child, parents, and family, as well as for the treating team. It also defines expectations about the treatment intervention itself, the issues that will be addressed in the current intervention, and the issues that may need longer-term work with a different clinician or clinical team. The contract establishes a common understanding of, and agreement concerning, the key ingredients needed for change. It also minimizes the likelihood that the child and family will encounter unpleasant surprises about the treatment process—which is especially important since the program is challenging, demanding, and confronting for both the child and the family. For example, it is helpful for parents to know upfront that the child will be attending her physiotherapy sessions, her psychotherapy sessions, and the hospital school on her own, without the presence of a parent.

If the family does not want to agree to the contract, if parents want to try providing treatment at home, or even if they change their mind about the treatment intervention midway, then the family can decline the intervention or withdraw the child from the program, and set up elsewhere (if at all) their own preferred way of working. The family always has the option of re-engaging with the program—with its particular structure and expectations—at some future time.

The Treatment Process: Effecting Change, Returning to Normal Function, and the Longer Journey to Maintain Health and Well-Being

Principle 16: The Treatment Is the First Step in a Longer-Term Process of Maintaining Health and Well-Being

Early during the treatment process for functional somatic symptoms, it can be useful to highlight that the treatment intervention offered by the clinical team is just the first step in a longer journey of maintaining health and well-being. That journey may involve ongoing therapeutic work on different system levels—individual, family, school, and so on. Common elements that need integration into the home routine include regular sleep and exercise, healthy eating, ongoing therapy for anxiety or depression, acquisition and maintenance of stress-management skills, improvement of family communication skills (e.g., via a family intervention), and system interventions that ensure resolution of ongoing stress in the family, school, and peer contexts. Ongoing attention to all these risk factors will build resilience, decrease the likelihood of relapse, and increase the probability of long-term health and well-being.

Principle 17: For the Treatment Intervention to Work, Everyone—Child, Family, and Multidisciplinary Team—Needs to Be Pushing in the Same Direction

All members of the multidisciplinary team, all members within the family unit (including, insofar as possible, grandparents and extended family), and all members of the school team need to share the formulation and support the treatment process. This same principle applies to interventions that take place within a health facility and those that take place in the community setting. In either setting, regular meetings and a written, updated treatment plan can be important tools in supporting a common understanding and in helping everyone involved in the child's care to *push in the same direction*. For example, an intervention will not work if the child's parents are supporting the child to complete her exercise program and her grandparents are simultaneously telling her that she should rest because her legs do not work normally and because she has pain and experiences fatigue.

Principle 18: Normal Activities Are Both the Treatment and the Goal

Many families hold the idea that the treatment process will first involve resolution of the child's symptoms and, second, resumption of normal activities. When treating functional somatic symptoms, resumption of normal activities—sometimes in a graded fashion—is part of the treatment itself, and this aspect of treatment begins alongside and at the same time as other interventions. As part of the conversation with the child and family, the clinician may also communicate that some symptoms—for example, pain, nausea, and fatigue—will typically resolve only *after* the child has been engaging in her normal activities for some period of time.

Principle 19: Promote Predictability, Control, and Mastery for the Child

The goals of predictability, control, and mastery (from the child's perspective) should guide the choice of treatment interventions alongside the specific areas of dysfunction identified by the clinician. Interventions that contribute to these goals promote health and well-being because they function to settle the stress system as well as to minimize activation of psychological processes on the mind system level that appraise the treatment intervention as threatening (see Chapter 12).

Principle 20: Self-Management Is Key to the Child Maintaining Stable, Long-Term Regulation of the Stress System

A crucial factor in recovery is the child's willingness—with the support of her parents—to work on mind-body strategies that enable her to down-regulate the stress system and, more broadly, to improve her capacity for neurophysiological regulation. Fundamentally, the child is the only person who can, moment to moment—on waking up, at school, on coming home, and so on—implement the mind-body strategies that will help her to settle her stress system and to shift it from defensive to restorative mode. Without the child's cooperation and engagement, no one can accomplish this change in body state. Consequently, there is much to gain in giving the child the choice as to which mind-body strategies she enjoys and therefore wants to prioritize in her treatment plan. Creativity, along with respect for the child's choices, results in a treatment program that is shaped—and *owned*—by the child. And when these efforts to regulate and to manage her own body meet with success, it promotes a sense of control, mastery, and motivation, which are essential for long-term progress and stability (see Principle 19). This approach is consistent with data from the pain literature suggesting that increases in children's readiness to self-manage pain are associated with decreased functional disability, depressive symptoms, and fear of pain, and with increased use of adaptive coping strategies (Walker et al. 2006).

***

In this chapter we have highlighted the overarching considerations that, under the stress-system model, structure and guide the treatment of children with functional somatic symptoms. We have also presented, in particular, some of the key principles that we, as clinicians, find helpful when working with these children. When colleagues ask for help with specific cases, we often find it useful to bring these principles to bear on the clinical situation. And when the going gets tough in our own clinical work, we often return to these principles to potentially realign our efforts and to check that we have not omitted some key element that could help the child and family back toward a path of health and well-being. In this way the principles function as a map that can be used to guide the treatment process or that provides guidance when the going gets tough.

References

Benedetti, F. (2011a). Meeting the Therapist: A Look into Trust, Hope, Empathy, and Compassion Mechanisms. In *The Patient's Brain*. Oxford: Oxford University Press.

Benedetti, F. (2011b). Receiving the Therapy: The Activation of Expectation and Placebo Mechanisms. In *The Patient's Brain*. Oxford: Oxford University Press.

Benedetti, F. (2013). Placebo and the New Physiology of the Doctor-Patient Relationship. *Physiological Reviews, 93,* 1207–1246.

Capra, F., & Luisi, P. L. (2014). *The Systems View of Life: A Unifying Vision.* Cambridge: Cambridge University Press.

Garralda, M. E. (2016). Hospital Management of Paediatric Functional Somatic Symptoms. *Acta Paediatrica, 105,* 452–453.

Gray, N., Savage, B., Scher, S., & Kozlowska, K. (2020). Psychologically Informed Physiotherapy for Children and Adolescents with Functional Neurological Symptoms: The Wellness Approach. *Journal of Neuropsychiatry and Clinical Neurosciences.*

Guite, J. W., Logan, D. E., Ely, E. A., & Weisman, S. J. (2012). The Ripple Effect: Systems-Level Interventions to Ameliorate Pediatric Pain. *Pain Management, 2,* 593–601.

Kozlowska, K., English, M., Savage, B., & Chudleigh, C. (2012). Multimodal Rehabilitation: A Mind-Body, Family-Based Intervention for Children and Adolescents Impaired by Medically Unexplained Symptoms. Part 1: The Program. *American Journal of Family Therapy, 40,* 399–419.

Porges, S. W., & Furman, S. A. (2011). The Early Development of the Autonomic Nervous System Provides a Neural Platform for Social Behavior: A Polyvagal Perspective. *Infant and Child Development, 20,* 106–118.

Ross, D. E. (2000). A Method for Developing a Biopsychosocial Formulation. *Journal of Child and Family Studies, 1,* 106.

Selye, H. (1956). *The Stress of Life.* New York: McGraw-Hill.

Tot-Strate, S., Dehlholm-Lambertsen, G., Lassen, K., & Rask, C. U. (2016). Clinical Features of Functional Somatic Symptoms in Children and Referral Patterns to Child and Adolescent Mental Health Services. *Acta Paediatrica, 105*, 514–521.

Walker, L. S., Williams, S. E., Smith, C. A., Garber, J., Van Slyke, D. A., & Lipani, T. A. (2006). Parent Attention Versus Distraction: Impact on Symptom Complaints by Children With and Without Chronic Functional Abdominal Pain. *Pain, 122*, 43–52.

Winters, N. C., Hanson, G., & Stoyanova, V. (2007). The Case Formulation in Child and Adolescent Psychiatry. *Child and Adolescent Psychiatric Clinics of North America, 16*(111–132), ix.

14

Treatment Interventions I: Working with the Body

Abstract From the perspective of the stress-system model, the treatment of functional somatic symptoms involves a system-level approach. The factors that contribute to stress-system dysregulation and the emergence of functional somatic symptoms operate, both proximally and over longer periods, on different system levels: body, mind, attachment and family relationships, academic expectations, and interactions and relationships at school with other children, teachers, and even health professionals. The treatment program will therefore require a multi-levelled, systems approach that is designed to meet the specific, but diverse, needs of each particular child and the family. In this way, the mental health clinician or, more usually, the clinicians that make up the multidisciplinary team work with the child to implement interventions on the body and mind system levels; with the family to

---

Electronic supplementary material The online version of this chapter (https://doi.org/10.1007/978-3-030-46184-3_14) contains supplementary material, which is available to authorized users.

293
K. Kozlowska et al., *Functional Somatic Symptoms in Children and Adolescents*, Palgrave Texts in Counselling and Psychotherapy, https://doi.org/10.1007/978-3-030-46184-3_14

implement interventions on the family system level; with the school to implement interventions on the school system level; with health staff to implement changes in the medical system; and so on. In this chapter we describe some of the treatment interventions that involve working with the child on the body and brain system level—what we call working from the *bottom up*.

Assessment leads into treatment. During the assessment process the mental health clinician (or more typically, the multidisciplinary team), the child (including adolescent), and family have worked together to co-construct a *formulation*, the story that integrates, in chronological order, all the factors, on multiple system levels, that contributed to the child's functional illness and her clinical presentation (see Chapter 3). Now the clinician uses the formulation to guide the choice of treatment strategies, techniques, and interventions to promote change. When working with children with functional somatic symptoms, the treatment starts with the body.

Bottom-Up Interventions and Regulation Strategies That Involve the Body System Level

In the broader literature, interventions that target the body system level—bottom-up regulation approaches—are also known as body-oriented, somatic, body mindfulness, bottom-up mindfulness, or biofeedback interventions (Bloch-Atefi and Smith 2015). Many of these approaches involve working with the *felt sense* of the body, in which attention is focused on body sensations. Attending to the felt sense of the body—the somatic or body narrative (Sharpe Lohrasbe and Ogden 2017; Levine et al. 2018)— is a skill that the child can practice with the guidance of a therapist or instructor. The child learns to attend to body sensations and learns to follow them. In this context, think of the rapidly evolving sensations that occur when drinking something with a lot of fizz, or the slow, repeating sensations in the nose, chest, or abdomen that can be felt with each breath.

The Neurobiology of Bottom-Up Interventions

Attention to body sensations involves activation of autonomic, interoceptive, proprioceptive, and classic sensory afferents. The activation of these afferents then influences the pattern of activation in three separate brain regions: subcortical regions that underpin homeostasis, arousal, and pain; cortical brain regions that are part of the limbic system (which also process information about homeostasis, arousal, pain, and emotional states); and temporal lobe regions that process internal representations about the self (Guendelman et al. 2017).

Currently available studies pertaining to programs implementing bottom-up interventions show that they result in neuroplastic (healing) changes in brain regions involved in processing body state and representations of self (see above). These interventions do not effect changes in regions of the prefrontal cortex that engage in top-down regulation of emotion via cognitive processes or changes in thinking and understanding (Guendelman et al. 2017). An example of a bottom-up intervention is Mindfulness-Based Stress Reduction (MBSR), a program that involves close attention to moment-to-moment experience, shifts in attention from one sensory modality to another, a body scan with attention to the transient nature of sensory experience, and various forms of meditation (breathing, eating, walking) (Goldin and Gross 2010; Kabat-Zinn 1990). In this book, for simplicity—and because of the need to use simple language when talking to children—we use the expression *brain stress systems* to refer to the complex network of regions involved in homeostasis, processing of information about body state, and responding to stress or threat (see Chapter 11 and Online Supplement 11). In this way, when bottom-up regulation strategies are implemented successfully, they facilitate a shift in body state and brain stress-system activation (reflected in biomarkers).

As we mentioned above, an important element of bottom-up regulation strategies is that they do not engage the prefrontal cortex and cortical regions that are usually implicated in top-down emotion regulation (Guendelman et al. 2017). They work directly with the body and do not require the child to use language, to be able to manipulate cognitions, or to have access to memory or cognitive information about stress or past events. Although interventions on the body system level do not target the mind system level per se, there are important ripple effects (see Chapter 13): the child increases her sense of mastery and control as she learns to observe and manage her body states and as she becomes increasingly more competent in averting states of incoherence, dysregulation, and dis-ease—for example, fainting episodes, non-epileptic seizures (NES), and exacerbations of pain—and in bringing about states of coherence, regulation, and well-being.

Begin the Treatment Process with Interventions That Target the Body

Bottom-up regulation approaches have particular utility in treating functional somatic symptoms. These approaches to regulation have an inherent acceptability for children and their families. Since the child is presenting with symptoms in the body, it seems natural to the child and family that treatment should start with the body. In this way, in day-to-day clinical practice, beginning the treatment intervention with bottom-up regulation approaches helps consolidate engagement and trust, and functions as a *safe* bridge that enables the child and family to move toward exploration of psychological issues that may also need to be examined and addressed. Interventions on the body system level can be used by the child to help decrease activation and dysregulation of her stress system—that is, to shift the stress system from defensive to restorative mode. If the child is able to shift her stress system from one mode to the other, then the neurophysiological conditions that support the production of functional somatic symptoms are no longer present, and the child's functional somatic symptoms should resolve.

Bottom-up interventions also provide a way of moving forward in circumstances where progress might otherwise be difficult: when the family is not yet ready to address other factors that contribute to stress-system activation and dysregulation; when factors that contribute to stress-system activation and dysregulation are beyond the capacity of therapy to address (e.g., death of an attachment figure); when meaning

making is difficult or impossible; when meaning making may potentially cause harm (see Online Supplement 12.1 about meaning making);
or when the child's level of activation is so intense that any attempts to
use a talking therapy or cognitive strategies are likely to fail because the
child's prefrontal cortex (along with her executive and problem-solving
skills) is unlikely to be functioning properly (Hermans et al. 2011;
Arnsten 2015). Because somatic interventions help the child to regulate,
they help the child to shift her body toward what Daniel Siegel (1999)
refers to as the *window of tolerance*—in which arousal is neither too high
nor too low—and what Stephen Porges refers to as the neurophysiological conditions, or *neural platform*, required for the child to utilize
talking, cognitive, or interpersonal interventions (Porges and Furman
2011). Likewise, somatic interventions may be the only way forward
to achieve regulation and well-being when working with children and
families who have a frank aversion of *psychological* interventions; in such
cases, adherence to treatment interventions that involve a large psychological component seems improbable.

How to Integrate Bottom-Up Interventions into the Treatment Program

Within the treatment program, bottom-up interventions on the body
system level are used in two different ways. When such interventions are
integrated into the child's daily routine, the child is learning, through
regular repetition, a means by which she can improve the regulation
of her stress system. They can also be used as part of the child's safety
plan (see below)—emergency strategies or stop-break strategies—to
interrupt the somatic sequence of activation that occurs in advance of
episodic functional somatic symptoms such as fainting, NES, or sudden exacerbations of pain, or that is associated with hyperventilation
or panic attacks. Initially, the child practices these emergency strategies
multiple times every day—to hone the skills of implementing them—
and she subsequently uses them preventively when she senses the specific changes in her body, her warning signs, that the somatic activation
sequence has been activated (see later subsection 'Tracking/Sequencing

Body Sensations'). Once the child has identified which bottom-up regulation approaches work for her, they become part of the child's mind-body toolkit (Kozlowska and Khan 2011).

Language for Talking About States of Body Activation with Children

When working with children we use the terms *activated, revved up, switched on, aroused,* and *in defensive mode* interchangeably to refer to the stress system or some component of the stress system being acti-vated (too much) or dysregulated. In our clinical practice we choose words that best match the child's presentation and that are appropri-ate for the child's developmental capacity and preference. For exam-ple, younger children understand the term *switched on* and like to use it in relation to tracking somatic sensations such as autonomic symp-toms of arousal (see Chapter 6), activation within the motor system (see Chapter 7), and activation of the pain system (see Chapter 9).

Interventions That Target the Body Itself

In this section we focus on interventions that target the body itself. The reader will see that many different interventions on the body system level can be integrated into the treatment intervention.

Stabilizing Sleep and the Circadian Clock

In Chapter 5, we saw that many children with functional somatic symp-toms have a dysregulated circadian clock: unrefreshing sleep, sleep that is interrupted, sleep that is too long, or a circadian rhythm that is out of alignment with the earth's revolutions around the sun. Because the cir-cadian clock coordinates activity and coherence in all other components of the stress system, the stabilization of sleep is often the first interven-tion that is implemented on a body system level (see Chapter 5). For some children, improved sleep brings an immediate improvement in subjective well-being, a decrease in the intensity or frequency of their somatic symptoms, and an increase in the child's capacity to engage with other treatment interventions. While stabilizing sleep may involve a combination of bottom-up (e.g., use of toys that can be heated up to provide comfort [akin to a hot water bottle]), behavioural (sleep hygiene), brain-level (e.g., use of melatonin), and top-down (e.g., hypnosis) interventions, we place the sleep intervention here because is it typically the first intervention—which children and families perceive as involving the body—that we implement with children and their families.

Documenting Somatic Symptoms on a Body Map

Given that sensations are difficult to communicate in words, the child should be encouraged to communicate to the clinician about them using non-verbal means, as by indicating colour, shape, or intensity (e.g., a light versus dark imprint) on a *body map* (see Fig. 14.1).

The body map intervention has multiple purposes.

- It ensures that no symptom has been missed.
- It enables the clinician to assess how skilled the child is at reading her body. Does she notice subtle changes in body state, or does she notice symptoms only once they have peaked? Does she notice the triggers that activate her body to produce her symptoms?
- The symptoms documented on a body map allow the child and therapist to compare what the child's body feels like when the child is activated versus when she is less activated—for example, after a relaxation exercise. This use of the body map to track a broad range of body states increases the probability that the child will be able to notice changes in body state—increases in activation—when these begin to occur.
- Some children find it helpful to depict their subjective experience of body state in this concrete fashion—the visual representation—because it helps them hone their skills in recognizing certain body states, in noticing changes in body state (e.g., states of activation), and in gaining confidence that these skills are within their reach.

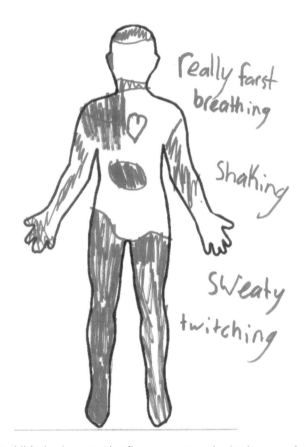

really farst breathing

Shaking

SWeaty twitching

Fig. 14.1 A child's body map. The figure presents the body map of an 11-year-old boy who presented with intermittent leg paralysis, fainting episodes, NES (which involved shaking of the entire body), and symptoms of dizziness, breathlessness, and fatigue. The body map shows his leg paralysis and his subjective experience of his body activating prior to the NES events (© Kasia Kozlowska 2017)

- Bringing attention to body sensations is a key skill in bottom-up mindfulness techniques—for example, the body scan meditation, or meditation while focusing on the breath—and, more generally, in bottom-up regulation strategies (see below).
- Sequential body maps are a means of tracking the degree to which the child's body has become less activated—shifted from defensive to

restorative mode—in response to treatment. These sequential maps are useful in marking treatment gains and in reinforcing the value of the program (e.g., 'See how well you're doing!').

• The clinician can use the map as part of psychoeducation (see Chapter 15) to explain again the connection between the symptoms, stress, and activation of the stress system—thereby repeating for the child some of the information that was given in the family assessment session. The process of drawing the body map also helps the child to feel understood in a tangible, embodied way.

Note that these maps are drawn and used as part of the child's individual therapy session, with the clinician using an interested, mindful stance that is very different from the anxious concern about symptoms and attention to symptoms that is typically shown by parents.

Tracking/Sequencing Body Sensations

Tracking somatic sensations—that is, identifying their occurrence—and then determining their temporal order, or sequence, are important tasks in some types of functional presentations, including hyperventilation-related somatic symptoms, NES, and pain presentations (see Online Supplement 14.1 for the different paths that therapists have travelled in coming to understand the value of tracking/sequencing body sensations). If the child and clinician can establish the recurring sequence of sensations, the child can practice identifying the sequence in its early stages—what we call the *warning signs*—and then implementing mind-body strategies that interrupt the sequence. The goal is to disrupt the sequence and to avert the functional somatic symptoms that otherwise would have resulted, as in the following vignette of Bella.

Bella, the 12-year-old girl presenting with NES whom we met in Chapter 7, experienced her NES as very stressful because she felt like she had no control over what happened to her body. She felt helpless and hopeless; she worried about her NES all the time; and she gave into her symptoms whenever they began to unfold. Soon after admission, during a session with her psychologist, Bella was able to identify some of her warning signs: 'spacing out' and not feeling real; a change in the quality of auditory and visual stimuli; a cold feeling in the chest and stomach; and feeling dizzy. In her next psychology session, Bella was able, with the guidance of her therapist, to implement a self-regulation strategy—slow breathing combined with images of safety and calm—when she first noticed the warning signs. In this way, she interrupted the pattern of activation and was able to avert the NES. Bella was excited by her achievement, and the therapist—together with the entire mind-body team—celebrated the achievement with her during ward rounds the next day. From a position of increasing competence, Bella now expected that if she practiced her regulation strategies, she would be able, in time, to manage her NES. In parallel, Bella's parents, rather than focusing on the NES per se, began to focus on the way that Bella was able to notice warning signs and to implement strategies that averted them (a focus-of-attention intervention with the family). Both her parents and the family system as a whole became less anxious and more regulated. As a consequence of her hard work—noticing her warning signs and implementing her strategy immediately—Bella's NES decreased in frequency and length, and then ceased altogether.

The following vignette, while similar in overall outline to the one above, illustrates the challenges of identifying the sequence of precursor symptoms and then developing an intervention that interrupts the sequence leading to the NES.

We first met Evie, a 15-year-old girl, in Chapter 2. As later discussed briefly in Chapter 12, her NES were triggered by acute chest pain (*precordial catch syndrome*), with the pain being so sudden and so distressing that she had no time to implement a regulation strategy. When the symptoms were tracked more carefully, however—that is, when the therapist asked Evie to track what happened in her body before the pain started—a regular sequence emerged. First, Evie felt a difference in temperature. She felt hot on the inside and cold on the outside. This change in temperature is consistent with sympathetic arousal, which causes increased energy use on the inside (feeling hot) and an increase in perspiration (feeling cold on the skin). Second, Evie experienced numbness and tingling in her left arm, blurring of vision, and shortness of breath—what she described as

'I can't breathe.' All these experiences are common symptoms of hyperventilation, the stress-related activation of the respiratory motor system
and skeletomotor muscles in the chest. Hyperventilation had previously
been documented in all of Evie's presentations to accident and emergency.
Third, alongside the symptoms of hyperventilation, Evie experienced a
burning and lump sensation in her throat—consistent with a tension pattern in skeletomotor muscles that make up the top third of the oesophagus—what is commonly known as a *globus sensation*. Sometimes this
sensation was accompanied by a burning sensation or an odd taste in the
mouth, presumably related to decreases in saliva secretion resulting from
sympathetic activation. Fourth, only at this point in the sequence would
Evie begin to experience the chest pain—starting initially at a low-grade
level of 3/10. Presumably, the chest pain reflected the progression of tension patterns of muscles and fascia within the mediastinum—what is
referred to as precordial catch syndrome (see Chapter 2). Fifth, the pain
would then rapidly progress in acuity, and any rating of > 5/10 would
be unbearable. Sixth, this unbearable, > 5/10 pain would then trigger an
NES. With practice, Evie found that if she could intervene with a regulation strategy (in her case a visualization strategy) in the early phases of
the sequence—when the feelings of heat and cold, the globus sensation,
the feeling of breathlessness, or the tinging in her arm or blurred vision
first emerged—then she was able to avert the subsequent phase of the
sequence. If she did not intervene early, the sequence would then inescapably progress to the chest pain and to an NES.

The Body Scan

The *body scan* was introduced into Western clinical practice by Jon
Kabat-Zinn, a professor of medicine who studied Buddhist practice under Zen Buddhist teachers (for early references and history, see
Online Supplement 14.1). The body scan is a bottom-up mindfulness
exercise that involves the child sitting or lying in a comfortable position
and slowly placing attention on various regions of the body, from the
feet to the head. The child is guided by a therapist or, if the exercise
is done in a group, an instructor, and audio recordings are also available for guidance. The body scan can be practiced at various speeds and
levels of precision, all with 'affectionate, openhearted [and] interested'

attention to the body (Kabat-Zinn 2005, p. 250). For children who enjoy movement or who find it difficult to stay still, an alternative to the body scan is to pay careful attention to the body during movement—for example, during a walking meditation or in the practice of Qigong—so that the movement is carried out in a conscious and deliberate manner. Another possibility is to engage them in group activities that involve synchronized movement. For a further discussion of Kabat-Zinn and the body scan, see Online Supplement 14.1.

In adults, mindfulness interventions based on Kabat-Zinn's MBSR program (Kabat-Zinn 1990)—which includes bottom-up interventions such as the body scan—have been found to down-regulate various components of the stress system: the hypothalamic-pituitary-adrenal (HPA) axis, autonomic system, immune-inflammatory system, pain system, and brain stress systems. For references see Online Supplement 14.1.

Slow-Breathing Interventions

Slow-breathing interventions, which have a long history in Eastern meditative traditions, are used in some biofeedback techniques and are integrated into most relaxation exercises. Slow-breathing interventions build on the human ability to control respiratory rate via skeletomotor muscles in the diaphragm and the intercostal muscles in the chest wall (Russo et al. 2017). A healthy inhalation pattern involves contraction (downward movement) of both the diaphragm and intercostal muscles, which work together to increase the size and decrease pressure within the chest cavity, enabling air to move into the lungs. Quiet expiration is a passive process that occurs when the muscles relax. Forceful expiration is an active process in which the abdominal and intercostal muscles work together to push the abdominal organs up against the diaphragm, thereby decreasing the size of the chest cavity, increasing pressure within it, and pushing air out of the lungs.

Because of coupling between the autonomic and respiratory motor systems (see Chapter 7), along with the interactions between the autonomic system and other components of the stress system—brain stress systems, immune-inflammatory system, and pain system—breathing at a slow rate is associated with myriad neurophysiological changes.

Key changes include increased vagal tone to the heart, increased neurophysiological coherence, down-regulation of energy-regulation systems, decreased energy use, down-regulation of brain stress systems, decreased subjective pain, and increased subjective well-being (for references see Online Supplement 14.1). In this way, slow-breathing interventions can be used as part of the child's daily routine to down-regulate the stress system and improve the child's overall health and well-being. In some children, slow-breathing interventions are also a useful *stop-break intervention* that the child can use to interrupt patterns of increasing arousal and motor activation that lead to panic attacks, fainting episodes, NES, or acute exacerbations of pain (Kozlowska et al. 2018).

Theoretically, formal assessment of the breathing rate that is associated with the highest vagal tone, also known as the *resonant-frequency breathing rate* (Lehrer et al. 2000), is helpful. This assessment can be done using biofeedback devices. The resonant-frequency breathing rate—usually around 6 breaths per minute in adults and 5–8 (median = 7) breaths per minute in children and adolescents (Richard N. Gevirtz, unpublished data)—is associated with the maximal heart rate variability, optimal baroreflex function, optimal gas exchange in the lungs, and coherence across body systems (Lehrer 2013; McCraty and Zayas 2014). This synchronization effect is also referred to as harmonic coupling between heart rate variability, respiration, blood pressure, and blood flow to tissues (Paccione and Jacobsen 2019). In clinical practice, however, children who present in a very activated state—with resting breathing rates that can be as high as 25–50 breaths per minute—can rarely achieve their resonant-frequency breathing rate. In this context, the child and clinician have to work with the lowest breathing rate that the child can achieve and comfortably train at. The option to formally measure the child's resonant-frequency rate and to make further gains from the slow-breathing intervention may be more achievable after the child has been able to achieve breathing rates within a normative range (Fleming et al. 2011) and after the child's skills for slowing down the breathing rate have improved (see, e.g., Chandra et al. [2017]).

The simplest way to achieve slow breathing is to have the child lying down on a mat on the floor with a paper cup or a toy on his or her abdomen, which enables both the child and the therapist to observe its movement. The clinician then counts slowly while the child breaths in through the nose and breathes out through the mouth. Theoretically, expirations should be longer than inspirations, but in reality, slow breathing that has a nice continuous rhythm (vs. jerky breathing) and that uses the diaphragm as the main muscle of breathing (so that the cup moves up and down in a smooth fashion) is a substantial achievement. Other techniques and resources for achieving diaphragmatic breathing, which readers can try out for themselves, are described elsewhere (see Online Supplement 14.1).

Alternatives to Breathing Interventions

Not all children can use breathing interventions. Sometimes the child is too young, and sometimes putting the focus on attention on the breath is activating; it increases the breathing rate and the probability of hyperventilation or a panic attack. Alternatives to the slow-breathing intervention include humming, *bee breathing* (see Online Supplement 14.1), and use of the *voo* sound (Brown and Gerberg 2005; Levine 2010). These techniques utilize the long, extended breath and activation of vagal afferents (from the vibration) to up-regulate vagal nerve function, thereby down-regulating autonomic arousal.

Grounding Interventions

Grounding interventions are used with children to help create 'a felt sense of connection to the ground' (Ogden and Fisher 2015, p. 18) and a sense of physical presence in the here and now. Grounding interventions include a body-focused activity coupled with attention to the felt sense of that activity. For example, the child may focus on the felt sense of heat, pressure, or movement associated with the activity (e.g., the feel of the breath moving when a hand is placed over the heart or over the belly) or the felt sense of the connection between the child's body and the outside world (e.g., the sensation associated with having one's feet placed firmly on the ground). In this way, grounding interventions help the child feel physically present, solid, centred, balanced, contained, connected to herself, and, in particular, connected to her body in the here and now (Ogden et al. 2006; Ogden and Fisher 2015; Jackson 2017). Commonly used grounding interventions also include feeling one's feet on the ground (which can be accentuated by having patients stomp their feet, massage their legs, or shift the body's weight to the toes, heels, and sides of the feet), feeling the chair pressing on one's back, feeling the firmness of the wall with one's hands, savouring the feel of cool water on one's face, noticing the colours of objects or the smells in the room, or noticing the feel and weight of a ball that is thrown from hand to hand or from child to parent and back. Mindful attention to an experience—for example, holding ice—is a useful emergency strategy that can be used as part of the child's safety plan (see Chapter 16).

Because grounding interventions are very concrete and can be implemented at any time in any context when working with children with functional somatic symptoms, they are useful early in the treatment process. Grounding strategies help the child hone her skills in shifting the focus of attention—for example, away from body states that she finds overwhelming or unmanageable, or from negative thoughts and feelings that activate the stress system. Grounding strategies can be added to the child's emergency strategies for states of escalating arousal that involve a sense of disconnection and *vagueing out*—states that sometimes occur, for example, in the sequence of feeling states that precede fainting episodes or NES. In this context, the grounding intervention is used to interrupt the sequence and to avert the fainting event or NES. What the child does first is to lower herself to the ground—to make sure she does not fall—as soon as she notices the onset of her warning signs. While on the ground, she may then practice a simple grounding intervention, such as demonstrating her 'capacity to direct somatic energy toward the ground' (Ogden and Fisher 2015, p. 325), so as to feel safe and held. Later on, slow breathing, visualization, and other interventions can be added to this simple grounding exercise.

Tensing the Muscles in the Legs

Tensing the large muscles in the legs (all together) in a rhythmical manner at ten-second intervals can induce an increase in heart rate variability (increase in parasympathetic activation) (Lehrer et al. 2009).

Tightening the lateral muscles of the thigh—the tensor faciae latae and the iliotibial tract—can be used to provide a sense of self-containment (Selvam and Parker n.d.): in the standing position the child digs her heels into the ground and attempts to raise her legs to the side, or in the sitting position she tries to spread her thighs, while at the same time, pushing her knees together with her hands (see Online Supplement 14.1 for other physical strategies suggested by Selvam and Parker). Children who prefer physical strategies—rather than cognitive strategies—often like these particular interventions.

Progressive Muscle Relaxation

In progressive muscle relaxation the child lies down; then, working from feet up or head down, and guided by a therapist, instructor (in a group setting), or audio recording, she reduces muscle tension by tensing a particular muscle group and then relaxing it. Most children can do this exercise; many enjoy it; and it is useful in helping the child to recognize what her body feels like when it is tense versus relaxed. Scripts for progressive muscle relaxation are widely available.

Completion of Self-Protective Motor Responses/Action Tendencies

Often when the child and therapist track body sensations, the child will report felt action tendencies—motor patterns that reflect the body's preparation for action to protect and defend itself (see vignette below). For example, when tracking sensations associated with a memory, the child may report a tightening in the hands (the action tendency that precedes the forming a fist and the action of hitting out with the hand) or the tensing of a foot (the action tendency that precedes the action of kicking out with the foot). Inhibiting action tendencies is like inhibiting negative thoughts and feelings—all of which can contribute to activation of the stress system (Pennebaker and Susman 1988). In this context, 'completion of the body's incomplete responses to protect and defend itself' can lead to symptom relief (Levine and Kline 2007, p. 419; Levine 2010). Completing motor responses is a key component of Peter Levine's psychotherapy approach, Somatic Experiencing (for more, see later subsection 'Trauma-Processing Interventions'). It is also used in the sensorimotor psychotherapy developed by Pat Ogden.

Betsy was a 13-year-old girl and a talented ballet dancer. She presented with NES in the context of cumulative stress: bullying at school, physical illness of her mother that needed hospitalization, illness of her father that needed hospitalization, academic difficulties, and difficulties in her relationship with her paternal grandmother. Amid all this stress, Betsy was most worried about her parents' health and most hurt by what she perceived to be emotional rejection by her grandmother. In the middle of a discussion with the family about an upcoming birthday and a visit by her grandmother, the therapist asked Betsy to scan her body to identify the sensations she felt at that moment in time. Betsy identified a large painful area in her chest, a tightness in her jaw, a tensing in her hands (which began to shape themselves into fists as she spoke), and a tensing in the legs, which Betsy said, felt like kicking. The therapist asked if one of the legs wanted to kick more than the other. Betsy identified the right leg. The therapist then asked Betsy to allow her leg to kick, but to do this in slow motion, against the resistance of a stuffed toy dog held by the therapist. After kicking in slow motion with the right leg and then the left—which Betsy did with immense force and precision, until the leg was fully extended—Betsy was asked to scan her body again. She reported that the painful area in her chest had gotten smaller and was less intense, that the tension in the jaw had dissipated, and that the impulse to strike out with the fist and the feet had gone. Betsy's parents, who had watched the intervention—and who were surprised by the extent of her movements (Betsy's leg kicked so far that it touched her face)—reported that they had never realized the extent of the hurt that Betsy experienced in being rejected by her grandmother.

Bottom-Up Mindfulness Practice

Many of the bottom-up regulation strategies mentioned in this section involve a bottom-up mindfulness practice: the practice of attending to body sensations, whether pleasant or unpleasant, with a curious, open stance. Because some children enjoy these bottom-up mindfulness practices, they are able to integrate a bottom-up meditation into their daily routines. Common bottom-up mindfulness meditations involve meditation with a focus on the breath, meditation while systematically focusing attention on different parts of the body (body scan), attending to body sensations via self-touch to the chest, abdomen, or kidney-adrenal region, and exercises that change the colour or shape of pain (for resources see Online Supplement 14.1). In the Eastern tradition, bottom-up mindfulness interventions also frequently involved the use of therapeutic touch by the healer. In Western practice, therapeutic touch is now being integrated into some forms of body-based psychotherapy (Yachi et al. 2018; Kain and Terrell 2018).

Regular Exercise

Voluntary regular exercise promotes regulation and coherence within and between multiple components of the stress system—the HPA axis, autonomic nervous system, immune-inflammatory system, and brain systems underpinning pain, arousal, and emotional states—via many complex mechanisms that are progressively coming into focus through current research (for references see Online Supplement 14.1). Through its effects on the immune-inflammatory system, exercise also prevents chronic pain (see Chapter 9) (Leung et al. 2016). In addition, exercise-induced alterations of the gut microbiota have implications not only for the gut but, via a complex array of mechanisms, the health of the body as a whole (Mailing et al. 2019; Bastiaanssen et al. 2020). In this context, when implemented (in stages) early in the treatment process, exercise functions as a key intervention for lowering arousal by modulating HPA-axis activity, the sympathetic nervous system, and brain systems underpinning pain, arousal, and emotional states. It also improves the child's physical resilience and day-to-day level of physical function. In the long term, regular exercise increases the child's whole-body health and resilience in response to stress. An exercise program should therefore be part of *every* child's intervention, regardless of symptom presentation.

Because arousal increases during exercise—even though the long-term goal and result of an exercise program is to decrease arousal—some children will need to start with gentle forms of exercise; otherwise, the sensations experienced during exercise may trigger panic or trauma-related responses such as innate defence responses (Kozlowska et al. 2015). Likewise, in children with chronic pain or with significant fatigue, exercise will need to be graded up slowly because it will, at least initially (see Fig. 16.1), exacerbate both pain and fatigue; the child will need to overcome this initial increase in symptoms in order to achieve the subsequent decrease in symptoms.

Physiotherapy

Children with functional neurological disorder (FND)—and especially those with loss of motor function or other functional neurological symptoms—require physiotherapy to help restore normal motor function (see vignette of Jai in Chapter 13). Physiotherapy for functional disorders is very different from standard physiotherapy because it is done in a way that does not focus attention on the symptoms (see vignette of Jai in Chapter 15) (Gray et al. 2020). The physiotherapist also assesses the child's safety in terms of balance on stairs, weight bearing on a painful foot, and so on.

Occupational Therapy

Some children who are disabled by their symptoms—and unable to manage skills of daily living on their own—may require input from an occupational therapist to help the children increase their day-to-day functioning. The occupational therapist can also contribute to the child's regulation strategies by introducing sensory strategies that the child can use to decrease arousal (Williams and Shellenberge 2012).

Releasing Trigger Points

Chronic activation of trigger points in muscle—as well as changes in the surrounding environment (fascia and connective tissue)—contributes to chronic pain in some presentations. Often, for example, chronic headache is maintained by tension in the muscles and trigger points of the neck, shoulders, and back. Manual therapies that release trigger points—all of which include some form of mechanical pressure—can be extremely helpful for some patients (Shah et al. 2015; Gevirtz [2020]).

Interventions That Target Key Brain Systems

Here we focus on interventions that aim to modulate the brain stress systems more directly, rather than by the bottom-up, body-based regulation strategies described above. These interventions include the following: pharmacotherapy for managing sleep, arousal, and anxiety and depression; various approaches to processing trauma; and neuromodulation, the use of electrical impulses or pharmaceutical agents that act directly upon the nervous system in an effort to alter its activity. In day-to-day clinical practice, these interventions are used, when indicated, alongside other indicated interventions on other system levels. For cautions when using pharmacotherapy with children and for sleep interventions, see Chapter 5.

Pharmacotherapy to Down-Regulate Arousal

Pharmacological treatments that help down-regulate arousal—clonidine, guanfacine, propranolol, selective serotonin reuptake inhibitors (SSRIs), and dual serotonin and noradrenalin reuptake inhibitors (SNRIs)—are thought to inhibit the amygdala and other limbic structures by acting on alpha, beta, GABA, or serotonin receptors in the amygdala, hypothalamus, or periaqueductal grey nucleus in the brainstem (Stahl 2013).

Pharmacological treatments to down-regulate arousal can be helpful in children whose stress systems are so activated that they are unable to utilize any of the non-pharmacological mind-body strategies described in this chapter. For many children, when their arousal is lessened somewhat—via pharmacotherapy—they are better able to learn and implement non-pharmacological regulation strategies for continued use in the long term.

Pharmacotherapy to Treat Comorbid Anxiety and Depression

Sometimes pharmacological treatment is needed to help in the treatment of anxiety and depression (see case of Jai in Chapter 5). Antidepressants (SSRIs and SNRIs) modulate neurotransmitter signalling in brain systems—serotonergic, noradrenergic, dopaminergic, GABAergic, and glutamatergic—that play a key role in arousal and mood regulation (Stahl 2013). Antidepressants—for example, SSRIs—also appear to have positive neuroplasticity effects (called *trophic effects*) that override the aberrant neuroplasticity changes that occur in the context of stress (Mann 2019). The experience of the first author (KK) is that SNRIs can be problematic in children because they often cause increases in arousal and that they are therefore often unhelpful in treating functional somatic symptoms, for which decreased arousal and activation are treatment goals.

Pharmacotherapy as a Neuromodulation Intervention

Antidepressants—tricyclics, SSRIs, and SNRIs—and atypical antipsychotic medications have complex actions that modulate multiple receptor systems involved in arousal, pain, and emotion regulation. In functional presentations that are very severe or difficult to treat, such medications may be used on a time-limited basis to manage sleep (see Chapter 5), pain, and extreme arousal by modulating key neurotransmitter signalling systems (for a review of mechanisms, see Tornblom and Drossman [2018]) (see, e.g., cases of Paula in Chapter 3 and Martin in Chapter 9).

Trauma-Processing Interventions

Some children presenting with functional somatic symptoms have specific trauma, loss, or stress events that need to be processed because these events contribute in an ongoing way to activation of the brain stress systems that may, in turn, disrupt motor and sensory processing or amplify subjective pain (see Chapter 11). The trauma-processing intervention with the largest evidence base is Eye Movement Desensitization and Reprocessing (EMDR) (for references see Online Supplement 14.1). EMDR was introduced into clinical practice by Francine Shapiro in the late 1980s (Shapiro 1989). In EMDR the child is asked to focus on the traumatic memory image while simultaneously attending to an alternate stimulus requiring brief eye movements (right and left) in sets of approximately 30 seconds. Recent studies suggest that when the processing is successful, the pattern of brain activation associated with the trauma memory shifts from activation of the brain stress systems to activation of cognitive-processing regions. More recently, EMDR using the flash technique has been introduced for individuals who are unable to tolerate access to the trauma memory for any period of time—for example, because they dissociate. The flash technique requires memory retrieval for very short periods of time with virtually no memory-related emotional arousal.

About the same time that Shapiro introduced EMDR, Peter Levine introduced Somatic Experiencing, a bottom-up psychotherapy approach for trauma (Levine 1997). In somatic experiencing, the direction of attention is on body sensations and how they change. Alongside the tracking of somatic sensations associated with a memory of an event—reflecting stress-system activation—somatic experiencing involves the tracking of action tendencies or latent action patterns (see below). If latent action patterns are identified, then the therapist may suggest interventions that may help the patient complete the latent patterns. For example, an impulse to run, heralded by a tensing in the legs, may be enacted in real time or in slow motion. Likewise, an effort to block something with the hand, heralded by a tensing in the hands, may be enacted in slow motion. In this way, defensive movements that the body was unable to enact, whether for a lack of time or for some other reason, may be enacted in slow motion, over and over again, until the body stress systems settle (as internally tracked by the patient). As previously noted, Pat Ogden uses a similar approach in her somatosensory approach to processing trauma memories (Ogden et al. 2006). For other references pertaining to somatic experiencing, see Online Supplement 14.1.

Amanda was a 9-year-old girl whose passion was playing rugby with her older brothers and their friends. During one game—with some older (and as they discovered, rougher) boys whom they did not know well—Amanda was tackled by one of the boys, and two other boys then kicked her and pushed her head into the ground, while yelling and swearing at her. Ever since the tackle, Amanda had been experiencing recurring headaches, sensitivity to light, and intermittent double vision. In the playground at school, she avoided the children who had attacked her. Sometimes, if she thought that they were trying to approach her, she would run and hide. Her sleep also deteriorated in quality, and she was waking multiple times during the night. The neurologist diagnosed Amanda's neurological symptoms as being functional and gave her the diagnosis of FND. Because Amanda had mentioned the recurring action tendency to run from the bullies, her therapist decided to use a somatic-experiencing intervention. With the aid of drawing materials, the therapist asked Amanda to show her exactly what had happened during the tackle. She also asked Amanda to show her—using her body—what her body would have done, had it had time and been able, to protect itself. Then the therapist (playing the boy who had tackled Amanda), a medical student (playing the other two boys), and Amanda's mother (playing a safe teacher) enacted the tackle in slow motion. In this slow-motion version of the tackle, Amanda was asked to put into effect all the protective actions that she had shown the therapist. On the fifth round Amanda reported that she had *got it right* and that she did not think that they needed to enact the scene again. Two weeks later Amanda's mother rang the therapist to report that all of Amanda's symptoms had resolved in the wake of the session.

More recently, other trauma-processing interventions—some of which also involve movement—have been introduced into clinical practice; the evidence base is slowly emerging (for references see Online Supplement 14.1). *Radical exposure tapping* combines elements of EMDR with various tapping sequences to create a memory-processing intervention that facilitates processing of the intense affect that accompanies some memories. In the *progressive counting technique*, the patient is asked to run a memory like a silent movie, over and over with their eyes closed, during progressively longer time periods while the therapist counts out loud. The patient starts and ends the 'movie' with a positive memory. The first author and her team have described the integration of radical exposure tapping and progressive counting into the treatment of functional somatic symptoms (Ratnamohan et al. 2018), and Laurie Mackinnon—a prominent Australian family therapist—uses these techniques routinely within a family therapy framework (MacKinnon 2014).

What is intriguing about some of the above-described trauma-processing interventions is the use of concurrent movement or sensory input as key elements of the interventions. Because action tendencies and somatic states are so closely tied to traumatic states, it is possible that engagement of motor and sensory systems facilitates changes in the processing of trauma-related material. Interestingly, imaging studies of trauma processing suggest that the healing process also engages motor systems (Santarnecchi et al. 2019).

Neuromodulation: A Treatment of the Future?

Advances in technology have led to the development of neuromodulation techniques that aim to change aberrant nervous system activation and patterns of connectivity between brain regions (for basic science references see Online Supplement 14.1). For example, in treating adults with chronic pain—and especially patients with chronic back pain—implantable spinal cord neurostimulators are now in widespread use (Sdrulla et al. 2018). Likewise, there is increasing interest in the use of neuromodulation devices—for example, transcranial magnetic stimulation—for treating FND. Topical, non-invasive neuromodulation devices—for example, the portable neuromodulation stimulator and transcutaneous auricular vagus nerve stimulator—that modulate subcortical brain regions have shown utility in patients undergoing rehabilitation interventions for motor symptoms related to brain injury, and they may be of use in treating children with severe functional impairment secondary to FND. We mention neuromodulation because this field is growing so rapidly and has demonstrated such potential.

* * *

In this chapter we have highlighted that within the stress-system model, the treatment of functional somatic symptoms involves the use of strategies, techniques, and interventions that target areas of activation, dysregulation, or difficulty on multiple system levels. What we have discussed are strategies that target the body, either with bottom-up strategies that target the body itself or with strategies that target brain systems bottom-up. These strategies can be used alone or in various combinations to assist the child in shifting her stress system back to a more regulated state, one that supports health and well-being and is incompatible with functional somatic symptoms. In the next chapter we turn to top-down strategies involving the mind.

References

Arnsten, A. F. (2015). Stress Weakens Prefrontal Networks: Molecular Insults to Higher Cognition. *Nature Neuroscience, 18,* 1376–1385.

Bastiaanssen, T. F. S., Cussotto, S., Claesson, M. J., Clarke, G., Dinan, T. G., & Cryan, J. F. (2020). Gutted! Unraveling the Role of the Microbiome in Major Depressive Disorder. *Harvard Review of Psychiatry, 28,* 26–39.

Bloch-Atefi, A., & Smith, J. (2015). The Effectiveness of Body-Oriented Psychotherapy: A Review of the Literature. *Psychotherapy and Counselling Journal of Australia, 3.* http://pacja.org.au/?p=2552.

Brown, R. P., & Gerbarg, P. L. (2005). Sudarshan Kriya Yogic Breathing in the Treatment of Stress, Anxiety, and Depression: Part I—Neurophysiologic Model. *Journal of Alternative and Complementary Medicine, 11,* 189–201.

Chandra, P., Kozlowska, K., Cruz, C., Baslet, G. C., Perez, D. L., & Garralda, M. E. (2017). Hyperventilation-Induced Non-epileptic Seizures in an Adolescent Boy with Pediatric Medical Traumatic Stress. *Harvard Review of Psychiatry, 25,* 180–190.

Fleming, S., Thompson, M., Stevens, R., Heneghan, C., Plüddemann, A., Maconochie, I., et al. (2011). Normal Ranges of Heart Rate and Respiratory Rate in Children from Birth to 18 Years of Age: A Systematic Review of Observational Studies. *Lancet, 19,* 1011–1018.

Gevirtz, R. (2020). Distinguishing Sources of Pain: Central vs. Peripheral Mediation. *Pelviperineology, 39,* 13–17.

Goldin, P. R., & Gross, J. J. (2010). Effects of Mindfulness-Based Stress Reduction (MBSR) on Emotion Regulation in Social Anxiety Disorder. *Emotion, 10,* 83–91.

Gray, N., Savage, B., Scher, S., & Kozlowska, K. (2020). Psychologically Informed Physiotherapy for Children and Adolescents with Functional Neurological Symptoms: The Wellness Approach. *Journal of Neuropsychiatry and Clinical Neurosciences.*

Guendelman, S., Medeiros, S., & Rampes, H. (2017). Mindfulness and Emotion Regulation: Insights from Neurobiological, Psychological, and Clinical Studies. *Frontiers in Psychology, 8,* 220.

Hermans, E. J., Van Marle, H. J., Ossewaarde, L., Henckens, M. J., Qin, S., Van Kesteren, M. T., et al. (2011). Stress-Related Noradrenergic Activity Prompts Large-Scale Neural Network Reconfiguration. *Science, 334,* 1151–1153.

Jackson, T. (2017). *Grounding: What to Do When You Feel Unstable.* https://tonijacksoncounselling.com/2017/08/24/Grounding-What-to-Do-When-You-Feel-Unstable/.

Kabat-Zinn, J. (1990). *Full Catastrophe Living: Using the Wisdom of Your Body and Mind to Face Stress, Pain, and Illness.* New York: Delta Trade Paperbacks.

Kabat-Zinn, J. (2005). *Coming to Our Senses: Healing Ourselves and the World Through Mindfulness.* New York: Hyperion.

Kain, K. L., & Terrell, S. J. (2018). *Nurturing Resilience: Helping Clients Move Forward from Developmental Trauma—An Integrative Somatic Approach.* Berkeley, CA: North Atlanta Books.

Kozlowska, K., Chudleigh, C., Cruz, C., Lim, M., McClure, G., Savage, B., et al. (2018). Psychogenic Non-epileptic Seizures in Children and Adolescents: Part II—Explanations to Families, Treatment, and Group Outcomes. *Clinical Child Psychology and Psychiatry, 23,* 160–176.

Kozlowska, K., & Khan, R. (2011). A Developmental, Body-Oriented Intervention for Children and Adolescents with Medically Unexplained Chronic Pain. *Clinical Child Psychology and Psychiatry, 16,* 575–598.

Kozlowska, K., Walker, P., Mclean, L., & Carrive, P. (2015). Fear and the Defense Cascade: Clinical Implications and Management. *Harvard Review of Psychiatry, 23,* 263–287. https://www.ncbi.nlm.nih.gov/pmc/articles/PMC4495877/.

Lehrer, P. (2013). How Does Heart Rate Variability Biofeedback Work? Resonance, the Baroreflex, and Other Mechanisms. *Biofeedback, 41,* 26–31.

Lehrer, P., Vaschillo, E., Trost, Z., & France, C. R. (2009). Effects of Rhythmical Muscle Tension at 0.1 Hz on Cardiovascular Resonance and the Baroreflex. *Biological Psychology, 81,* 24–30.

Lehrer, P. M., Vaschillo, E., & Vaschillo, B. (2000). Resonant Frequency Biofeedback Training to Increase Cardiac Variability: Rationale and Manual for Training. *Applied Psychophysiology and Biofeedback, 25,* 177–191.

Leung, A., Gregory, N. S., Allen, L. A., & Sluka, K. A. (2016). Regular Physical Activity Prevents Chronic Pain by Altering Resident Muscle Macrophage Phenotype and Increasing Interleukin-10 in Mice. *Pain, 157,* 70–79.

Levine, P. A. (1997). *Waking the Tiger: Healing Trauma.* Berkeley, CA: North Atlantic Books.

Levine, P. A. (2010). *In an Unspoken Voice: How the Body Releases Trauma and Restores Goodness.* Berkeley, CA: North Atlantic Books.

Levine, P. A., Blakeslee, A., & Sylvae, J. (2018). Reintegrating Fragmentation of the Primitive Self: Discussion of "Somatic Experiencing". *Psychoanalytic Dialogues, 28,* 620–628.

Levine, P. A., & Kline, M. (2007). *Trauma Through a Child's Eyes.* Berkeley, CA and Lyons, CO: North Atlanta Books and ERGOS Institute Press.

Mackinnon, L. (2014). Deactivating the Buttons: Integrating Radical Exposure Tapping with a Family Therapy Framework. *Australian and New Zealand Journal of Family Therapy, 35,* 244–260.

Mailing, L. J., Allen, J. M., Buford, T. W., Fields, C. J., & Woods, J. A. (2019). Exercise and the Gut Microbiome: A Review of the Evidence, Potential Mechanisms, and Implications for Human Health. *Exercise and Sport Sciences Reviews, 47,* 75–85.

Mann, J. (2019). *Brain Plasticity: The Effects of Antidepressants on Major Depression.* https://www.bbrfoundation.org/Event/Brain-Plasticity-Effects-Antidepressants-Major-Depression.

McCraty, R., & Zayas, M. A. (2014). Cardiac Coherence, Self-Regulation, Autonomic Stability, and Psychosocial Well-Being. *Frontiers in Psychology, 5,* 1090.

Ogden, P., & Fisher, J. (2015). *Sensorimotor Psychotherapy: Interventions for Trauma and Attachment.* New York: Norton.

Ogden, P., Minton, K., & Pain, C. (2006). *Trauma and the Body: A Sensorimotor Approach to Psychotherapy.* New York: Norton.

Paccione, C. E., & Jacobsen, H. B. (2019). Motivational Non-directive Resonance Breathing as a Treatment for Chronic Widespread Pain. *Frontiers in Psychology, 10,* 1207.

Pennebaker, J. W., & Susman, J. R. (1988). Disclosure of Traumas and Psychosomatic Processes. *Social Science and Medicine, 26,* 327–332.

Porges, S. W., & Furman, S. A. (2011). The Early Development of the Autonomic Nervous System Provides a Neural Platform for Social Behavior: A Polyvagal Perspective. *Infant and Child Development, 20,* 106–118.

Ratnamohan, L., MacKinnon, L., Lim, M., Webster, R., Waters, K., Kozlowska, K., et al. (2018). Ambushed by Memories of Trauma: Memory-Processing Interventions in an Adolescent Boy with Nocturnal Dissociative Episodes. *Harvard Review of Psychiatry, 26,* 228–236.

Russo, M. A., Santarelli, D. M., & O'Rourke, D. (2017). The Physiological Effects of Slow Breathing in the Healthy Human. *Breathe (Sheffield, England), 13,* 298–309.

Santarnecchi, E., Bossini, L., Vatti, G., Fagiolini, A., La Porta, P., Di Lorenzo, G., et al. (2019). Psychological and Brain Connectivity Changes Following Trauma-Focused CBT and EMDR Treatment in Single-Episode PTSD Patients. *Frontiers in Psychology, 10,* 129.

Sdrulla, A. D., Guan, Y., & Raja, S. N. (2018). Spinal Cord Stimulation: Clinical Efficacy and Potential Mechanisms. *Pain Practice, 18,* 1048–1067.

Selvam, R., & Parker, L. A. (n.d.). *Restoration of Body Resources Lost in Trauma.* https://www.dropbox.com/s/xrbb5i1b288rwz2/File%205%20Body%20Resources%20Lost%20in%20Trauma.doc?dl=0.

Shah, J. P., Thaker, N., Heimur, J., Aredo, J. V., Sikdar, S., & Gerber, L. (2015). Myofascial Trigger Points Then and Now: A Historical and Scientific Perspective. *PM & R, 7,* 746–761.

Shapiro, F. (1989). Eye Movement Desensitization: A New Treatment for Post-traumatic Stress Disorder. *Journal of Behavior Therapy and Experimental Psychiatry, 20,* 211–217.

Sharpe Lohrasbe, R., & Ogden, P. (2017). Somatic Resources: Sensorimotor Psychotherapy Approach to Stabilising Arousal in Child and Family Treatment. *Australian and New Zealand Journal of Family Therapy, 38,* 573–581.

Siegel, D. J. (1999). *The Developing Mind: How Relationships and the Brain Interact to Shape Who We Are.* New York: Guilford.

Stahl, S. M. (2013). *Stahl's Essential Psychopharmacology: Neuroscientific Basis and Practical Application.* New York: Cambridge University Press.

Tornblom, H., & Drossman, D. A. (2018). Psychotropics, Antidepressants, and Visceral Analgesics in Functional Gastrointestinal Disorders. *Current Gastroenterology Reports, 20,* 58.

Williams, M. S., & Shellenberge, S. (2012). *How Does Your Engine Run? A Leader's Guide to the Alert Program for Self-Regulation.* Albuquerque, NM: Therapy Works.

Yachi, C. T., Hitomi, T., & Yamaguchi, H. (2018). Two Experiments on the Psychological and Physiological Effects of Touching-Effect of Touching on the HPA Axis-Related Parts of the Body on Both Healthy and Traumatized Experiment Participants. *Behavioral Sciences (Basel, Switzerland), 8,* 95.

15

Treatment Interventions II: Working with the Mind

Abstract Cognitive and other psychological processes on the mind level of operations are amenable to conscious manipulation, and they provide a therapeutic window for change. These psychological processes can have a powerful top-down effect, with the capacity to contribute to the child's efforts to regulate her stress system, her body more generally, and her thoughts, feelings, and beliefs. In this chapter we briefly discuss a variety of interventions on the mind level of operations. These interventions are helpful for interrupting illness-promoting psychological processes that activate the stress system and that trigger or maintain functional somatic symptoms, and also for fostering health-promoting psychological processes that down-regulate the stress system and abate functional somatic symptoms.

In this chapter we turn to regulation strategies that involve working with the mind, which is to work from the top down. As we saw

Electronic supplementary material The online version of this chapter (https://doi.org/10.1007/978-3-030-46184-3_15) contains supplementary material, which is available to authorized users.

in Chapter 12, cognitive and other psychological processes—those involving the mind—have a powerful top-down effect, with the capacity both to activate and to down-regulate the stress system. Top-down interventions are meant to address ongoing processes that do not necessarily match the actual degree of threat that a child (including adolescent) is exposed to. In some cases, though, the child is actually at risk of harm—for example, from abuse within the family or from cyberbullying—in which case the thought processes relating to threat may match the actual degree of threat. In that case, addressing the threat via the appropriate *protective intervention* is the proper course of treatment. Assuming, however, that the child or adolescent is safe in her actual family and school contexts and that real-life threats do not need to be addressed, top-down mind interventions can be used alongside interventions on other system levels to down-regulate the stress system.

Top-down emotion-regulation strategies are those in which the child utilizes intentional efforts to increase her attention and awareness capacities for better control of thoughts and feelings (Guendelman et al. 2017). From the neuroscience perspective, successful implementation of top-down self-regulation strategies involves activation of the executive control system and deactivation of brain regions that are part of the brain stress systems and that play a role in regulating physiological arousal (Guendelman et al. 2017). The executive control system involves a network of regions—midline frontal areas (anterior cingulate and ventral prefrontal cortex), lateral prefrontal cortex, and posterior brain regions (posterior cingulate cortex and parts of the parietal cortex)—that operate as a unit on any task involving high-level cognition (Posner 2012; Williams 2016).

Expectations and the Placebo Effect

The child's and family's expectations, as well as the placebo effect, play an important part in the child's therapeutic response to each treatment intervention and to the treatment intervention as a whole (Benedetti 2013; Koyama et al. 2005). As noted by Tor Wager and Lauren Atlas (2015), all treatments are delivered in a context that includes social and physical cues, verbal suggestions and treatment history. This context is actively interpreted by the brain and can elicit expectations, memories and emotions, which in turn can influence health-related outcomes in the brain and body. Placebo effects are thus brain-body responses to context information that promote health and well-being. (Wager and Atlas 2015, p. 2)

Consequently, the total therapeutic effect of the systemic intervention for functional somatic symptoms includes both the neurophysiological effects from the actual treatments and the (neurophysiological) placebo effect. The expectations held by the child and the family—which are shaped by the conversations and non-verbal communications that take place between the child, family, and the clinician (clinical team)—are a fundamental component of treatment. If the expectations are positive, they will propel the child toward health and well-being (with a placebo effect). If they are negative, they will potentially propel the child toward ill health and the maintenance of functional somatic symptoms (with a nocebo effect) (see also Chapter 12).

Positive expectations were part of each morning's daily ward rounds with Jai, the 14-year-old boy with painful dystonia, weakness and lack of coordination in the legs, and disrupted circadian clock whom we met in Chapters 5 and 11. When the focus of treatment was to stabilize Jai's sleep—he was sleeping only 3–4 hours a night—the first author (KK) made repeated positive suggestions: 'As your sleep gets better and better, your brain will be able to take a rest from the pain at nighttime, and you will be able to manage the pain better and better during the daytime. We are getting there, bit by bit, step by step.' The suggestions aimed both to maintain Jai's morale and to increase the therapeutic effect of the nighttime medication by activating the placebo effect.

Psychoeducation and Giving the Child (and Parents) Space for Questions

The manner in which the therapist, at the outset, discusses the neurobiology of the symptoms and integrates this information with the story of the child's symptoms was described in Chapter 3. Over time, the child and her therapist, as well as the family and therapist, may need to engage in additional conversations about the formulation, the many different factors (or triggers) that can activate the stress system, or the many ways in which the body responds to threat. Likewise, some neurologists and paediatricians with a special interest in functional somatic symptoms use education about the symptoms as a key element in their medical interventions (Carson et al. 2015).

> Johnny, the 9-year-old boy whom we met in Chapter 12, presented with layer upon layer of functional somatic symptoms. He experienced an aha! moment when the therapist explained the formulation: 'I see! They [the danger systems/circles in the stress-system diagram] are trying to protect me, but they keep switching on when they shouldn't. I thought I had cancer and I was going to die.' Two years later, after a relapse of leg paralysis, and after the therapist reiterated the need for Johnny to keep working on his regulation strategies, Johnny exclaimed, 'It's like before. I need to settle down my body when it first starts to switch on. Then I won't get the [functional neurological disorder].'

The following vignette, told by a clinical psychologist, highlights the healing power of psychoeducation—in this case through a lecture (by the first author) about functional somatic symptoms that arise in the context of the body's innate responses to threat (Kozlowska et al. 2015). In the vignette the speaker, Johan, describes his experience (years earlier) of *tonic immobility* after being shot in the neck by his cousin Thor (the pseudonym refers to Thor, the Norse god who was known to favour violence when he solved problems). In the paediatric context, children presenting with tonic immobility—who habitually activate this innate defence mechanism in response to memories of past maltreatment—may come to the attention of the neurologist and may be given a diagnosis of non-epileptic seizures (Ratnamohan et al. 2018).

As background for the vignette, Johan, a young clinical psychologist who had just finished his training, was working at his local hospital. One day, his cousin Thor, with whom he was close and whom he had known all his life, assaulted him in front of the hospital. Thor refused to tell Johan the reason for the assault. Ten days later, Johan saw Thor passing time outside the hospital and went out to talk to him, hoping to find out what the problem was. Thor was, by then, standing right outside the door, with his back to it. And then, reports Johan:

When I said his name, Thor turned around and lifted his right arm, pointing it at my face. There was a plastic shopping bag around his hand. His hand completed the arc and when it pointed at my face, the bag exploded. From there on everything happened very, very slowly … I remember falling, like I was slowly sailing through the air. I ended on my back on the icy tarmac in front of the stairs leading up to the door. The thought I had was, 'This is unbelievable. He is killing me. And my desk is in such a mess.' I remember touching my throat with my right hand, and it felt sticky. I looked at it, and it was all red. There were no feelings about these facts. No pain, no sadness, no fear, nothing. Just like some sort of total emotional numbness. Thor watched me for a few seconds, then turned and left. I tried to get up, but I could not move. It felt like I spent an eternity flat on my back waiting for help.

For a long time afterward, I tortured myself with the idea that the shooting communicated the message that I was so worthless and despicable that there was nothing left for Thor to do but to kill me—like you do a rabid dog. He was arrested in his apartment after two hours of very good police work. The first thing he told the officers was that he was proud and relieved that he had eliminated me. He had been told by hundreds of voices (psychotic breakdown as part of a paranoid schizophrenia illness) to kill me because I was the leader of an organization that was out to get him and his daughter. It really was his intention to kill me, and he thought he had succeeded. He still had the gun and one spare cartridge in his pocket. So yes, the body's ancient defences really saved me, by making me look dead. For many years I wondered why I just did not scream or shout to get help or try to get away. I felt worry and shame for not having done anything to save myself that morning. It was not until I attended your lecture in Oslo in 2017 that I understood why my body had responded the way it did on that awful morning. You can't imagine the relief I felt. This ancient defence—tonic immobility—had saved me.

328 K. Kozlowska et al.

Changing the Focus of Attention

Changing the focus of attention can be used by some children in an explicit, conscious, and mindful manner to manage symptoms of pain, fatigue, nausea, discomfort, and so on. Focusing attention on a piece of music, on an artwork/craftwork that is in the process of being completed, on the breath, or on the child's favourite regulation strategy—and away from the symptoms—are methods that children commonly choose and that become part of their toolboxes. As we have seen elsewhere, the focus of attention is also managed implicitly in the treatment program via the structure of the program, via the way that conversations are conducted, via the manner in which all interventions are implemented, and via the family intervention, all of which focus attention onto the plans and goals of the day, and away from the symptoms themselves. The following vignette of Jai highlights this principle in the physiotherapy component of the treatment intervention. The vignette describes how the physiotherapist maintained the focus of attention on a particular goal (e.g., reaching a particular distance), on a conversation (e.g., about an unrelated topic), or on some other external stimulus (e.g., the beat of a song), and *not* on the affected limb or the symptom itself.

Fourteen-year-old Jai presented with multiple functional somatic symptoms—painful fixed dystonia in the neck, motor weakness and lack of coordination in the legs, and a pain-related curve of the body to the left. Toward the end of his admission, when Jai had progressed to mobilizing with walking sticks, his physiotherapist managed the focus of attention very carefully during sessions. Sometimes, when practicing to walk with the sticks, she would chat with Jai about how impressed she was that he had managed to walk up steps earlier in the session, rather than noting or acknowledging in any way that he was dragging his left foot while walking. Any direct focus on the dragging foot would have made the symptom worse.

At other times, when Jai was practicing walking with the sticks, the physiotherapist would ask him—he was very musical—to step to a beat, rhythm, or piece of music. They routinely played a song that Jai loved and that had a moderate tempo, to which he could move step by step. By focusing on the song's beat and not on the clearance of his dragging foot, Jai was able to achieve the required clearance in the swing phase of his gait.

Being an adolescent, Jai was also motivated to build up his strength and conditioning using gym equipment. The physiotherapist would focus on and positively reinforce Jai's *increasing strength* during activities such as a boxing, squats, calf raises, and abdominal crunches. While the explicit focus of attention was Jai's strength, all these activities also involved practice in standing, body control, and positioning. Immersed in the task and focused on his strength, Jai would override the motor patterns associated with his functional neurological disorder. For example, he would complete a boxing set in a standing position. If he had been asked to practice standing for a few minutes on his own, he would have been unable to do so. (This particular material on physiotherapy with Jai is drawn from the first author's materials for her teaching workshops [© Kozlowska 2019]).

Cognitive-Behavioural Interventions

Children with functional somatic symptoms often suffer from comorbid anxiety. A key feature of their anxiety is a tendency to anticipate negative outcomes (anticipatory anxiety), to appraise situations in a negative way, and to ruminate, catastrophize, and engage in negative self-talk. All these psychological processes, which activate the stress system in a top-down fashion, can trigger, amplify, or maintain functional somatic symptoms (see Chapter 12 for vignettes). Standard cognitive interventions—those known as *second-wave cognitive-behavioural therapy* (CBT)—are useful in addressing these unhelpful psychological processes.

There are many good resources describing standard CBT interventions that have been developed for working with children (Chansky 2008; Rapee et al. 2000). In addition, Nicole Williams and Sara Zahka provide a detailed description of second-wave CBT in the treatment of children with functional somatic symptoms (Williams and Zahka 2017), and the New South Wales (Australia) Pain Management Network has developed *Painbytes*, an online program that encourages children to develop self-management for pain skills through physical activity and cognitive approaches (Pain Management Network 2020). For a description of the three waves of CBT, see Online Supplement 15.1.

Top-Down Mindfulness Interventions

Jon Kabat-Zinn (2003, p. 145) defined mindfulness as 'the aware-ness that emerges through paying attention on purpose, in the present moment, and nonjudgmentally to the unfolding of experience moment by moment'. In our own work with children with functional somatic symp-toms, we mostly use bottom-up mindfulness strategies. These strategies focus attention on the body, promote deactivation of the brain stress sys-tems, and do not engage the executive control system (see Chapter 14). It is also possible, however, to use top-down mindfulness strategies. These strategies engage the child's cognitions and thought processes, help the child to employ intentional efforts to increase her attention and awareness capacities (in particular, for better regulation and control of emotions), and activate the executive control system (Guendelman et al. 2017). Top-down regulation strategies have been incorporated into third-wave CBT interventions such as acceptance and commitment therapy (ACT) and dialectical behaviour therapy (DBT).

As noted earlier in the chapter, many children presenting with func-tional somatic symptoms amplify their symptoms via psychological pro-cesses that have become dysfunctional. In this context, some children find that top-down mindfulness interventions—ones that help them observe thoughts and feelings nonjudgmentally and with curiosity and compassion, and that enable them to hold onto memories lightly—are a useful addition to their toolboxes. Some of our favourite top-down mindfulness exercises include the following: asking children to be aware of their feelings and to notice where those feelings reside in their bodies, and placing stressful thoughts and feelings that come to mind onto a leaf floating down a stream, or onto a balloon or into clouds that float away. For resources see Online Supplement 15.1.

Chantal, a 15-year-old girl, had presented to hospital with different functional somatic symptoms—leg weakness and lack of coordination, non-epileptic seizures, and jaw dystonia—on each of three different occasions. In all three admissions the triggering circumstance was some combination of a loss, threatened loss, and activation of past memories of loss or trauma. As part of Chantal's therapy, she and her therapist engaged in a trauma-processing intervention (radical exposure tapping) (MacKinnon 2014), processing each memory in turn. During this intervention, the therapist noticed that Chantal was holding onto her memories and not letting them go. After each memory had been processed, so that it no longer caused such a high level of activation in Chantal's body, the therapist asked her to practice—between sessions, holding the memory lightly when it came to mind, 'like a cloud that came and went'. She also suggested that Chantal could verbalize the compassion phrase that came at the end of each tapping sequence, 'I deeply and completely accept myself' to remind her that she could remember the memory lightly and with compassion. Chantal practiced this top-down mindfulness strategy and added it to her toolbox of strategies.

Visualization Exercises

Some children enjoy and are able to utilize visualization exercises as a means of down-regulating arousal and attaining a relaxed body state. In this scenario it is useful to keep a range of visualization scripts available so that the child can choose those that she likes most. Alternatively, the imagery script can be based on the child's lived experience of attachment figures who are safe and comforting or on her imagination of what is safe and comforting. The script that the therapist will use during the visualization can be co-constructed with the child. The scripts can be recorded onto the child's telephone by the therapist during a session so that the child can use the script independently at bedtime or during scheduled slots for practicing her regulation strategies. For resources see Online Supplement 15.1.

An emerging literature—which is clustered under the construct of *attachment security priming*—suggests that guided imagery or visualization of a security-enhancing interaction has beneficial outcomes on both subjective and objective (stress-system biomarkers) measures of well-being (Gillath and Karantzas 2019; Norman et al. 2015).

Hypnosis

Hypnosis is also a top-down regulation strategy that involves activation of the executive control system and increased top-down control of the brain regions processing pain and body states, deactivation of the brain stress systems, and deactivation of the regions involved in attentional control; the overall effect is to enable the hypnotizable subject to suspend critical judgment and immerse herself in a task, while reducing awareness of alternatives (Jiang et al. 2017). A growing evidence base supports the use of hypnosis in treating children with functional somatic symptoms (see commentary by the third author [HH] in 'Twisted in Pain: The Multidisciplinary Treatment Approach to Functional Dystonia' [Khachane et al. 2019]). Hypnosis can be used in two different ways: as therapeutic suggestions that are part of ordinary conversation and as a formal procedure involving a formal induction process.

Therapeutic suggestions are part of all therapeutic conversations. In this context, the therapist uses language in a way that makes positive suggestions, promotes hope, and harnesses the placebo effect in a maximal way. Both the first and third authors have been influenced by the work of Milton Erickson, an American psychiatrist who specialized in medical hypnosis and family therapy, and who saw 'deeds [as the] offspring of hope and expectancy' (Erickson 1954, p. 261; Haley 1973), meaning that the individuals' hopes and expectations have a profound influence on their actions. Positive hopes and expectations lead into positive actions, and negative hopes and expectations lead into negative actions. Using words, metaphors, and suggestion to put down stepping stones and create a path ahead for each patient, Erickson hoped to steer the patients toward healthy actions and healthy future outcomes. In the same way, all members of our multidisciplinary teams integrate positive suggestions—suggestions that point the child in the right direction— into our conversations.

> In a ward conversation we might say something like, 'How exciting that you were able to do the slow-breathing exercise all by yourself last night. You really have the skills you need—don't you! As you practice your breathing exercise more and more, your breathing rate will get slower and

slower, and your pain will get less and less—even in periods of the day when you are not practicing—all by itself. Isn't that interesting!'

When used more formally, with individuals who are hypnotizable, a formal induction process is used to help the child enter the hypnotic state, a brain state involving activation of the executive control system and increased connectivity between the executive control system and brain regions processing information about body state, coupled with deactivation of attention control regions. Children who are able to enter the hypnotic state—to '"switch" connectivity patterns' (Jiang et al. 2017, p. 4088)—are then able to respond to verbal suggestions to elicit pronounced changes in pain perception, level of arousal, and motor and sensory function.

Some children enjoy hypnosis as a means of decreasing arousal and practicing a state of relaxation accompanied by vivid imagery. Once they are able to do self-hypnosis—they practice using an audio recording of a hypnosis session by their hypnotherapist—they can integrate this skill into the program that they take home or use it to help them fall asleep at night or to settle themselves if they wake up at night. Some children are able to use self-hypnosis to manage their chronic pain. As described in the following vignette, the first author's team also used hypnosis alongside physiotherapy and occupational therapy to help mobilize—in essence, straighten out—a boy with fixed dystonia and comorbid chronic pain (see Chapter 5 for details of Jai's presentation).

Jai, the 14-year-old boy we met in Chapter 5, presented with a painful fixed dystonia in the neck, a pain-related twisting of his body to the left, with the consequence that, when sitting in the wheelchair, he twisted over the side in an arc. He had also lost power and coordination in his legs. He experienced constant pain, and any attempt at movement caused contracture of the muscles in the neck that were unbearably painful. Jai's pain prevented all physiotherapy and occupational therapy interventions that would assist him to mobilize him or to begin the process of correcting his body posture. The breakthrough came when it became apparent that Jai was highly hypnotizable. Hypnosis was added to Jai's treatment program to manage the pain. With hypnotic suggestions, Jai was able to disconnect from the pain and was able to imagine his body bending and moving like a reed or a tree. While Jai imagined the movement, the physiotherapist would reposition him into a straighter posture. In addition, the hypnotherapist made suggestions that, with time, Jai's brain would readjust and that his body would be straight and tall like a young tree.

After completing the program, Jai continued to use the hypnosis strategies with the assistance of audio recordings that he took home. For a detailed account of the intervention with Jai, see Khachane and colleagues (2019). For references to hypnosis in working with children, see Online Supplement 1.3.

Pain Coping Skills

We include pain coping skills as a separate heading because pain is a common symptom in functional presentations. Pain coping skills were developed in the 1980s by therapists working in the second-wave CBT tradition for use with patients with chronic medical conditions. At that time these skills included the following: involving oneself in distracting activities; attempting to ignore or reinterpret pain sensations; changing activity level; praying or hoping; and use of calming self-statements (Keefe et al. 1987). Later on, as the importance of pain catastrophizing became better understood, cognitive strategies also came to be used to manage that catastrophizing. More recently, both bottom-up (see Chapter 14) and top-down (this chapter) mindfulness strategies have been added to the pain coping strategies that are taught to patients with chronic pain or with certain medical conditions. For a current review of pain coping skills and strategies used with children with chronic pain and their parents, see Harrison et al. (2019).

> Jai, the 14-year-old boy with a painful dystonia, often used distraction as a pain-management strategy. After experimenting with a range of activities, he decided that what worked especially well was to distract himself from the pain by playing his favourite songs on the keyboard or by composing new songs with the help of the keyboard.

***

In this chapter we have touched upon some of the cognitive and psychological interventions that pertain to the mind level of operations and that can be integrated by the clinician into the systemic intervention for functional somatic symptoms. These top-down interventions can be integrated alongside interventions on other system levels to help the child shift her stress system back to a more regulated state, one that supports health and well-being and is incompatible with functional somatic symptoms.

References

Benedetti, F. (2013). Placebo and the New Physiology of the Doctor-Patient Relationship. *Physiological Reviews, 93,* 1207–1246.

Carson, A., Lehn, A., Ludwig, L., & Stone, J. (2015). Explaining Functional Disorders in the Neurology Clinic: A Photo Story. *Practical Neurology, 16,* 56–61.

Chansky, T. E. (2008). *Freeing Your Child from Negative Thinking: Powerful, Practical Strategies to Build a Lifetime of Resilience, Flexibility, and Happiness.* Cambridge, MA: Da Capo Press.

Erickson, M. (1954). Pseudo-orientation in Time as a Hypnotherapeutic Procedure. *Journal of Clinical and Experimental Hypnosis, 2,* 261–283.

Gillath, O., & Karantzas, G. (2019). Attachment Security Priming: A Systematic Review. *Current Opinion in Psychology, 25,* 86–95.

Guendelman, S., Medeiros, S., & Rampes, H. (2017). Mindfulness and Emotion Regulation: Insights from Neurobiological, Psychological, and Clinical Studies. *Frontiers in Psychology, 8,* 220.

Haley, J. (1973). *Uncommon Therapy: The Psychiatric Techniques of Milton H. Erickson, M.D.* New York: Norton.

Harrison, L. E., Pate, J. W., Richardson, P. A., Ickmans, K., Wicksell, R. K., & Simons, L. E. (2019). Best-Evidence for the Rehabilitation of Chronic Pain Part 1: Pediatric Pain. *Journal of Clinical Medicine, 8,* E1267.

Jiang, H., White, M. P., Greicius, M. D., Waelde, L. C., & Spiegel, D. (2017). Brain Activity and Functional Connectivity Associated with Hypnosis. *Cerebral Cortex, 27,* 4083–4093.

Kabat-Zinn, J. (2003). Mindfulness-Based Interventions in Context: Past, Present, and Future. *Clinical Psychology: Science and Practice, 10,* 144–156.

Keefe, F. J., Caldwell, D. S., Queen, K. T., Gil, K. M., Martinez, S., Crisson, J. E., et al. (1987). Pain Coping Strategies in Osteoarthritis Patients. *Journal of Consulting and Clinical Psychology, 55,* 208–212.

Khachane, Y., Kozlowska, K., Savage, B., McClure, G., Butler, G., Gray, N., et al. (2019). Twisted in Pain: The Multidisciplinary Treatment Approach to Functional Dystonia. *Harvard Review of Psychiatry, 27,* 359–381. https://pubmed.ncbi.nlm.nih.gov/31714467/.

Koyama, T., McHaffie, J. G., Laurienti, P. J., & Coghill, R. C. (2005). The Subjective Experience of Pain: Where Expectations Become Reality. *Proceedings of the National Academy of Sciences of the United States of America, 102,* 12950–12955.

Kozlowska, K. (2019, February). *Making Sense of Somatic Symptoms: The Neurobiology of Bodytalk.* Workshop, Children's Hospital at Westmead, Sydney, Australia.

Kozlowska, K., Walker, P., McLean, L., & Carrive, P. (2015). Fear and the Defense Cascade: Clinical Implications and Management. *Harvard Review of Psychiatry, 23,* 263–287. https://www.ncbi.nlm.nih.gov/pmc/articles/PMC4495877/.

MacKinnon, L. (2014). Deactivating the Buttons: Integrating Radical Exposure Tapping with a Family Therapy Framework. *Australian and New Zealand Journal of Family Therapy, 35,* 244–260.

Norman, L., Lawrence, N., Iles, A., Benattayallah, A., & Karl, A. (2015). Attachment-Security Priming Attenuates Amygdala Activation to Social and Linguistic Threat. *Social Cognitive and Affective Neuroscience, 10,* 832–839.

Pain Management Network. (2020). *Painbytes.* https://www.aci.health.nsw.gov.au/chronic-pain/painbytes.

Posner, M. I. (2012). *Attention in a Social World.* New York: Oxford University Press.

Rapee, R., Wignall, A., Hudson, J., & Schniering, C. A. (2000). *Treating Anxious Children and Adolescents.* Oakland, CA: New Harbinger Publications.

Ratnamohan, L., MacKinnon, L., Lim, M., Webster, R., Waters, K., Kozlowska, K., et al. (2018). Ambushed by Memories of Trauma: Memory-Processing Interventions in an Adolescent Boy with Nocturnal Dissociative Episodes. *Harvard Review of Psychiatry, 26,* 228–236.

Wager, T. D., & Atlas, L. Y. (2015). The Neuroscience of Placebo Effects: Connecting Context, Learning and Health. *Nature Reviews Neuroscience, 16,* 403–418.

Williams, L. M. (2016). Defining Biotypes for Depression and Anxiety Based on Large-Scale Circuit Dysfunction: A Theoretical Review of the Evidence and Future Directions for Clinical Translation. *Depression and Anxiety, 34,* 9–24.

Williams, S. E., & Zahka, N. E. (2017). *Treating Somatic Symptoms in Children and Adolescents.* New York: Guilford Press.

16

Treatment Interventions III: Working with the Family and Implementing Behavioural Interventions

Abstract Children are born into a family and shaped by the relationships, interactions, beliefs, stories, and experiences within the family system. In this way, the health of the family and the health of the child are closely interconnected, and interventions with children presenting with functional somatic symptoms must always involve the family. All the interventions presented in this chapter—and those presented in Chapter 14 (bottom-up interventions working with the body) and Chapter 15 (top-down interventions working with the mind)—are best effected if they are supported and sustained by the family, are integrated into family processes and ways of being, and enable the family to engage in its own process of change.

The process of working with the family takes place together with and alongside the work with the child (including adolescent) and alongside the implementation of interventions from other system levels. The family

---

Electronic supplementary material The online version of this chapter (https://doi.org/10.1007/978-3-030-46184-3_16) contains supplementary material, which is available to authorized users.

339

K. Kozlowska et al., *Functional Somatic Symptoms in Children and Adolescents*, Palgrave Texts in Counselling and Psychotherapy, https://doi.org/10.1007/978-3-030-46184-3_16

is part of the family assessment interview—the process of co-constructing a formulation, discussing a treatment plan, and negotiating a treatment contract (see Chapter 3). In this way, from the very beginning, the family is part of the storytelling process that identifies past events that contributed, as well as current matters that are still contributing, to the child's stress and distress, and, in turn, to the activation of her stress system. The natural flow-on from this approach is that, at the outset, the clinician emphasizes the importance of the family in the therapeutic process. Early in this process, the clinician works with the parents to support them in the task of supporting the child as she engages in the treatment program (see interventions outlined in Chapters 14 and 15). Later, as the treatment progresses, the clinician may need to work with the family—or arrange family work via an appropriate referral—to address any residual issues on the parental or family system level that are continuing to stress the child or otherwise slowing her progress. In the sections that follow, we outline some of the family interventions that we use to support children with functional somatic symptoms.

Interventions to Establish a Foundation for Moving Forward

Advocating for the Family in the Health Care System

When initially presenting for assessment to the mental health clinician—or more commonly the multidisciplinary team—many families are confused about the medical process that preceded the referral. Often they do not quite understand the results or implications of the clinical examination and investigations done by the paediatrician:

- How have those results excluded organic illness?
- On what basis has the paediatrician made a positive diagnosis of a functional disorder?
- How is the family to make sense of the different terminologies that different health professionals have used to talk about functional problems?
- Why has a referral has been made to a mental health professional?

In the hospital setting, helping to address these shortfalls—and advocating for the family to have them addressed—may be one of the first interventions undertaken by the team or clinician. The advocacy may involve any or all or the following:

- A call to the paediatrician while the family is in the room to clarify the diagnosis and medical findings
- A joint consultation with the paediatrician and family in which the medical process and diagnosis are explained again
- Completion of tests that should have been done and were not
- A referral for a second opinion so that the parents can feel confident about the diagnosis and can move on to engage with the treatment process
- An explanation of the entire process in words that the family can understand.

This intervention helps the family move from a medical model to the systems (biopsychosocial) model of understanding and treating functional somatic symptoms. If this step is not completed, the child and family are unable to shift gears, as it were—from the medical model to the systems model—and unable to engage in the treatment process. Importantly, too, the family are not positioned to help their child get well. Instead, they are likely to go doctor shopping and to take the child down the spiral of chronicity that was described in Chapter 2. In this way, this initial family intervention is a make-it or break-it intervention. If it fails, the entire intervention never gets off the ground.

Identifying the Level of Capacity When Working with the Family

Early in the assessment process—based on the family's responses and interactions within the family assessment interview—the clinician needs to make an assessment of the family's capacity or lack of capacity to think about their contribution to the child's functional somatic symptoms, and their readiness for a family intervention. This judgment will influence whether the clinician includes family interventions upfront and early in the treatment process or whether the clinician implements family interventions slowly or even indirectly, while trust between the clinician and family—the secure base from which they work (Byng-Hall 1995)—is being further established. In any event, the clinician will begin working on system levels that the family can tolerate, and will progress from there to interventions on the system levels that are more challenging for the family. In this way, the clinician builds a secure base from which to work, bit by bit. Nonetheless, the need to address these different system levels should be raised at the outset so that the child and family are aware, from the very beginning, that all components of the intervention are important.

An advantage of this multi-levelled, systems approach is its flexibility and adaptability. It enables the clinician, child, and family to determine interventions that can, even at first, be used to good effect and that, building upon the trust thereby established, enable the treatment to move onto system levels that the child or family may previously have resisted as too difficult or anxiety provoking. What this means in practice is that the treatment is less likely to get 'stuck'; creative, flexible approaches to the choice of intervention at any particular time are likely to enable treatment to proceed in a positive direction. A less systemic approach—one that locates difficulties at a particular system level, such as the child only or the family only—is much more likely to encounter dead ends, with no obvious options for new, potentially useful interventions along pathways not previously considered.

Using the Body as a Beacon to Track Stressful Events Within the Family and Child's Social Context

One way to identify the family's capacity early in the assessment process is to use the body as a beacon to track stressful events within the family and child's social context—in particular, by initially asking questions about the symptoms and asking questions that help build a context around the symptoms (see case of Paula in Chapter 3). This way of gathering information can help to clarify quite quickly whether the family can manage any direct questions about family function and family emotional processes, whether the family will spontaneously offer any relational information, and whether gathering information via direct questions is too threatening.

Containing Anxiety in the Family System: The Therapist as a Container of Anxiety

The notion that the clinician functions as a *container of anxiety* comes from the 1940s and 1950s, from the psychotherapy tradition. According to Linda Finlay (2015a, p. 64; 2015b), 'the concept of *containing* is based on Jung's (1946) idea that the therapy process can be likened to an alchemical container in which the chemicals are the thoughts and feelings of both patient and analyst which have to be held safely'. The notion of the clinician as a container of anxiety is also implicit in John Bowlby's conceptualization of the therapeutic relationship as a secure base (Bowlby 1988; Byng-Hall 1995) (see also Chapters 2 and 3).

In working with children and families, *the clinician as container* refers to the holding or containment—the secure base—that the clinician provides in the therapeutic relationship with the child and family. According to attachment theorist Patricia Crittenden, the sense of connection that babies experience in attachment relationships is built up in two different ways: connection via *shared feelings* (affective states) and connection via *doing* (shared action) (Crittenden 2007). In our experience in working with children with functional somatic symptoms, these two ingredients are likewise important in the therapeutic relationship and in the clinician's role as therapeutic container. While it is important to the family that the clinician connects with the family on *the feeling level*, enabling the family to feel understood, it is equally important that the clinician connect with the family on *the doing level*, enabling the family to engage in the course of therapeutic action that they and the clinician need to take. Along the same lines, Edward Bordin, an American psychologist who saw the therapeutic relationship as the cornerstone of the patient's change through psychotherapy, described that relationship as involving different elements, including feelings, beliefs and understandings, and actions (Bordin 1979).

Most parents are earnest in supporting the child in her effort to get well, and they are eager to learn what they can do to support the child during the treatment process. But they often feel helpless in the face of the symptoms; they need to rely on the therapist to point the way forward.

Because the behaviours—the doings—that are required of the parents are sometimes counterintuitive, the therapist needs to explain how and why their attention to the child's pain or other symptoms has the unfortunate consequence of triggering and amplifying both the pain and other symptoms. For many parents this is an aha! moment, and they are dismayed that other health professionals failed to provide them with the information that some of what they were doing with the child—in an effort to be supportive and caring—was counterproductive.

Once a common understanding has been achieved, the *doing* ingredient of the therapeutic relationship necessitates that the clinician be explicit—and sometimes prescriptive (as in giving the family homework tasks)—in asking the family to practice new ways of being with the child; these ways need to become part of family interactions in order for the child to get well. The therapist also needs to work and collaborate with the family to help them begin implementing the *doing* part of therapy immediately. Connecting with the family via *feeling together* and via *doing together* contains anxiety. For more detail see later subsections 'Stepping Back and Giving the Child Space' and 'Changing the Focus of Attention'.

Facilitating Healing from Adverse Experiences in the Health Care System

As discussed in Chapter 3, some children and families have experienced unhelpful—and sometimes frankly abusive—interactions in their efforts to obtain help for the child via the health care system. Sometimes the child and family feel dismissed or emotionally battered because of inappropriate, mean, or ignorant comments made by health workers (see Chapter 3). An important intervention during the assessment process is to probe for such negative experiences, listen to what happened, acknowledge the child and family's pain, confusion, and anger, and highlight the dearth of knowledge about functional symptoms in the medical and paramedical world. Usually, this sort of frank acknowledgment about what has happened enables the family to leave it behind and to connect with the treating team in a positive way. Sometimes, the emotional damage has been so significant that it may be necessary to implement trauma-specific interventions with the child or even a family member, potentially around specific memories or events (see 'Trauma-Processing Interventions' in Chapter 14).

Starting the Intervention with a Working Formulation

Some children and families are forthcoming with information, and others are not. Separate from these initial attitudes toward disclosure, some children and families provide the clinician with rich information; others omit information because they do not realize that it is important or because they are unaware that events in the child's life have affected the child adversely; still others, at least at first, do not trust the process and choose not to share what they know. Sometimes additional sensitive information is offered by the child or family once trust has been established. In this context, and with the information that is available at the time, the clinician and family need to co-construct a working formulation and, if agreed, to start treatment. With time, as more information becomes available, the working formulation evolves, and treatment interventions can be updated in turn.

> Peppa was a 12-year-old girl with sudden-onset functional paralysis of both legs and episodic whole-body shaking. Peppa was a high achiever. Prior to her illness she had been an elite dancer and had ranked academically at the top of her class two years in a row. Peppa reported that she had grown up in a loving and kind family. She maintained that her growing up was 'the best' and that she had never once been angry with her parents. Akin to Peppa, her parents were unable to identify any stress or difficulties that may have contributed to their daughter's illness. But the

team's experience of the emotional interactions within the family was inconsistent with the family story. During the first half of Peppa's admission, her father, frustrated by some aspect of her clinical care, accosted the female resident—the most junior member of the team—with a volley of questions. A week later, and coinciding with the new rotation of residents, the father repeated this behaviour, picking out the new female resident who had insufficient knowledge to respond to his questions and points of dissatisfaction. The resident felt sufficiently rattled that she subsequently made sure to protect herself by going to the ward with a colleague. The same pattern of interaction was observed with other professionals on several other occasions. It was through these interactions that the team understood that Peppa needed to be a good girl and needed to use a Type A attachment strategy—one that prioritized compliance, performance, inhibition of negative affect, and expression of false-positive affect—to facilitate a close relationship with her father and to ensure that she obtained his love and approval and was not the object of his anger. (For attachment strategies see Crittenden [1999], Farnfield et al. [2010], and Online Supplement 4.1.)

Structural Interventions Involving the Family

Stepping Back and Giving the Child Space

Most parents are distressed about their child's symptoms and would do anything possible to fix those problems. In this context, it can be difficult for parents to step back and support the child as she engages in treatment. But she is, after all, the only person who can track her body from the inside and the only person who can implement body-based strategies to help down-regulate her stress system. Parents whose child has been ill for a prolonged period find this stepping back especially difficult because the process of adapting to the illness has resulted in changes in both the parent-child relationship and family dynamics (see the spiral into chronicity in Chapter 2).

Parents also need to step back from other aspects of the program— for example, physiotherapy sessions—to give the child space to work without parental attention to her symptoms.

Some parents find it helpful to know that the child's symptoms are most likely to first settle when the child is participating in enjoyable activities that take place in contexts where the parent and the treating team's therapists are not present—for example, when she is enjoying learning activities at school, interactions with the adolescent group, or physical activities with the physiotherapist. Others find it helpful to know that their attention to symptoms will amplify them. Yet others are encouraged to learn that their stepping back and giving the child space is a treatment intervention in itself. In this context, providing parents a clear explanation for why the clinician is asking them to step back (i.e., that the child is learning to take responsibility for her own body) can help the parents to do so without feeling blamed for the child's symptoms. Providing regular emotional support to the parents can also be helpful—for example, by calling them on a daily basis and giving them updates as to how the child is going in their absence, especially in the early stage, when the parents are still adjusting to the need to step back.

Changing the Focus of Attention

Many parents are distressed when they discover that their attempts to look after the child—for example, by frequently asking the child about her pain—have actually made the situation worse, contributing to the intensity and frequency of the child's symptoms. In this context, parents usually work hard to change their focus of attention. One way for them to change the focus of attention is by talking to the child about the progress that she is making with her mind-body strategies. This shifts the focus of attention from the symptoms themselves to what the child is doing about them. It also changes the focus of attention to the child's capacity to regulate her body, thereby increasing her sense of self-efficacy and control. Another way to change the focus of attention is for the parents to make sure that, when they spend time with the child, they engage in activities that are enjoyable for everyone—that is, that they connect by *doing together*.

Unfortunately, some symptoms—for example, non-epileptic seizures (NES)—necessitate action. During a seizure, the parents are asked to make sure that the child is safe and comfortable. If music is one of the strategies that help the child to regulate, parents might, for example, pop an earphone into the child's ear and play some music or the relaxation script that the child uses to help her down-regulate. Otherwise, parents need to sit quietly by the child, waiting or reading. Once the event is over, parents may coach the child to engage in her mind-body strategies to down-regulate her stress system. Once the child is settled, they will encourage the child to continue with what she was doing before the onset of the NES.

Whatever the symptom, changing the focus of attention is difficult for parents; when their efforts at managing this aspect of the treatment program are going well, it is helpful to provide them with feedback and encouragement to that effect.

> The mother of Paula—the 15-year-old, bed-bound adolescent girl we met in Chapter 3—was very distressed when she found out that constantly asking Paula about her pain functioned to amplify the pain. She wondered why no one had told her that before. In this context, she and Paula's father accepted the therapist's suggestion that the hospital admission provided an opportunity to step back (see also above), to allow Paula to manage the therapeutic components of the admission on her own (free of her parents' attention), and to practice not asking Paula about her pain—for example, by asking Paula (during their evening visit) about what she had done or achieved that day.

Timetabling Activities: Getting on with Normal Activities as Much as Possible

Outside of the treatment program, parents are encouraged to persevere with, and timetable in (see also later subsection 'Daily Timetable'), any normal activities that the child is able to engage in. The key message given by the family to the child is that life goes on and that resumption of normal activities is treatment. In the initial phase of treatment, these activities may be graded to ensure that the child isn't overdoing it (see Figs. 16.1 and 16.2). Many families struggle to find the balance between doing too little (leading to slower progress and potentially frustration with the pace of improvement) and doing too much (causing

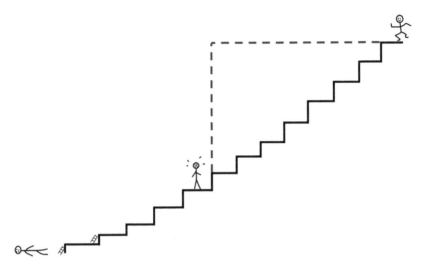

Fig. 16.1 Staircase metaphor for the treatment process. This illustration of the stairs is a metaphor for how in the initial phase of treatment the activities that make up treatment—self-care, physiotherapy, going to school—may be graded to ensure the child is not overdoing it and to avoid a crash. In other words, the treatment process for functional somatic symptoms is like a staircase made up of many small steps. Treatment starts with very, very small steps and continues with small steps. Over time the steps add up to mark significant progress (see dotted line). If at any point the steps are too hard, they can be further broken down into smaller steps (represented by the ladder). The drawing shows that when the child is very ill (depicted by the figure at the bottom of the stairs), the goals for the activity will be modest (the small low stairs at the bottom of the staircase), and that sometimes it will even be necessary to use a ladder to get up the small stairs (depicted by the ladder). When the child gets better and has more energy and capacity, the stairs will be correspondingly bigger. For example, going to school may start with a few hours a day in a wheelchair, build up to more hours and transferring out of the wheelchair, and then build up to even more hours and leaving the wheelchair in the school office. For some children, if the principle of gradual increase (one small step at a time) is not explained clearly, then the child sees just one big staircase (depicted in the broken line)—and thinks 'I cannot do this'—which can provoke anxiety and trigger significant increases in arousal (© Trond H. Diseth 1991. Reprinted with permission)

the child to crash, a potentially serious setback). The timetable—which is upgraded as the child's capacity improves—aims to find the right balance. Finally, with coercive children, the timetable is a key element of the behavioural intervention (Sells 1988; Kozlowska 2016).

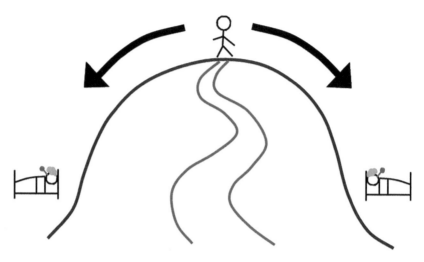

Fig. 16.2 Path on the mountain metaphor for the treatment process. This line drawing shows that the treatment process for functional somatic symptoms involves a balancing act that can be likened to the child walking on a narrow path on the ridge of a mountain. If the interventions that make up the treatment program are not challenging enough, the child will slide down one side of the mountain and will remain sick. If the interventions that make up the program are too challenging, the child will slide down the other side of the mountain and will retreat back into bed, into the sick state. When the treatment program is just right, the child progresses slowly—along the narrow path—to a state of health and well-being (© Kasia Kozlowska 2019)

Intra-familial Issues and Interventions

Learning Skills to Identify and Talk About Stress and Distress

The therapeutic process of helping the child and family to make links between stressful life events and escalations of the child's symptoms is crucially important. A family that acquires this skill will be better able to support the child in the face of future stress. Because most families have conceptualized the child's symptoms as distinct phenomena and have not made the connection between the symptoms and the events in the child's life, these skills are ones that the family needs to learn. In this context, the clinician works to support the child to communicate to her parents when she notices that her stress system is activating, to support the parents to communicate to the child when they notice her stress system is activating, and to support the family as a whole to notice what events or situations the child finds stressful. For some parents, an emotional-coaching intervention may be helpful (Gottman and DeClaire 1997; Owenz 2017).

> Betsy, the 13-year-old girl with NES whom we met in Chapter 14, always told her parents that she was fine. On weekend leave from the Mind-Body Program, Betsy had had a good weekend with few NES. However, on coming back to hospital, Betsy had a series of NES. Betsy admitted that she hated being in hospital, so the link between Betsy's NES and her distress pertaining to the return to hospital was made. A week later, on the afternoon of discharge for the school holidays—the Mind-Body Program does not run during holidays—Betsy also had a series of NES. The therapist asked the family what had happened to trigger the NES. Betsy's mother said that earlier in the afternoon, Betsy had phoned her and sounded frantic. In the phone call Betsy had told her mother that after she had packed up her things for the trip home, the nurses had put her temporarily into the treatment room—a room that was full of medical gadgets. In that room Betsy had imagined needles going into her arm. Her anxiety and arousal had escalated, and she had triggered her NES. The therapist noted that the treatment room episode—like that of coming back to hospital—were excellent examples of how, when Betsy became very aroused or anxious, her NES were triggered. She suggested that Betsy and the family were getting better at noticing the circumstances in which Betsy's body activated.

Addressing Health Issues in the Family System

Quite often the child's distress pertains to the well-being of her parents. In this context, ensuring that parental health issues are being addressed can be an important component of the intervention. This can involve addressing areas of both physical and mental health.

Addressing Other Family Issues

The storytelling process often elicits other family issues that may need to be addressed. Common issues that contribute to activation of the child's stress system include family or parental conflict, breakdown of important relationships, and differences in parenting. For example, if the formulation is that the child's stress system is activated because of sustained parental conflict, then this needs to be raised with the parents in a way that they can tolerate and hear, because with unremitting conflict the child will not get well or will keep relapsing with new health problems (see case of Rudi in Chapter 9). However, because these issues are not specific to working with children with functional somatic symptoms, we do not discuss them in detail here. For helpful resources for working with such issues in family therapy, see Rhodes and Wallis (2011) and the many other wonderful family therapy resources available in the literature (e.g., Dallos and Draper 2010).

Working with Behavioural Interventions

Behavioural interventions are a basic component in treating functional somatic symptoms. Whether the child is managed in the community or in the hospital setting, the treating team and family need to implement a structure—a behavioural program—around the child that facilitates normal daily activities and that helps the child move toward health and well-being. The members of the family are, indeed, key players in all behavioural interventions; they support, sustain, and maintain those interventions whenever the child goes home. Common behavioural interventions that we use day in and day out are included below.

Daily Timetable

The daily timetable visually sets out the patient's activities from waking up to going to bed. It includes bedtime and waking time, eating times, activity times, the time and frequency of the regulation strategies that the child is practicing daily to down-regulate her stress system, and also time to rest. The third author (HH) and the multidisciplinary team she works with view the timetable as a *dosette box* for a treatment whose 'ingredients' are the specified activities—carefully chosen and 'tailored' to the individual child—and their total effects.

For both the patient and the multidisciplinary team, the timetable is an important tool that, for either a day or a week at a time, organizes the treatment program. For the *child*, the timetable provides predictability and promotes the sense of control and mastery. These factors may help to lower the child's arousal and worries/anxiety—which is an intervention in itself and also important for maintaining the child's motivation. For *cooperative* children, the timetable provides scaffolding for the day and establishes a predictable rhythm for it. For *uncooperative* children, the timetable provides the treating team and family with a way to check whether a child is actually taking responsibility by engaging in the interventions that will make her better.

For the multidisciplinary team and also the family, the timetable is an important management tool ensuring that everybody involved knows exactly what the treatment plan is and that they all *push in the same direction*. And since the child's schedule is set in advance for the day regardless of her symptoms, having the timetable in hand preempts the need to start each day by querying the patient about her symptoms ('How are you feeling?' 'How is your pain or energy level?' 'Will you be able to do this and that?')—a sure way to exacerbate them.

Goal Setting

Setting small tangible goals in skills of daily living, physiotherapy, psychological work, reintegration to school, and so on is imperative to ensure that the child continues to progress.

Managing Avoidance Behaviours

Avoidance behaviours are common in children with functional somatic symptoms. Usually children will avoid certain activities because they are associated with pain or fatigue, or because the child might be afraid of having an NES, and so on. Many children also avoid certain activities because of anxiety: negative anticipatory thoughts, catastrophizing, and so on. The overall treatment program is designed as a behavioural intervention that includes all the activities that the child needs to re-engage in and re-master—such as getting up in the morning, exercising, going to school, and engaging with peers.

The Traffic Light Safety Plan

We include safety planning as a behavioural intervention because the child may need to use it as a reference point on a daily basis and, when necessary, to act as the plan requires. The *traffic light safety plan* is used as a way of identifying, and of implementing an immediate response to, low mood, suicidal ideation, and thoughts of self-harm (see Online Supplements 16.1 and 16.2). Also, in children with NES, who face the risk of falling and injuring the head, identifying the antecedents of NES events enables them to protect their physical safety by immediately assuming a sitting position (the first action documented on the safety plan). The first author (KK) and her team use a *traffic light system* developed by mental health clinician Danae Laskowski. Using that system, the child develops the safety plan with her individual therapist and summarizes it in a visual representation, with events or states coded as green (safe and stable), orange (beginning to activate; use mind-body techniques to settle), or red (high risk) (see Online Supplement 16.2). The safety plan is shared with the family, school, and other persons who implement the plan. The parents can carry a copy of the safety plan with them in case they need to take the child to the emergency department. The safety plan is updated as the child learns additional strategies to manage perturbations in body state, arousal, thought processes, and mood.

Using a Bike/Rugby Helmet to Protect the Head from Falls

Children with fainting episodes or NES are potentially at risk of injuring themselves from falls until they have gained control over these episodes (usually by recognizing the antecedents [warning signs], lowering themselves safely to the ground, and then engaging in mind-body techniques to lessen their arousal). When such a risk is present, we have, at times, used bike or rugby helmets to protect these children's heads.

Betsy, the 13-year-old girl and ballet dancer with NES whom we met earlier in the chapter, had NES that were very difficult to manage. Betsy found it difficult to notice warning signs, and after the NES she had no memory of them. At first, she thought everyone was trying to keep her in hospital for no reason at all. She broke down wailing when she saw one of her events on her mother's phone. When an NES occurred, Betsy would fall. In the first author's room, she fell face down, narrowly missing the metal rail of the chair. In the hospital she sustained multiple injuries—sometimes by falling off the toilet—despite being nursed one to one. During one event she fell into her food, and her face and hair were covered with vomited watermelon. On a gate pass home, she cut open her head and bled profusely onto the bathroom floor. During the latter part of her admission—and on integration to school—Betsy wore a rugby helmet.

Working with Other System Levels: Don't Forget the School

There are also other system levels that are important when working with children with functional somatic symptoms. The most important of these are the school system, the health care system, and, when children live in small communities, leaders within those communities. While each of these areas of work could be the subject of another chapter (as could other topics), we need to keep this particular book within manageable limits. With regard to the school system level, we have provided the reader with some ideas in Online Supplement 16.3.

***

In this chapter we have discussed interventions pertaining to the family system level. Family interventions are a fundamental component of the treatment intervention because they enable parents and families to support the child with functional somatic symptoms in her efforts to get well. We have described commonly used behavioural interventions that are typically collaboratively implemented by the child, family, and clinician. Family interventions aim to increase regulation within the child's stress system, to create safety in the child's family and social contexts (because safe contexts do not require activation of the stress system), to strengthen nurturing relationships (because mammals regulate better in the context of close relationships), and, by doing all these things, to increase the child's capacity for managing stress and distress, thereby building resilience so as to buffer the child from future stress.

References

Bordin, E. S. (1979). The Generalizability of the Psychoanalytic Concept of the Working Alliance. *Psychotherapy: Theory, Research and Practice, 16,* 252–260.

Bowlby, J. (1988). *A Secure Base: Clinical Applications of Attachment Theory.* London: Routledge.

Byng-Hall, J. (1995). *Rewriting Family Scripts.* London: Guilford Press.

Crittenden, P. M. (1999). Danger and Development: The Organization of Self-Protective Strategies. *Monographs for the Society for Research on Child Development, 64,* 145–171.

Crittenden, P. M. (2007). *Care-Index: Infant Coding Manual.* Miami, FL.

Dallos, R., & Draper, R. (2010). *An Introduction to Family Therapy: Systemic Theory and Practice.* Maidenhead, Berkshire, UK: Open University Press.

Farnfield, S., Hautamaki, A., Nørbech, P., & Sahar, N. (2010). DMM Assessments of Attachment and Adaptation: Procedures, Validity and Utility. *Clinical Child Psychology and Psychiatry, 15,* 313–328.

Finlay, L. (2015a). Holding, Containing and Boundarying. In *Relational Integrative Psychotherapy: Engaging Process and Theory in Practice.* Chichester, Sussex: Wiley.

Finlay, L. (2015b). *Holding, Containing and Boundarying: Handouts: Chapter 5—Therapeutic Holding and Containing.* http://relational-integrative-psychotherapy.uk/chapters/holding-containing-and-boundarying/.

Gottman, J., & Declaire, J. (1997). *Raising an Emotionally Intelligent Child.* New York: Simon and Schuster.

Kozlowska, K. (2016). The Body Comes to Family Therapy: Utilizing Research to Formulate Treatment Interventions with Somatising Children and Their Families. *Australian and New Zealand Journal of Family Therapy, 37,* 6–25.

Owenz, M. (2017). *How to Strengthen Your Child's Emotional Intelligence.* https://www.gottman.com/blog/strengthen-childs-emotional-intelligence/.

Rhodes, P., & Wallis, A. (2011). *A Practical Guide to Family Therapy: Structured Guidelines and Key Skills.* Hawthorn, VIC: IP Communications.

Sells, S. P. (1988). Setting Clear Rules and Consequences: The Basic Work of Therapy. In *Treating the Tough Adolescent: A Family-Based, Step-by-Step Guide.* New York: Guilford Press.

17

Conclusion

Abstract In this brief conclusion we take a step back and reflect on the continuing need for health professionals and health care systems to develop a more holistic (systemic), mind-body approach to diagnosing and managing functional somatic symptoms in children and adolescents. And as we have seen, specialized multidisciplinary, multimodal programs are necessary when these symptoms are severe, causing significant impairment. We also need to recognize that our current knowledge in this field remains approximate, though the evidence base continues to grow. In the interim, especially given the diversity of functional symptoms and presentations, we need to be creative and to move beyond established silos and settled approaches to research and treatment. And because these symptoms are so common in children and adolescents, we encourage readers to take an educational and leadership role in their own professional communities.

When the final chapters of this book were being completed, the first author (KK) was engaged in an ongoing, trans-Pacific email conversation with a parent who happened to be a well-known professor at a major

© The Author(s) 2020   **359**
K. Kozlowska et al., *Functional Somatic Symptoms in Children
and Adolescents*, Palgrave Texts in Counselling and Psychotherapy,
https://doi.org/10.1007/978-3-030-46184-3_17

US university. His 13-year-old daughter had been hurt in an outdoors accident, and she remained unwell despite the family's proximity and access to a world-renowned medical centre. After recovering from her concussion, she continued to experience a barrage of progressive trauma-related symptoms: non-epileptics seizures (NES) (see Chapter 11), vocal cord adduction (see Chapter 7), disturbed sleep (see Chapter 5), anxiety and panic attacks, and post-traumatic re-experiencing. The NES, which were occurring so frequently as to disrupt all family routines, were triggered by exercise or environmental cues reminiscent of the accident. Cognitive-behavioural therapy—the therapy with the best evidence base for NES—had not been particularly successful. At the time of the correspondence, the hospital-based clinical care involved neurology, the ear, nose, and throat team, psychiatry and clinical psychology, and the ambulance service.

Robert, the father, described the experience as being one

trapped in a void between medical specialties. Once the neurologists determined the events were NES, they didn't have anything neurological to add, either in terms of diagnosis or treatment. Our daughter's psychiatrist didn't have any expertise with NES, nor did, apparently, the psychiatrist's pediatric colleagues. And none of the specialists had ever encountered NES complicated by vocal fold closure. Fourteen months of CBT with a skilled provider had little impact, with the NES actually developing out of what were initially only panic attacks during this treatment. Clinicians in private practice—who offer alternative ways of working—have declined to see my daughter because of her NES and the fear that a seizure might occur in their offices. As far as I can tell, this void between specialities is simply a function of historical divisions of labor and discipline, with little defensible intellectual basis given how we now (since the early 90s) think about mind, brain, and body. But particularly in our country, 'mind-body' medicine is still considered alternative, and no one seems to tackle problems like my daughter's with a multidisciplinary approach. A lot of researchers are looking at brain networks (and using very cool machines), but the clinical impact, especially with children, is slight to non-existent. And though data bases such as UpToDate, DynaMed, and Clinical Evidence have some useful information and frameworks regarding adults, none of it relates to children, and in any event, the clinical usefulness is no better than thin. On my reading, it seems that what is missing is work that is more neuroscientifically engaged, and clinically concrete. It's a huge gap that needs to be filled.

This book is about that gap, that void. This book is our attempt to share with mental health clinicians, paediatricians, and other health professionals our clinical journey and what we have learnt in helping hundreds of children (including adolescents), along with their families, who presented to our hospital settings with functional somatic symptoms. Like the clinicians in Robert's story, we began our journey in the void, with little information to guide us and with no sure idea of how to fill the gap between existing medical specialties or between mind and body. Slowly, in a journey of many years, drawing on our clinical observations and the research literature—and in particular, George Chrousos's concept of the stress system (Chrousos et al. 1988) (see Chapter 1)—we began to gain insight into the functional presentations that we encountered. Like Robert, his daughter, and family, we had to search for alternative treatment options and pathways whenever accepted therapeutic techniques fell short of what we—and the patient—needed.

Throughout this book, using the lens of contemporary neuroscience and applying a systems approach, we have considered the complex, reciprocal influences of the brain, body, and mind—as well as the role of the relational and social contexts that define each person's immediate environment—in the biology of stress and in the emergence of functional somatic symptoms. The key point emerging in this book is that brain, body, and mind are deeply integrated in the person and do not follow Cartesian dualism; for our purposes, there is no distinction between physical and psychological stress. Mind and body are inseparable, as are, in effect, the phrases *embodied mind* and *minded body*. No matter how stress is generated, when it becomes cumulative, chronic, uncontrollable, or associated with extreme distress, it can dysregulate the stress system and affect the well-being and health of the individual child.

Using this systems approach, we have presented what we refer to as the *stress-system model for functional somatic symptoms*. Under this model, functional somatic symptoms are conceptualized as emerging when the person's stress system is activated in response to stress that exceeds the person's capacity to cope. Accordingly, from the perspective of the stress-system framework, the treatment of functional somatic symptoms involves interventions that help the child shift her stress system back to a more regulated state, one that supports health and well-being and is incompatible with functional somatic symptoms.

In many ways, writing this book is an act of courage. When our *science* colleagues read this book, they may cringe at the simplicity of our metaphors for what is very complicated science. When our *evidence-based* colleagues read the book, they may see the material as (for the present) lacking the evidence base that they require for inclusion in evidence-based reviews and publications. When our *medical* colleagues read the book, they may find the material confronting because it steps outside of and between medical specialties and because we utilize systems thinking, shifting from system level to system level, in a way that ignores the neat silos of contemporary medicine. When our *psychology* and *mental health* colleagues read the book, they may see the book as too medical, too biological, and too focused on processes that take place in the human body, with only two chapters about the mind as such. And when *philosophers* read the book, they might find it too concrete, too rooted in biology rather than the mind.

So, in the end, we just have to focus on who we are and what we do, and to communicate our work to other clinicians in the clearest way possible. We—the first and third (HH) authors—are clinicians who work on multidisciplinary teams using a systems (biopsychosocial) framework in collaboration with our medical and mental health colleagues. We treat children with functional somatic symptoms and give particular attention to the circumstances (familial, social, educational) in which the symptoms arose. When we initially meet with the children and families, we provide a careful assessment and reach a formulation that guides our choice of treatment interventions on multiple system levels: body, brain, mind, family, and school. Working systemically, we expect that our interventions will have a synergistic effect—that the overall effect of working on multiple system levels at once will be greater than the effects of the separate treatments. Likewise, we expect that the interventions will shift the child's stress system from an activated and dysregulated state to a more regulated state not compatible with functional somatic symptoms. And we have documented our outcomes—in three research cohorts—with studies published in mainstream medical journals (see Online Supplement 2.1). From this data we know that the majority of children whom we treat return to health and well-being.

The writing of this book has been an exercise of stepping outside the box or of stepping out on a limb of a tree. Here we are comforted by Fritjof Capra's words that all knowledge is approximate (Capra 1997); the knowledge in this book is, inescapably, approximate. It describes what we know today, in full recognition that we shall know more, and with better evidence, tomorrow. We are also comforted by Desmond Sheridan's analysis of evidence-based medicine, as both best practice and restrictive dogma (Sheridan 2016). We are conscious that the evidence base in the field of functional somatic symptoms is still taking shape, though we should note that the published research of the first author, in particular, constitutes an important part of the existing evidence base. We (the first and third authors, in particular) should also note that this work, here and elsewhere, has been markedly improved by the contributions of the second author (SS), who, in a role approximating that of participant-observer, has brought his background in philosophy, psychiatry, consulting, and publications to bear on this project. He has, among other things, facilitated the process of reaching what we all see as an effective accommodation between theory and practice, and to communicate our knowledge in a way that is actually accessible to, and useful for, readers.

In the time that we have been working with children with functional somatic symptoms, the era of talking therapies, with an emphasis on psychoanalytic paradigm, has been largely displaced by a cognitive-behavioural paradigm. But that newer paradigm has been oversold as the fix-all therapy, and we have found it to be of only limited use in ameliorating the functional somatic symptoms of our child patients. Clinicians working more directly with the body—many of whom are quoted in the pages of this book—have been pioneering other ways of understanding and working with somatic symptoms, including those of our patients. More broadly in the therapy world, clinicians have come to recognize that working on the mind system level (see Chapter 15) is one therapeutic option among others and that working with the body harnesses healing properties of the body/mind/person that might not otherwise be available (see Chapter 14). Clinicians have also recognized that, in actual clinical practice, targeted interventions from multiple system levels can be combined to address stress-system dysfunction, functional impairment, psychological distress, relational difficulties/issues, and issues within the family and school systems. Even more broadly, this shift in our understanding of the interconnections between mind and body has been moving into the mainstream, as is apparent in David Brooks's 2019 *New York Times* column entitled 'The Wisdom of Your Body' (Brooks 2019).

The need to move beyond established silos and settled approaches to research and treatment is not unique to the field of functional somatic symptoms. We note, for example, that in response to frustrating failures to develop new curative treatments in mental health, the *Harvard Review of Psychiatry* has started a new feature, 'Disruptive Innovations'. The aims are to catalyse clinical translation of cutting-edge science and expert perspectives, 'to challenge orthodoxy in thoughtful and well-reasoned ways, and [to] propose new ideas, approaches, and methods to tackle intractable problems in psychiatry' (Roffman 2019, p. 275). The need to step outside the box is also known to our medical colleagues interested in the long-term effects of early-life stress on health and well-being across the lifespan—or as some researchers put it, 'searching outside the streetlight' (Bush and Aschbacher 2020, p. 17).

A recurring theme from all these clinicians, researchers, and writers is that the pathway beyond the void—the space where healing can be found—requires one to step outside the box, out on a limb, past what's visible under the streetlight. We need to be comfortable with approximate knowledge, to avail ourselves of information from multiple system levels, and to use that information in a fluid and flexible way, all in an effort to work collaboratively and productively with our patients and their families. And because what we know now is only approximate, we need to remain forever curious about body and mind, about the way that the body regulates itself, and about how the stress system (and for our purposes, each child) responds to the challenges of daily living—the *stress of life* (see Online Supplement 1.2).

We hope that mental health clinicians, paediatricians, and other health professionals will enjoy the book and use it as a helpful resource for their day-to-day clinical practice. We hope that, in our clinical vignettes, they will recognize the children and families that they work with in their own practices. And we hope that in describing our clinical work, we have provided sufficient detail for readers to implement our approach in their own work with the children—and their families— who come asking them for treatment of functional somatic symptoms.

Finally, we hope that readers will come to see themselves not only as having a role in treating their own patients but as having the capacity to educate their own colleagues about functional somatic symptoms. Mental health professionals, as a group, have only recently come to have the tools available—as presented here—for working productively with children with functional somatic symptoms. Readers can, themselves, play an important role in increasing professional awareness of these problems, of spreading knowledge of the available treatment interventions, and of helping to ensure that children with functional somatic symptoms are identified early and obtain effective treatment.

References

Brooks, D. (2019, November 28). The Wisdom Your Body Knows. You Are Not Just Thinking with Your Brain. *New York Times*.

Bush, N. R., & Aschbacher, K. (2020). Immune Biomarkers of Early-Life Adversity and Exposure to Stress and Violence—Searching Outside the Streetlight. *JAMA Pediatrics, 174*, 17–19.

Capra, F. (1997). *The Web of Life: A New Synthesis of Mind and Matter*. London: Flamingo.

Chrousos, G. P., Loriaux, D. L., & Gold, P. W. (1988). Preface. In G. P. Chrousos, D. L. Loriaux, & P. W. Gold (Eds.), *Mechanisms of Physical and Emotional Stress*. New York: Plenum Press (Advances in Experimental Medicine and Biology, Vol. 245).

Roffman, J. L. (2019). Reaffirming Core Scientific Values in Psychiatry Research. *Harvard Review of Psychiatry, 27*, 275–278.

Sheridan, D. J. (2016). *Evidence-Based Medicine: Best Practice or Restrictive Dogma*. London: Imperial College Press.

Index of Vignettes by Name, with Principal Problems

FND = functional neurological disorder; NES = non-epileptic seizures; POTS = postural orthostatic tachycardia syndrome.

Index of Concepts, Problems, and Processes, with Relevant Vignettes

FND = functional neurological disorder; NES = non-epileptic seizures; POTS = postural orthostatic tachycardia syndrome.

© The Editor(s) (if applicable) and The Author(s) 2020
K. Kozlowska et al., *Functional Somatic Symptoms in Children and Adolescents*,
Palgrave Texts in Counselling and Psychotherapy,
https://doi.org/10.1007/978-3-030-46184-3

Main Index

© The Editor(s) (if applicable) and The Author(s) 2020
K. Kozlowska et al., *Functional Somatic Symptoms in Children and Adolescents*,
Palgrave Texts in Counselling and Psychotherapy,
https://doi.org/10.1007/978-3-030-46184-3

Printed by Printforce, the Netherlands

PALGRAVE TEXTS IN COUNSELLING AND PSYCHOTHERAPY

Series Editors: **Arlene Vetere · Rudi Dallos**

"This book, at the intersection of mind-body medicine, is a must-read … The authors have masterfully linked together the emerging, cutting-edge biology with case-based discussions and practical suggestions for treating functional somatic disorders in children and adolescents. This book is a major advance in bringing this set of conditions out of the shadows and into the mainstream."
—**David L. Perez**, Massachusetts General Hospital, Harvard Medical School, USA

"Uniquely creative, well-informed, and authoritative, the authors' stress-system model is integrated into an overarching clinical framework that, complemented by the extensive use of clinical vignettes, will prove useful for trainees and the broad range of clinicians addressing these problems in their own practices."
—**Elena Garralda**, Emeritus Professor of Child and Adolescent Psychiatry, Imperial College London, UK

This open access book sets out the stress-system model for functional somatic symptoms in children and adolescents. In addition to providing a new understanding of how such symptoms emerge, the book explores the initial encounter between the paediatrician, child, and family, describes the assessment process, and presents wide-ranging interventions for settling the child's dysregulated stress system. The overarching goal is to help the child and family find an effective path back to health and well-being.

Kasia Kozlowska is a child and adolescent psychiatrist at The Children's Hospital at Westmead and Clinical Associate Professor, Sydney Medical School, Australia.

Stephen Scher is Senior Editor, *Harvard Review of Psychiatry*, and Lecturer in Psychiatry at McLean Hospital/Harvard Medical School, USA.

Helene Helgeland is a child and adolescent psychiatrist at Oslo University Hospital and head of Norway's National Advisory Unit on Complex Psychosomatic Disorders in Children and Adolescents.

ISBN 978-3-030-46183-6

9 783030 461836

palgrave
macmillan

www.palgrave.com